Lymph Node Cytopathology

ESSENTIALS IN CYTOPATHOLOGY SERIES

Dorothy L. Rosenthal, MD, FIAC, Series Editor

For other titles published in this series, go to
http://www.springer.com/series/6996

Stefan E. Pambuccian

University of Minnesota, Minneapolis, MN, USA

Ricardo H. Bardales

Outpatient Pathology Associates, Sacramento, CA, USA

Lymph Node Cytopathology

Springer

Stefan E. Pambuccian
University of Minnesota
Department of Lab. Medicine
& Pathology
C422 Mayo MMC 76
420 Delaware St. SE.
55455 Minneapolis, Minnesota
USA
pambu001@umn.edu

Ricardo H. Bardales
Outpatient Pathology Associates
3301 C Street, Suite 103C
95816 Sacramento California
USA
rhbardales@aol.com

ISBN 978-1-4419-6963-7 e-ISBN 978-1-4419-6964-4
DOI 10.1007/978-1-4419-6964-4
Springer New York Dordrecht Heidelberg London

Library of Congress Control Number: 2010935190

Printed on acid-free paper

Springer is part of Springer Science+Business Media (www.springer.com)

Series Preface

The subspeciality of cytopathology is 60 years old and has become established as a solid and reliable discipline in medicine. As expected, cytopathology literature has expanded in a remarkably short period of time, from a few textbooks prior to the 1980s to a current and substantial library of texts and journals devoted exclusively to cytomorphology. *Essentials in Cytopathology* does not presume to replace any of the distinguished textbooks in cytopathology. Instead, the series will publish generously illustrated and user-friendly guides for both pathologists and clinicians.

Building on the amazing success of *The Bethesda System for Reporting Cervical Cytology*, now in its second edition, the *Series* will utilize a similar format, including minimal text, tabular criteria, and superb illustrations based on real-life specimens. *Essentials in Cytopathology* will, at times, deviate from the classic organization of pathology texts. The logic of decision trees, elimination of unlikely choices, and narrowing of differential diagnosis via a pragmatic approach based on morphologic criteria will be some of the strategies used to illustrate principles and practice in cytopathology.

Most of the authors for *Essentials in Cytopathology* are faculty members in The Johns Hopkins University School of Medicine, Department of Pathology, Division of Cytopathology. They bring to each volume the legacy of John K. Frost and the collective experience of a preeminent cytopathology service. The archives at Hopkins are meticulously catalogued and form the framework for text and illustrations. Authors from other institutions have been selected on the basis of their national reputations, experience, and enthusiasm for cytopathology. They bring to the series complementary viewpoints and enlarge the scope of materials contained in the photographs.

The editor and the authors are indebted to our students, past and future, who challenge and motivate us to become the best that we possibly can be. We share that experience with you through these pages, and hope that you will learn from them as we have from those who have come before us. We would be remiss if we did not pay tribute to our professional colleagues, the cytotechnologists and preparatory technicians who lovingly care for the specimens that our clinical colleagues send to us.

And finally, we cannot emphasize enough throughout these volumes the importance of collaboration with the patient care team. Every specimen comes to us as questions begging an answer. Without input from the clinicians, complete patient history, results of imaging studies and other ancillary tests, we cannot perform optimally. It is our responsibility to educate our clinicians about their role in our interpretation, and for us to integrate as much information as we can gather into our final diagnosis, even if the answer at first seems obvious.

We hope you will find this series useful and welcome your feedback as you place these handbooks by your microscopes and into your book bags.

Baltimore, MD *Dorothy L. Rosenthal*

Acknowledgements

To the memory of my father, who guided my first steps in pathology.
To my wife Corina and my son Felix.
My gratitude to my mentors Harry L. Ioachim, Yener Erozan, and Dorothy L. Rosenthal.

Stefan E. Pambuccian

To my parents, my first teachers.
To Angela, Angie, and Ricky from whom I continue learning.
To my mentors, residents, and fellows.

Ricardo H. Bardales

Contents

1 Introduction

Historical Overview

Lymph nodes are some of the most common targets for fine needle aspiration (FNA) as persistent lymphadenopathy is a common finding. It is therefore not surprising that the first description of what we now call FNA biopsy was made in 1904 by two British marine officers, Captain E.D.W. Greig and Lieutenant A.C.H. Gray who reported their findings on the aspiration of lymph nodes in sleeping sickness. They could demonstrate motile trypanosomes in the "node juice" obtained by aspirating from swollen neck lymph nodes of patients in Uganda with hypodermic needles. The following year, German physicians Fritz Schaudinn and Erich Hoffmann, were able to identify *Treponema pallidum*, which they had previously identified as the causative agent of syphilis, in inguinal lymph node aspirates by using dark-field microscopy.

The first uses of lymph node FNA in the diagnosis of tumors occurred in 1914 by an English physician, Gordon R. Ward who was able to diagnose "lymphoblastomas" (i.e., lymphomas) by this method. In 1921, Dr. C.G. Guthrie, head of the department of Clinical Pathology at the Johns Hopkins Hospital, successfully made the diagnosis of Hodgkin lymphoma by "gland puncture," and the patient received treatment based solely on that diagnostic procedure.

S.E. Pambuccian and R.H. Bardales, *Lymph Node Cytopathology*,
Essentials in Cytopathology 10, DOI 10.1007/978-1-4419-6964-4_1,

However, the most influential in establishing needle aspiration of lymph nodes as a valid diagnostic measure was Dr. Hayes E. Martin from the Head and Neck Service of the Memorial Hospital for Cancer and Allied Diseases in New York (currently the Memorial Sloan Kettering Cancer Center). With the help of Edward B. Ellis, the chief histotechnologist and Fred W Stewart, the surgical pathologist responsible for interpreting the smears, Dr. Martin proposed needle aspiration of cervical lymph nodes to replace excisional biopsies in 1926.

The rapidly accumulated experience with 2,500 tumors aspirated by 1933 allowed Dr. Fred Stewart to formulate the principles of needle aspiration cytology, which are still valid today, emphasizing sample preparation, clinical correlation, histologic correlation, attention to both smear pattern and individual cell cytomorphology, and awareness of the limitations of the method. One of the limitations that he noticed was in the diagnosis of primary lymph node lesion, where the diagnosis was difficult even when tissue sections were available. This skepticism was appropriate at a time when diagnostic criteria and ancillary studies were lacking, and very high rates of histopathologic misdiagnosis were occurring, as demonstrated by the amazing 50% reclassification rate (most often to benign conditions) of cases originally diagnosed histologically as Hodgkin disease found by Dr. W.S.C. Symmers in 1968.

After being almost abandoned in USA, the needle aspiration technique was revived and improved in the 1950s in Europe (especially in the Netherlands and Sweden) by clinical hematologists who used Romanovsky-type stains instead of the hematoxylin and eosin stain used by Dr. Fred Stewart, and smaller needles that were less likely to result in complications or tumor implantation. The technique, which became known as FNA, was used most often for cytologic diagnosis of metastatic lesions, an indication for which it rapidly gained widespread acceptance and worldwide dissemination.

However, skepticism about the possibility of accurate lymphoma diagnosis in aspiration smears persisted in the pathology community despite a 1980 publication documenting the diagnosis of over 1,000 lymphomas diagnosed by FNA by one of the pioneers of FNA, Dr. Lopes-Cardozo, and other papers on the subject.

FNA in the initial diagnosis of lymphomas became more widely accepted only in the 1990s, when ancillary studies (especially immunophenotyping) became routinely used in the diagnosis of lymph node aspirates suspected of lymphoma, and the classification of lymphomas was modified with more emphasis placed on cytomorphology (rather than histologic/architectural pattern), immunophenotypic, and cytogenetic features in the revised European American classification (REAL) of 1994, and the World Health Organization (WHO) classifications of 2001 and 2008.

Indications for Fine Needle Aspiration of Lymph Nodes

Currently, FNA, whether performed on superficial lymph nodes by palpation or performed under ultrasound, transesophageal endoscopic ultrasound (EUS), endobronchial ultrasound (EBUS), or computerized tomography (CT) guidance is used to:

1. Establish the cause of lymphadenopathy
2. Stage a known lymphoid, or nonlymphoid malignancy
3. Monitor for recurrence of lymphoid, or nonlymphoid malignancies, and for potential progression or transformation of lymphoid malignancies

Lymph Node Pathology Diagnosed by Fine Needle Aspiration

In patients presenting with lymphadenopathy without a history of malignancy, more than half of lymph node aspirates represent a variety of reactive, inflammatory, infectious, and granulomatous disorders; about a third are metastatic malignancies and less than 10% are lymphomas. Benign conditions are even more common in pediatric lymphadenopathies, where about 80% of aspirated lymph nodes prove to be benign. The relative frequency of aspirates diagnostic of malignancy varies according to the nodal site biopsied. The most commonly aspirated lymph node region, the cervical lymph nodes is the least likely to be malignant, and the likelihood of a malignant diagnosis increases for inguinal, axillary, intraabdominal, retroperitoneal, and supraclavicular lymph nodes.

As with fine needle aspirates from other sites, the reported specificity of lymph node aspirates is very high, between 98 and 100% as false positive diagnoses are very rare. The sensitivity of FNA of lymph nodes, on the contrary, depends heavily on the population studied and case mix. The sensitivity for metastatic malignancies causing lymph node enlargement is over 95%, while the sensitivity for lymphomas varies from 80 to 90%, with a typing accuracy of about 70% and higher when flow cytometry is routinely used in fine needle aspirates of lymph nodes. The sensitivity of FNA in lymphoma diagnosis is heavily dependent on the relative representation of T- vs. B-cell lymphomas, and small-cell vs. large-cell lymphomas, the former being more difficult to diagnose than the latter.

Benefits of Lymph Node FNA

Lymphadenopathy is most commonly superficial and palpable, and therefore easily accessible to sampling by palpation or ultrasound-guided FNA, which usually results in a fast, reliable, and relatively inexpensive diagnosis. A variety of ancillary studies (cultures, immunohistochemistry, EM, flow cytometry, cytogenetics, and molecular diagnostics) can be performed on the aspirate and the choice of ancillary studies is determined during the on-site evaluation of the aspirate.

Excisional biopsy is not necessary when inflammatory or reactive conditions, or metastases are diagnosed. The management of patients with lymphoma initially diagnosed by FNA combined with flow cytometry or other immunophenotyping studies is controversial, but in most institutions, an excisional biopsy is performed to confirm the diagnosis after weighing the potential benefits that histologic assessment of the lymph node would give against the risks of the procedure. Excisional biopsy will be performed in most cases diagnosed as lymphoma, or suspicious for lymphoma in FNA of superficial lymph nodes. However, the definitive diagnosis of lymphoma on fine needle aspirates or core biopsies of deep lymph nodes such as retroperitoneal lymph nodes is usually not followed by excisional biopsies due to the higher risks of the surgical procedure. The advantages of needle core biopsies as opposed to fine needle aspirates obtained by imaging-guided procedures are probably overstated, since the presence of some minimal architectural features has to be weighed against the frequent presence of extensive crush artifact that may render the morphologic interpretation difficult and lower the yield of ancillary studies. When such core biopsies are performed, it is always useful to prepare gentle touch imprints or "roll-preps" of the cores during the procedure to serve for both the evaluation of adequacy and triage of the specimen, and for morphologic correlation with the core biopsy histology, as these cytologic preparations frequently allow better evaluation of morphologic features.

It has been calculated that FNA of lymph nodes avoids at least 86% of lymph node excisional biopsies. Cases in which FNA fails to establish a definitive diagnosis, as well as cases in which the lymph node enlargement persists 1–3 months after the FNA was interpreted as benign/reactive, should undergo excisional biopsy to rule out a potentially missed pathology.

Difficulties and Limitation of FNA Diagnosis

FNA biopsy of lymph nodes is arguably one of the most difficult areas of cytopathology as lymph nodes can harbor a bewildering array of benign and malignant conditions Over 50 types of lymphomas are included in the latest (2008) WHO classification (Table 1.1), some of them are so rare that they may be encountered only once in a pathologist's career. In addition, lymph nodes can be the site of metastases from virtually any malignancy. The difficulty of correctly interpreting lymph node FNAs is increased by the minimal degrees of cytologic atypia that some low-grade lymphomas exhibit and the potential overlap between the cytologic features of some high-grade lymphomas and metastatic malignancies. This makes the use of ancillary techniques (immunohistochemistry, flow cytometry, fluorescence in situ hybridization, and molecular techniques) more important to achieve an accurate FNA diagnosis than in any other site. Accurate subtyping of lymphoid malignancies according to the current classification of lymphoid neoplasms, the 2008 WHO classification that relies heavily on immunophenotypic, cytogenetic, and molecular features, is virtually impossible without the use of ancillary studies. We will follow the 2008 WHO

TABLE 1.1. WHO classification of lymphoid neoplasms (2008), including only neoplasms potentially encountered in fine needle aspiration of lymph nodes and mediastinum.

Precursor lymphoid neoplasms
B lymphoblastic leukemia/lymphoma NOS
T lymphoblastic leukemia/lymphoma
Mature B-cell neoplasms
Chronic lymphocytic leukemia/small lymphocytic lymphoma
Lymphoplasmacytic lymphoma/Waldenstrom macroglobulinemia
Plasma cell myeloma
Extraosseous plasmacytoma
Extranodal marginal zone B-cell lymphoma of mucosa-associated lymphoid tissue (MALT) type
Nodal marginal zone lymphoma
Follicular lymphoma
Mantle cell lymphoma
Diffuse large B-cell lymphoma, NOS
T-cell/histiocyte-rich type
Diffuse large B-cell lymphoma with chronic inflammation
Primary mediastinal large B-cell lymphoma
Intravascular large B-cell lymphoma
ALK+ large B-cell lymphoma
Plasmablastic lymphoma
Large B-cell lymphoma associated with HHV8+ Castleman disease
Primary effusion lymphoma
Burkitt lymphoma
B-cell lymphoma, unclassifiable, Burkitt-like
B-cell lymphoma, unclassifiable, Hodgkin lymphoma-like
Mature T-cell & NK-cell neoplasms
Adult T-cell lymphoma/leukemia
Extranodal T-cell/NK-cell lymphoma, nasal type
Mycosis fungoides
Peripheral T-cell lymphoma, NOS
Angioimmunoblastic T-cell lymphoma
Anaplastic large cell lymphoma, ALK+ type
Anaplastic large cell lymphoma, ALK− type
Hodgkin lymphoma
Nodular lymphocyte-predominant Hodgkin lymphoma
Classic Hodgkin lymphoma
Nodular sclerosis Hodgkin lymphoma
Lymphocyte-rich classic Hodgkin lymphoma
Mixed cellularity Hodgkin lymphoma
Lymphocyte depletion Hodgkin lymphoma

(continued)

TABLE 1.1. (continued)

Posttransplant lymphoproliferative disorders (PTLD)
Plasmacytic hyperplasia
Infectious mononucleosis-like PTLD
Polymorphic PTLD
Monomorphic PTLD (B & T/NK cell types)
Classic HD-type PTLD
Histiocytic and dendritic cell neoplasms
Histiocytic sarcoma
Langerhans cell histiocytosis
Langerhans cell sarcoma
Interdigitating dendritic cell sarcoma
Follicular dendritic cell sarcoma
Fibroblastic reticular cell tumor
Indeterminate dendritic cell sarcoma
Disseminated juvenile xanthogranuloma

Classification of Tumors of Hematopoietic and Lymphoid Tissues throughout this book, unless otherwise stated.

The purpose of this book is to describe the application of FNA to the assessment of lymphadenopathy, with particular emphasis on the utility, limitations, and potential pitfalls of FNA. It will adopt an algorithmic diagnostic approach, starting from the cytomorphologic pattern of the lymph node aspirate, focusing on the appropriate and effective use of ancillary studies, and integration of their results into the final diagnosis.

The book will present the cytopathologic features and differential diagnoses for the major cytologic patterns in lymph node FNA. The entities typically falling within each of these patterns will be discussed with illustration of the spectrum of cytologic features, differential diagnoses, and pitfalls. The cytologic diagnosis of lymph node aspirates, even when combined with ancillary studies, has definite limitations in the diagnosis of some conditions. Awareness of these limitations helps avoid some potential diagnostic pitfalls. Lymph node aspirates should be interpreted in the clinical context; aspirates where the cytomorphology does not explain the clinical findings or where the cytomorphologic findings or ancillary test results are not entirely characteristic are best diagnosed descriptively with a recommendation for excisional biopsy.

We have attempted to cover the full spectrum of benign and malignant primary conditions of the lymph nodes, with emphasis on common disorders. Discussion of metastatic conditions will be restricted to those that are relevant to the differential diagnosis of primary lymphoid disorders.

Suggested Reading

Das DK (1999) Value and limitations of fine-needle aspiration cytology in diagnosis and classification of lymphomas: a review. Diagn Cytopathol 21(4):240–249

Frable WJ, Kardos TF (1988) Fine needle aspiration biopsy. Applications in the diagnosis of lymphoproliferative diseases. Am J Surg Pathol 12(suppl 1):62–72

Ioachim HL, Medeiros LJ (2009) Ioachim's lymph node pathology, 4th edn. Wolters Kluwer Lippincott Williams & Wilkins, Philadelphia

Katz RL (1997) Controversy in fine-needle aspiration of lymph nodes. A territorial imperative? Am J Clin Pathol 108(4 suppl 1):S3–S5

Lopes Cardozo P (1980) The significance of fine needle aspiration cytology for the diagnosis and treatment of malignant lymphomas. Folia Haematol Int Mag Klin Morphol Blutforsch 107(4):601–620

Sandhaus LM (2000) Fine-needle aspiration cytology in the diagnosis of lymphoma. The next step. Am J Clin Pathol 113(5):623–627

Serrano Egea A, Martinez Gonzalez MA, Perez Barrios A, Alberti Masgrau N, de Agustin de Agustin P (2002) Usefulness of light microscopy in lymph node fine needle aspiration biopsy. Acta Cytol 46(2):364–368

Skoog L, Tani E (2009) Historical aspects. Monogr Clin Cytol 18:1–4

Söderström N (1966) Fine-needle aspiration biopsy used as a direct adjunct in clinical diagnostic work. Grune & Stratton, New York

Swerdlow SH, Campo E, Harris NL, Jaffe ES, Pileri SA, Stein H, Thiele J, Vardiman JW (2008) WHO classification of tumours of haematopoietic and lymphoid tissues, 4th edn. IARC, Lyon

Ultmann JE, Koprowska I, Engle RL Jr (1958) A cytological study of lymph node imprints. Cancer 11(3):507–524

Van Heerde P, Meijer CJLM, Noorduyn LA, Van der Valk P (1996) An atlas and textbook of malignant lymphomas: cytology, histopathology and immunochemistry Harvey Miller Publishers/Manson Publishing, Oxford University Press, London

Wakely PE Jr (2000) Fine-needle aspiration cytopathology in diagnosis and classification of malignant lymphoma: accurate and reliable? Diagn Cytopathol 22(2):120–125

2
Overview of Ancillary Methods in Lymph Node FNA diagnosis

Ancillary tests are critically important tools in the assessment of lymph node aspirates, as they can help establish the etiology of infectious lymphadenopathies, determine the type and primary site of metastatic malignancies, diagnose and subclassify lymphomas, and exclude malignancy in reactive lymphadenopathies. In addition, ancillary tests can also be used to provide prognostic information in certain neoplasms and help predict treatment response.

Clinical correlation is *always* essential when employing ancillary tests and their results should *only* be interpreted in the cytomorphologic context to prevent potential pitfalls.

The decision on which of the ancillary tests are available to use in the individual case depends on the clinical context, characteristics of the lymph node aspirated, and the on-site examination of the aspirate. Some of the ancillary studies that are most useful in the evaluation of lymph node FNA, such as cultures, flow cytometry (FC), and cytogenetic testing, require fresh (not fixed) samples. FC and cytogenetics also require the presence of viable neoplastic cells. It is therefore important that the specimen is triaged and aliquots are taken during the on-site evaluation of lymph node fine needle aspirates. Aspirates showing predominantly neutrophils and/or granulomas should be submitted for the appropriate microbiologic cultures, whereas aspirates from enlarged lymph nodes showing a predominantly lymphoid population in adults should be submitted to immunophenotyping by FC. Care should be taken

S.E. Pambuccian and R.H. Bardales, *Lymph Node Cytopathology*,
Essentials in Cytopathology 10, DOI 10.1007/978-1-4419-6964-4_2,

that sufficient sample is available for performing adequate studies and the appropriate medium (culture or transport media and RPMI) is used. If no on-site evaluation was performed and no fresh sample is available, cell block preparations should be routinely performed, as studies not requiring fresh samples, such as immunohistochemistry and fluorescent in situ hybridization, can frequently be performed on such cell blocks.

The following is a brief overview of ancillary techniques that are useful in the diagnosis of lymph node aspirates. The use of some of these methods will be further discussed in the following chapters. The suggested references contain a more extensive discussion of these ancillary methods. Ancillary tests used in the diagnosis of lymph node aspirates can be divided according to their usefulness into the following:

1. Ancillary methods useful for establishing the etiologic agent of lymphadenitis;
2. Ancillary methods useful for establishing the clonality of a lymphoid process and characterizing the clonal proliferation;
3. Ancillary methods useful for establishing the nature and potential site of origin of a metastatic malignancy.

Ancillary Methods Useful for Establishing the Etiologic Agent of Lymphadenitis

Special Stains and Immunohistochemical Stains

Special stains, such as the Gram stain for bacteria, acid-fast stains (Ziehl–Neelson, Fite, auramine-rhodamine) for mycobacteria, Gomori's methenamine silver (GMS), PAS, and mucicarmine stains for fungi, Warthin Starry stain for cat-scratch disease (*Bartonella henselae*) and spirochetes can be applied to either the FNA smears or cell block preparations. However, the sensitivity of these stains is, rather low, especially for mycobacteria (40–60%, depending on the mycobacterial species), and the interpretation of the stains may be difficult and time consuming. Immunoperoxidase stains are commercially available against some infectious agents that are otherwise difficult to identify, such as *Bartonella henselae, Listeria monocytogenes, Mycobacterium tuberculosis, Aspergillus, CMV, Herpes simplex, HHV8, Pneumocystis jiroveci, and Toxoplasma gondii*, and can be used when clinical and/or morphologic findings suggest these organisms. Since immunohistochemical stains for *M. tuberculosis* are superior in sensitivity and specificity to conventional acid-fast stains and are easier to interpret, they can be used as an alternative method to the conventional stains.

Special stains are useful in the diagnosis of fungi identified in lymph node aspirates (Table 2.1).

As the morphologic identification of fungi may sometimes be difficult, in situ hybridization can be used to determine definitively the species of fungi identified on GMS stains. This method allows the specific identification of yeasts (*Blastomyces dermatitides, Coccidioides immitis, Cryptococcus neoformans, Histoplasma capsulatum, and Sporothrix schenkii)* based on the sequence differences of their 18S and 28S rRNA, and of filamentous fungi (*Aspergillus, Fusarium, and Pseudoallescheria*) based on the sequence differences of their 5S, 18S, and 28S rRNA.

Cultures

Cultures of lymph node aspirates are performed if the clinical or imaging findings suggest an infection, or if neutrophilic or granulomatous inflammation is identified during the on-site evaluation. Depending on the clinical presentation and the presence or absence of granulomas, aerobic and anaerobic, mycobacterial and fungal cultures are submitted in the appropriate media.

Cultures obtained on fine needle aspirates of lymph nodes may be positive for a variety of microorganisms, especially for pyogenic organisms such as *Staphylococcus aureus* or *Streptococcus pyogenes*, and the culture may be useful in choosing the right antibiotic, especially due to the increasing prevalence of methicillin-resistant *S. aureus*. Anaerobes such as *Peptostreptococcus* and *Bacteroides* species may also be cultured singly or in mixed cultures with aerobes. Other organisms may rarely be the cause of suppurative lymphadenitis (*Actinomyces israeli, Francisella tularensis, Yersinia* spp, *Corynebacterium* spp, *Brucella* spp, *Listeria monocytogenes, and Bacillus anthracis*).

Bartonella henselae, the causative agent of cat-scratch disease, is a small, Gram-negative bacillus, detectable by silver stains

TABLE 2.1. Differential diagnostic findings in FNA of fungal lymphadenitis.

Fungus	Size (μm)	Morphology	Budding	Stains typically positive
Histoplasma capsulatum	2–5	Small yeast, often within macrophages	Single bud	GMS
Coccidioides immitis	20–200 (spherules) 2–5 (endospores)	Large spherules with or without endospores	Endospores	GMS, PAS, Fontana-Masson
Blastomyces dermatitidis	8–15	Spherical yeasts with thick (double contoured) walls	Single, broad-based bud	GMS, PAS, Congo red
Cryptococcus neoformans	2–15	Variably sized yeasts, thick capsule	Single, narrow-based bud	GMS, PAS, Mucicarmine, Fontana-Masson
Sporothrix shenkii	2–8	Pleomorphic round, oval, or elongate, cigar-shaped yeasts	Narrow-based, "teardrop" buds; may be multiple	GMS, PAS

(Warthin–Starry silver impregnation). Although the organism can be identified by culture, it is more commonly identified by special stains, immunohistochemistry, or molecular methods as culture is slow and lacks sensitivity.

Cultures from lymph node FNAs may also be positive for mycobacteria, especially for nontuberculous mycobacteria (*M. avium-intracellulare, M. scrofulaceum, and M. kansasii*) in young children and patients who are immunosuppressed or have hematologic malignancies, and *M. tuberculosis* mostly in nonimmunosuppressed adults

Cultures for fungal diseases are rarely positive but should be undertaken in granulomatous lymphadenitis, especially in mediastinal granulomata.

The limitations of cultures are twofold: they are slow and final results may be available only after 4–6 weeks as in the case of mycobacteria, and they may be falsely negative. This may occur either due to the submission of nonrepresentative samples, especially if multiple passes were performed and one pass was entirely submitted for cultures. Performing a single smear from the aspirate submitted for cultures with care not to contaminate the specimen may be useful. Other causes of falsely negative culture results are the compromise of bacterial, mycobacterial, or fungal viability due to delays, inappropriate transportation media, and empiric antibiotic treatment received by the patient prior to the FNA. Finally, the significance of some cultured organisms requires clinical correlation, as they may represent skin contaminants.

Molecular Tests for Microorganisms

Molecular diagnoses for infectious agents can be useful if no specimen was sent for culture, if cultures are negative but the clinical suspicion for infection is high, or clinical therapeutic decisions have to be made before final culture results. Tests based on PCR, real-time PCR, or alternative exponential amplification methodologies can be used for many causative agents of lymphadenitis such as viruses, *Bartonella henselae, F. tularensis, Tropheryma whipplei, M. tuberculosis*, fungi, and protozoa (*T. gondii, Leishmania, etc.*).

Compared to culture, these tests are fast and have a high sensitivity and specificity; however, the sensitivity is frequently lower in fixed specimens. A limitation is the inability to perform susceptibility testing.

Establishing the Clonality of a Lymphoid Process and Characterizing the Clonal Proliferation

Flow Cytometry

FC is probably the ancillary method that is most helpful in the diagnosis of lymph node aspirates. Its increasing use during the last two decades in conjunction with the cytomorphologic evaluation of fine needle aspirates has made lymph node FNA more acceptable in the primary diagnosis of lymphomas by increasing the sensitivity and accuracy of the subclassification of lymphomas on aspirates. As submitting all FNA samples from enlarged lymph nodes may be impractical, some institutions have developed guidelines on which samples should be submitted for immunophenotyping. One of these is the "rule of twos": aspirates from lymph node, which have been enlarged for over 2 months, measure over 2 cm in patients over 20 years of age should be submitted for FC in addition to any aspirates in which the lymphoid population appears atypical during on-site evaluation.

Aspirates from lymph nodes placed in RPMI are an ideal sample for FC, since FC is performed on single cell suspensions. FC usually detects surface antigens, but may also detect cytoplasmic or nuclear antigens after permeabilization of the cell membranes. A relatively high number of cells are needed for accurate FC results, in the range of 300,000–1,000,000; however, this number is easily achieved by placing needle rinses from three successful cellular FNA passes in RPMI or other media.

After the cells have been conjugated with fluorochrome-tagged antibodies, FC evaluates for the simultaneous presence and absence of multiple specific antigens on each individual cell that passes in front of a laser beam. The emitted immunofluorescence signals from all cells in suspension are captured and presented as histograms by the instrument's software. In addition, FC gives information about the size of the cells in the form of forward scatter (FSC) and the complexity of the cells (including the granularity of the cytoplasm and nuclear shape) in the form of side scatter (SSC).

The number of "colors" (fluorochromes) of a FC denotes the maximal number different antibodies that can be applied simultaneously to the cells. Most FC laboratories use at least three, allowing five-parameter analysis (three colors plus forward and side scatter), but 4-color, 8-color, and even 11-color flow cytometers are used by some laboratories. Fewer cells are needed when more colors are used, since the cells can be marked simultaneously with more antibodies, thus reducing the number of tubes used.

FC not only allows the simultaneous assessment of multiple antigens on a cell population, but can also quantify the intensity of antigen expression (e.g., dim vs. moderate vs. bright), a feature that may be important in the classification of some lymphoid proliferations.

In addition to determining what markers the cells express, FC can be helpful by allowing an objective measurement of the abnormal lymphoid population by its FSC, and by allowing ploidy and S-phase measurements.

The most important first step in the flow cytometric immunophenotyping analysis of a lymph node aspirate is *gating* the populations of interest. Gating refers to the selections of subsets of cells based on their levels of expression of one or more markers and/or their light scatter properties. The most important gating strategies employed in fine needle aspirates of lymph nodes are as follows:

1. By cell size in the FSC vs. SSC histograms (FSC vs. SSC) (Fig. 2.1). Lymphoid populations usually have low FSC and low SSC as they are small, and show little nuclear or cytoplasmic complexity. Large cell lymphoma cells usually show intermediate FSC and higher SSC than reactive lymphocyte populations and may be gated on the FSC vs. SSC histogram for further analysis.
2. By cell distribution in the CD45 vs. SCC histogram (Fig. 2.2). This gating strategy is more useful in specimens that include mixed cell populations like bone marrow samples, but can be useful in the assessment of lymph node aspirates. Lymphocytes are usually brightly CD45 positive and show low SSC. Almost all lymphoid malignancies, except Hodgkin lymphoma, plasmablastic lymphomas, and plasma cell neoplasms express CD45, although in some the expression may

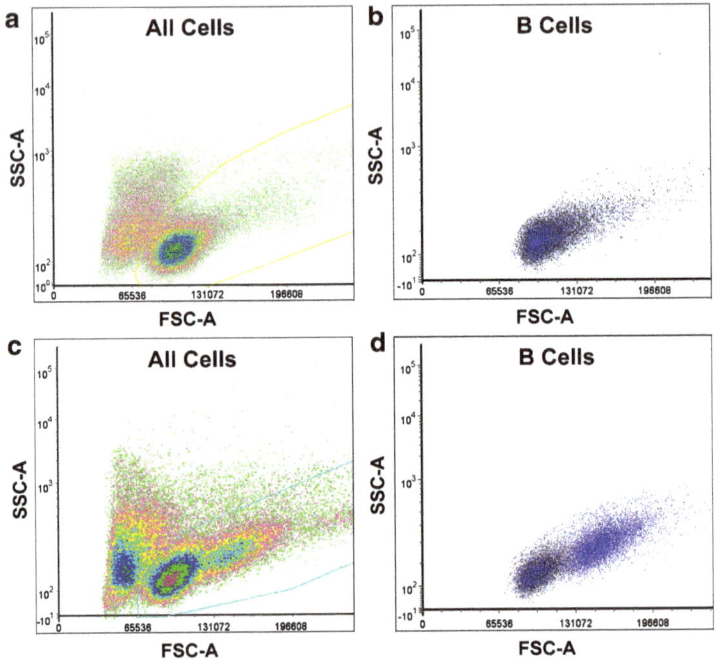

FIGURE 2.1. Histograms of side scatter (SSC) vs. forward scatter (FSC) can help detect the presence of a large cell (neoplastic) lymphoid population. (**a**, **b**) Reactive lymph node aspirate: no significant large cell lymphoid population is present when all cells are considered (**a**) or when gating only on CD19+ B-cells (**b**). (**c**, **d**) Diffuse large B-cell lymphoma (DLBCL) aspirate showing the presence of a larger cell population (increased FSC) when all cells are considered (**c**) or when gating only on CD19+ B-cells (**d**) (courtesy of Timothy P. Singleton, M.D. and Dan McKeon, Flow Cytometry Laboratory, Department of Laboratory Medicine and Pathology, University of Minnesota).

be reduced. This strategy is also useful to identify and exclude nonhematopoietic cell populations such as metastatic malignancies which do not express CD45.

3. By cell lineage-specific antigens. This strategy is useful in the determination of clonality.

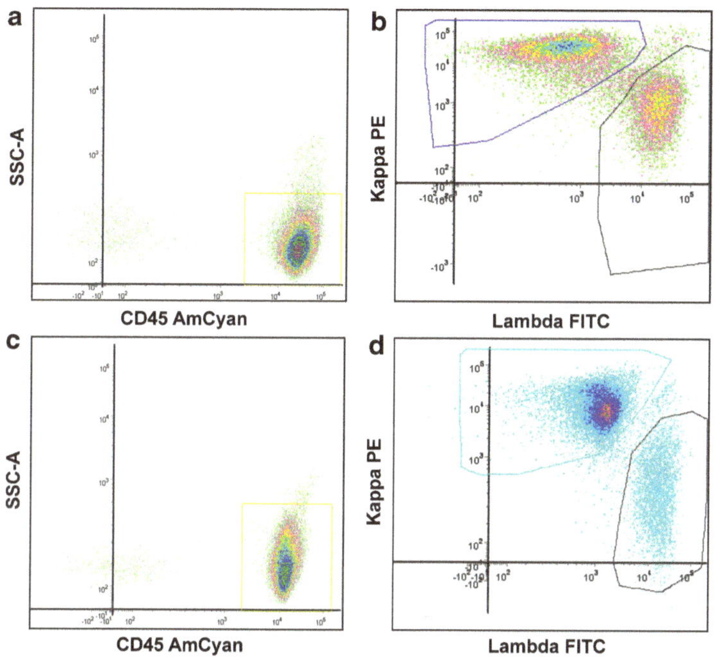

FIGURE 2.2. Histograms of SSC vs. CD45 can help determine if the cells fall in the lymphocyte gate (CD45 bright and low SSC); histograms of kappa vs. lambda can determine the presence of light chain restriction. (**a**, **b**) Reactive lymph node aspirate: most cells fall within the leukocyte gate (CD45 bright and low SSC) and show both kappa and lambda expression (kappa to lambda ratio of 2/1). (**c**, **d**) DLBCL aspirate most cells fall within the leukocyte gate. The cells show light chain restriction (kappa to lambda ratio of 11/1) (courtesy of Timothy P. Singleton, M.D. and Dan McKeon, Flow Cytometry Laboratory, Department of Laboratory Medicine and Pathology, University of Minnesota).

Establishing Clonality

Establishing B-Cell Clonality

B-cells express immunoglobulins on their surface, except in very early phases of their differentiation and when terminally differentiated (plasma cells). The latter express only cytoplasmic immunoglobulins. Since individual B-cells express *either* kappa or lambda light chains, clonal populations of B-cells (i.e., cells derived from the same progeny) show light-chain restriction, i.e., their cells express only one type of light chains (kappa or lambda), in contrast to polyclonal populations, where some cells express kappa and some lambda light chains.

In lymph nodes, blood, and other tissues, kappa-light chain expressing cells usually outnumber lambda-expressing cells by a mean of 2/1 (range 1/1 to 3/1). Kappa/lambda ratios higher than 4/1 or lower than 1/3 are rarely found in reactive lymph nodes and these numbers are frequently used as cut-off points to determine clonality when all B-cells are analyzed. However, cut-off values for kappa/lambda ratios are determined by each laboratory by trying to achieve the best balance between sensitivity and specificity.

When adequately *gated* on the *abnormal* B-cell population showing larger size (higher FSC), inappropriate marker coexpression, or abnormal intensity of marker expression, most lymphomas show much higher light chain ratios (kappa/lambda or lambda/kappa), and values lower than 6/1 should be accepted with care as indicators of clonality. Rare reactive B-cell populations, especially those from reactive germinal centers and Hashimoto thyroiditis, may have light chain ratios over 6/1. In such cases, correlation with other markers determined by FC and with cytomorphologic findings will establish the correct diagnosis.

Some neoplastic B-cell proliferations fail to mark for surface immunoglobulins due to abnormal immunoglobulin synthesis; sometimes applying different antibodies directed against another epitope will successfully determine the presence of the immunoglobulin and the light chain restriction. However, in some cases, no expression of immunoglobulins can be detected and the identification of an abnormal B-cell proliferation has to rely on the demonstration of inappropriate coexpression of differentiation or activation antigens, such as the expression of myeloid antigens (CD13 or CD33) in lymphoplasmacytic lymphoma or of Bcl-2 by CD10-positive B-cells in follicular lymphoma.

Normal B-cells express CD19, which is the most sensitive marker and defines their B-cell lineage. CD20 and CD22 are also expressed by all but the very early B-cells. However, terminally differentiated plasma cells do not express any of these markers, but usually express CD38 and CD138. CD79a may also be used to determine B-cell lineage.

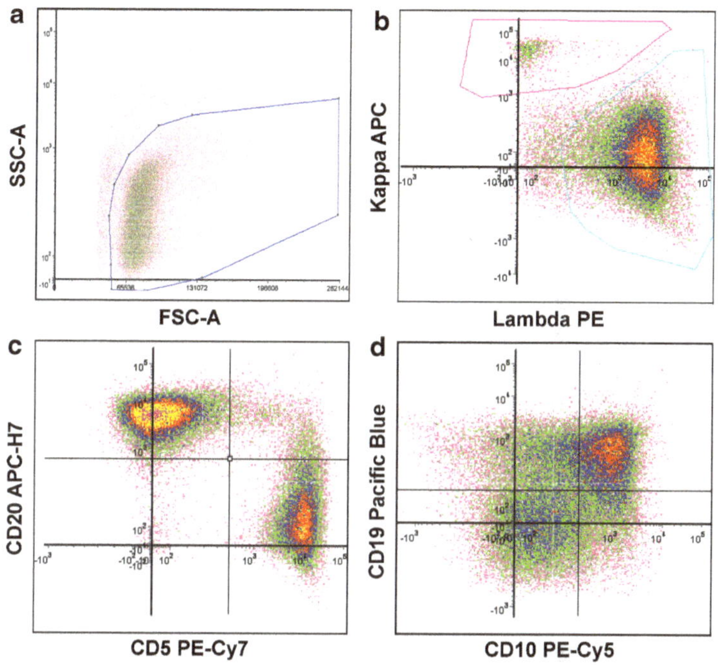

FIGURE 2.3. Flow cytometry (FC) from an aspirate of a patient with grade 1 follicular lymphoma. FC allows the determination of light chain restriction/clonality and the lack of a large cell component on FSC may help excluding a DLBCL. The diagnosis requires clinical and cytologic correlation. (**a**) SSC vs. FSC histogram showing that most cells show low FSC and SSC consistent with small lymphocytes. No large cell population is present. (**b**) Kappa vs. lambda histogram shows overwhelming predominance of lambda-positive cells, demonstrating light chain restriction. (**c**) CD20 vs. CD5 histogram shows lack of CD5 expression on the lambda monotypic B-cells. (**d**) CD20 vs. CD10 histogram shows CD10 expression on the lambda monotypic B-cells (courtesy of Timothy P. Singleton, M.D. and Dan McKeon, Flow Cytometry Laboratory, Department of Laboratory Medicine and Pathology, University of Minnesota).

CD10 is expressed by both B-cell and T-cell lymphoid progenitor cells, and on follicular germinal center B-cells; however, CD10 expression on a large percentage of B-cells needs to be further investigated, as it may represent follicular lymphoma (Fig. 2.3).

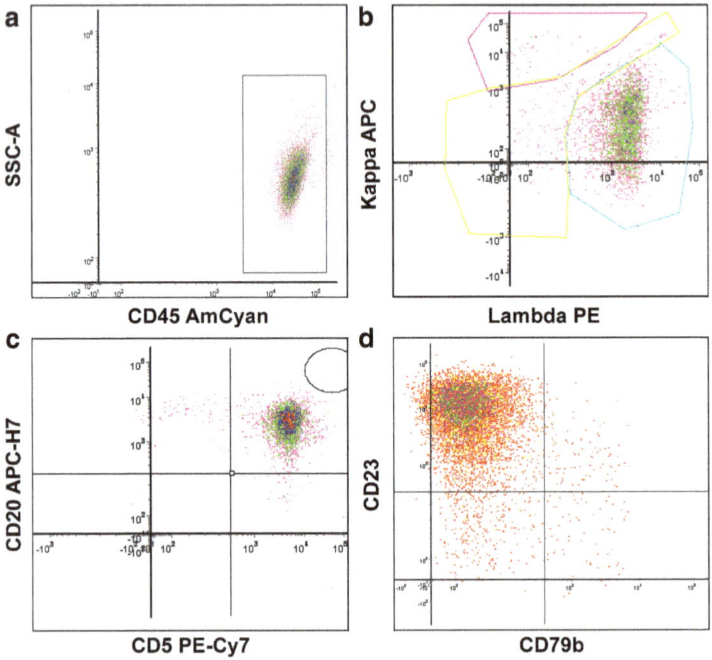

FIGURE 2.4. Flow cytometry from an aspirate of a patient with small lymphocytic lymphoma (CLL/SLL). The flow cytometric findings are characteristic. (**a**) CD45 vs. SSC histogram showing that the cells are hematolymphoid (CD45+) and are present within the lymphocyte window. (**b**) Kappa vs. lambda histogram shows overwhelming predominance of lambda-positive cells, demonstrating light chain restriction. (**c**) CD20 vs. CD5 histogram showing coexpression of CD5 on B-cells. CD20 expression is usually low (dim) in CLL/SLL. (**d**) CD23 vs. CD79b histogram showing expression of CD23 and absence of CD79b expression, which are characteristic for CLL/SLL, as is the absence of FMC7 expression (courtesy of Timothy P. Singleton, M.D. and Dan McKeon, Flow Cytometry Laboratory, Department of Laboratory Medicine and Pathology, University of Minnesota).

The T-cell markers CD5 and CD43 may normally be expressed in a small percentage of B-cells; however, their expression on a large percentage of B-cells is abnormal and may be seen in low-grade B-cell lymphomas (Fig. 2.4).

In about 15-25% of diffuse large B-cell lymphoma (DLBCL) FC results are nondiagnostic due to the presence of nonviable or apoptotic cells, or of fragile cells that are preferentially lost during transportation, storage, or processing. In addition, mechanical factors, such as sclerosis, which is more commonly encountered in DLBCL, can lead to mechanical disruption of neoplastic cells. All of these factors lead to underrepresentation of neoplastic cells in the FC sample (Fig. 2.5).

For similar reasons, lymphomas with low numbers of neoplastic cells such as Hodgkin lymphoma, T-cell-rich B-cell lymphoma, and anaplastic large cell lymphoma (ALCL) frequently lead to nondiagnostic FC results. If the presence of one of these types of lymphoma is suspected during on-site evaluation, it is preferable to submit the specimen remaining after the smears are made for cell block preparation rather than for FC.

Establishing T-Cell and NK Cell Clonality

T-cell clonality is more difficult to determine by FC. The demonstration of an abnormal phenotype on a large percentage of T-cells is a useful, albeit indirect indicator of T-cell clonality. Cytomorphologic correlation is essential for the diagnosis once an aberrant immunophenotype has been found, but additional studies, including cytogenetics, and molecular studies, especially T-cell receptor (TCR) gene rearrangement studies, may sometimes be necessary for the diagnosis.

Normal peripheral T-cells express CD2, CD3, CD5, CD7, and either CD4 or CD8, while thymic T-cells express both CD4 and CD8. In normal T-cells, the percentage of cells expressing CD2, CD3, CD5, and CD7 is similar, and approximates the sum of CD4- and CD8-expressing cells. Peripheral T-cell lymphomas frequently show loss of or dim expression of one or more of these pan-T antigens; absence or presence of both CD4 and CD8 on a large proportion of nodal T-cells; and diminished CD45 (leukocyte common antigen) expression. These abnormalities are frequently associated with increased FSC. Abnormal CD4/CD8 ratios, especially above 15/1, also occur frequently in peripheral T-cell lymphomas, but are not specific as they are also found in Hodgkin lymphomas, viral infections, DLBCLs, dermatopathic lymphadenopathy, and atypical T-cell proliferations associated with phenytoin

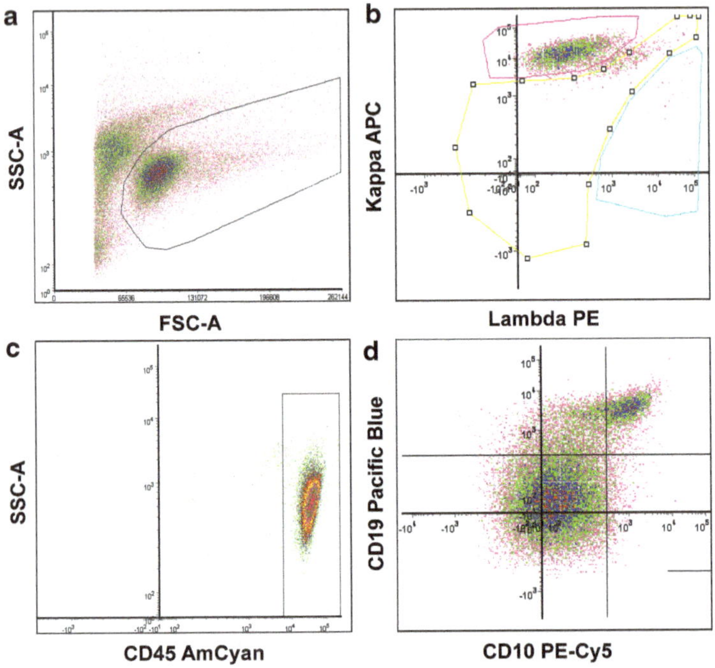

FIGURE 2.5. Flow cytometry from a lymph node aspirate of a patient with DLBCL. FC allows the determination of light chain restriction/clonality but the immunophenotype is not specific, as follicular lymphomas and Burkitt lymphomas may show the same immunophenotype and the diagnosis requires cytologic correlation. (**a**) SSC vs. FSC histogram showing that most cells show low FSC and SSC consistent with small lymphocytes. A population of larger cells (higher FSC) is also present. Larger cells are underrepresented due to loss during processing. (**b**) Kappa vs. lambda histogram shows overwhelming predominance of kappa-positive cells, demonstrating light chain restriction. (**c**) CD45 vs. SSC histogram showing that the cells are hematolymphoid (CD45+) and are present within the lymphocyte window. (**d**) CD19 vs. CD10 histogram shows CD10 expression in a subset of cells (courtesy of Timothy P. Singleton, M.D. and Dan McKeon, Flow Cytometry Laboratory, Department of Laboratory Medicine and Pathology, University of Minnesota).

treatment. Most T-cell lymphomas have a CD4+ phenotype; some T-cell lymphomas also express other characteristic markers such as CD25 in adult T-cell leukemia/lymphoma, CD10 in angioimmunoblastic lymphoma, and CD30 in ALCL.

T-cell clonality may also be determined by the flow cytometric analysis of the TCR's Vβ repertoire.

NK cells and their proliferations express markers also expressed by T-cells (CD2, CD7, and CD8) but do not express surface CD3 and CD4, and frequently express CD56, and CD57.

Classification of Lymphoma

According to the current (2008) World Health Organization classification, non-Hodgkin lymphomas are defined by their morphology, immunophenotype, cytogenetics, and sometimes also by their clinical features. Therefore, it is essential to establish the immunophenotype of a neoplastic lymphoid proliferation by FC (preferably) or immunohistochemistry. This immunophenotype, interpreted in the clinical and cytomorphologic context, is essential in the accurate classification of lymphomas on FNA specimens.

The more common nodal B-cell non-Hodgkin lymphomas can be divided according to their expression of CD5 and CD10 into the following:

1. CD5-positive, CD10-negative
   (a) Chronic lymphocytic leukemia/small lymphocytic lymphoma (CLL/SLL)
   (b) Mantle cell lymphoma (MCL)
   (c) Diffuse large B-cell lymphoma, including Richter transformation of CLL
   (d) Lymphoplasmacytic lymphoma
2. CD5-negative, CD10-positive
   (a) Follicular lymphoma (FL)
   (b) Diffuse large B-cell lymphoma (DLBCL)
   (c) Burkitt lymphoma (BL)
3. CD5-negative, CD10-negative
   (a) Marginal zone lymphoma (MZL) (Fig. 2.6)
   (b) Lymphoplasmacytic lymphoma

While these are the typically encountered immunophenotypes, follicular lymphoma, DLBCL, and MCL lymphoma can also have a CD5+/CD10+, or a CD5−/CD10− phenotype, Burkitt lymphoma can be CD5+/CD10+, and MZL can be positive for CD5.

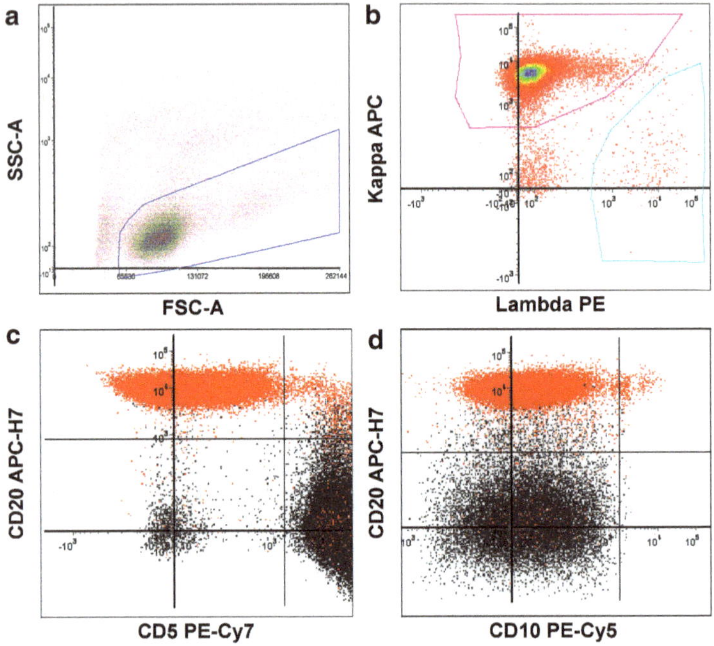

FIGURE 2.6. Flow cytometry from an EUS-guided fine needle aspirate of a perigastric lymph node of a patient with marginal zone lymphoma. FC allows the determination of light chain restriction/clonality but there are no specific surface markers for this lymphoma and the diagnosis is based on the absence of immunophenotyping features characteristic for other lymphomas, clinical and cytologic correlation. (**a**) SSC vs. FSC histogram showing that most cells show low FSC and SSC consistent with small lymphocytes. (**b**) Kappa vs. lambda histogram shows overwhelming predominance of kappa-positive cells, demonstrating light chain restriction. (**c**) CD20 vs. CD5 histogram shows lack of CD5 expression on the kappa monotypic B-cells. (**d**) CD20 vs. CD10 histogram shows lack of CD10 expression on the kappa monotypic B-cells (courtesy of Timothy P. Singleton, M.D. and Dan McKeon, Flow Cytometry Laboratory, Department of Laboratory Medicine and Pathology, University of Minnesota).

The typical phenotype of each lymphoma will be presented in the following chapters together with their characteristic cytomorphology and cytogenetic findings.

Immunocytochemical and Immunohistochemical Methods

Immunocytochemistry on Cytospin Preparations

In some laboratories, immunophenotyping is performed on cytospin preparations. This technique has some advantages over FC, since it requires fewer cells, and the presence and intensity of markers can be correlated with cytomorphology. It may also allow immunophenotyping in cases where FC is unsuccessful due to the fragility of the neoplastic cells. However, the disadvantage of this technique is that it does not allow the simultaneous assessment of multiple markers on the same cell.

Immunohistochemistry on Cell Block Specimens

Immunohistochemical stains for a variety of markers can also be performed on cell block preparations. These immunohistochemical stains can be useful in the classification of lymphoid proliferations, and the differential diagnosis between lymphoid and nonlymphoid neoplasms.

In the diagnosis of lymphoid proliferations, this method has some definite disadvantages over FC, because the number of antibodies available is smaller than for FC, the simultaneous assessment of multiple markers on the same cell is not possible, and kappa and lambda stains are difficult to interpret, thus limiting its usefulness in the determination of clonality. It is therefore important to submit routinely the needle rinses from 2 to 3 passes for FC and possibly submit the majority of cells obtained in an additional FNA pass for cell block preparation, since immunohistochemistry also has some advantages. Apart from the possibility to correlate the stains with the cytomorphology, immunohistochemical stains frequently react with nonviable "ghost" cells. It also allows the use of some markers that are not routinely available for FC, such as cyclin D1. In addition, immunohistochemistry is the method of choice for lymphoid proliferations showing rare neoplastic cells such as Hodgkin lymphoma, ALCL, and T-cell-rich B-cell lymphomas, despite recent advances with multicolor FC in these conditions.

Because each immunohistochemical stain is performed on a separate section and the material available is limited, panels of immunostains are sequentially performed to reach a complete characterization of the lymphoid proliferation.

A general panel that can be used when non-Hodgkin lymphoma is suspected is composed of CD20, which identifies most B-cells and their neoplasms; CD3, which identifies most T-cells (membranous staining) and natural killer cells (cytoplasmic staining); CD5 and CD43, T-cell markers frequently aberrantly expressed in B-cell lymphomas; CD10 and Bcl6, markers of germinal center B-cells; and Bcl2, which marks many neoplastic B-cells but not normal germinal center B-cells and Cyclin D1.

As normal lymph node aspirates show a marked predominance of T-cells, a suspicion of B-cell lymphoma is raised if a large proportion of the aspirate is composed of CD20+ B-cells. Coexpression of CD5 and/or CD43 on a large proportion of these cells is an indicator of lymphoma (CLL/SLL), as is the presence of Bcl2 staining on CD10 or Bcl6-staining cells (follicular lymphoma), or staining for Cyclin D1 of a large proportion of lymphoid cells (MCL).

In addition to markers also available for FC, there are a number of unique immunohistochemical markers that may be useful in characterizing lymphoid proliferations. Pax-5, a B-cell marker expressed in normal B-cells (but not plasma cells) and most B-cell lymphomas, is useful especially in situations when CD20 is negative in recurrences of B-cell lymphomas after rituximab therapy. Awareness of the fact that Pax-5 is also expressed in small cell carcinomas, Merkel cell carcinomas, and alveolar rhabdomyosarcomas that may enter the differential diagnosis is essential to prevent pitfalls. Other potential pitfalls are the expression of CD5 in smooth and skeletal muscles and their tumors, and the expression of TdT in Merkel cell carcinoma.

B-cell light chain restriction by kappa and lambda light chain immunoperoxidase stains, or in-situ hybridization studies can only rarely establish clonality; however, they may be useful in characterizing aspirates with a prominent plasma cell component.

A variety of other immunohistochemical markers may be used, including Ki67 (MIB1), either as diagnostic or as prognostic markers. Almost 100% expression of Ki67 in Burkitt lymphoma is helpful in its differentiation from other high-grade lymphomas.

A general first panel that can be used when Hodgkin lymphoma is suspected is composed of CD20, CD3, CD15, CD30, CD45RB

(LCA), EMA, and ALK-1. Their use in the differential diagnosis between Hodgkin lymphoma and non-Hodgkin lymphomas and in the classification of Hodgkin lymphoma will be addressed in Chap. 11.

Immunoperoxidase stains for LMP-1 and in situ hybridization for EBER can also detect EBV, which is present in infectious mononucleosis, immunosuppression-associated lymphoproliferations, Burkitt lymphoma, immunoblastic/plasmablastic tumors, Hodgkin lymphoma, angioimmunoblastic T-cell lymphoma, and NK-cell neoplasms. Immunohistochemical detection of HHV8 with an antibody against the latent nuclear antigen (LNA-1) may be useful in the diagnosis of multicentric Castleman disease (MCD), plasmablastic lymphoma (PBL) arising in MCD, and primary effusion lymphoma (PEL).

FISH and Conventional Cytogenetics

Both conventional cytogenetics (G-banding) and FISH can be used to demonstrate the characteristic recurrent cytogenetic abnormalities found in some lymphomas (see Table 2.2).

Conventional cytogenetic studies can also demonstrate additional abnormalities that may be of prognostic importance. For the evaluation of FNA biopsy samples, FISH is preferable to conventional cytogenetics because it is faster, does not require a fresh sample (although fresh tissue is preferred), and can be performed on smears, cytospins, or cell block preparations. Because FISH is usually performed on interphase (nondividing) nuclei, low proliferative rates do not preclude analysis.

Several types of FISH probes can be used in the evaluation of lymphoid proliferation. Probes that hybridize to specific centromeres are useful for detection of polysomies such as trisomy 12 in CLL/SLL (Fig. 2.7a–c), and fusion or break-apart probes are useful in the detection of translocations.

Break-apart probes hybridize to a specific region on a single chromosome, flanking the breakpoint region with a green and a red probe (i.e., the 3′ region is labeled in either red or green, and the 5′ region is labeled in the other color). In a fluorescence microscope, overlapping or closely apposed red and green signals appear yellow; thus, the pattern in a normal interphase nucleus is two yellow signals (the red and green components of this yellow fusion signal

TABLE 2.2. Characteristic cytogenetic abnormalities in lymphomas.

Lymphoma	Cytogenetic abnormalities	Frequency (%)	Genes involved	Diagnostic or prognostic use	FISH type
SLL/CLL	Trisomy 12	25		Diagnostic	Centromeric enumeration
SLL/CLL	del 13	40–60	*RB1*	Positive prognostic	Locus specific
SLL/CLL	del 11	10–20	*ATM*	Negative prognostic	Locus specific
SLL/CLL	del 17	10	*p53*	Negative prognostic	Locus specific
MCL	t(11;14)	Over 95	*IGH/BCL1*	Diagnostic	Break-apart, dual-fusion
FL	t(14;18)	70–80	*IGH/BCL2*	Diagnostic	Break-apart, dual-fusion
MZL	t(11;18)	15–30	*API2/ MALT1*	Diagnostic	Break-apart, dual-fusion
BL	t(8;14)	80	*IGH/CMYC*	Diagnostic	Dual fusion, break-apart
DLBCL	t(14;18)	30	*IGH/BCL2*	Diagnostic	Break-apart, dual fusion
ALCL	t(2;5)	70	*ALK/NPM*	Diagnostic Positive prognostic	Break-apart, Multicolor

SLL/CLL small lymphocytic lymphoma/chronic lymphocytic leukemia; *MCL* mantle cell lymphoma; *FL* follicular lymphoma; *MZL* marginal zone lymphoma; *BL* Burkitt lymphoma; *DLBCL* diffuse large B-cell lymphoma; *ALCL* anaplastic large cell lymphoma

are sometimes visible). A translocation will break apart the 3′ and 5′ probes flanking the breakpoint, thus resulting in the following signal pattern: one yellow (the normal chromosome homolog), one red, and one green signal (representing the now separated 3′ and 5′ portions of the involved gene) (Fig. 2.8a–c).

Break-apart probes are useful in determining rearrangement of "promiscuous" genes that have a number of different partner genes. Although such a signal pattern indicates the presence of a translocation, it does not identify the other partner chromosome. For example, the *IGH* gene is involved in translocations with several different partners in a large percentage of B-cell lymphomas. Using an *IGH* break-apart probe will identify the presence of an *IGH*

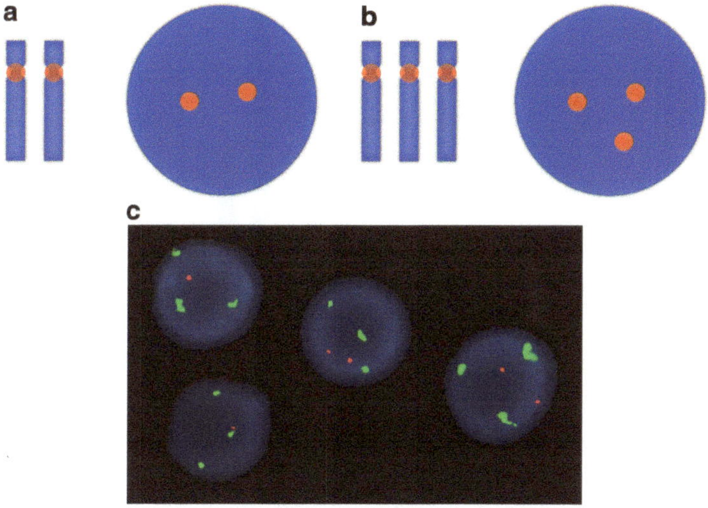

FIGURE 2.7. FISH with chromosome enumeration probes to determine trisomy. (**a**, **b**) Schematic representation with normal (**a**) and abnormal (**b**) results of FISH. (**c**) FISH result in a case of CLL/SLL with trisomy 12 in all four cells (*green signals*) and loss of D13S319 (13q14) (*red signals*) in two cells (courtesy of Michelle Dolan, M.D., Cytogenetics Laboratory, and Jonathan Henriksen, Department of Laboratory Medicine and Pathology, University of Minnesota).

gene rearrangement, but a specific dual-fusion translocation probe (e.g., *IGH*/BCL2 or *IGH*/CCND1) would be needed to identify the partner chromosome.

The most sensitive FISH probes to detect reciprocal translocations are dual fusion probes. Each of the genes or loci of interest is labeled in either red or green, and each probe extends both proximal and distal to the breakpoint (i.e., the labeled region spans the breakpoint). In normal cells, two distinct red and two distinct green signals are present. In a reciprocal translocation, the chromosomal regions distal to the breakpoints are exchanged, thus bringing together red and green probes on each of the involved derivative chromosomes. Thus, the signal pattern in a cell with a translocation is one red and one green (representing the normal, uninvolved chromosomes) signal, and two yellow fusion signals (representing

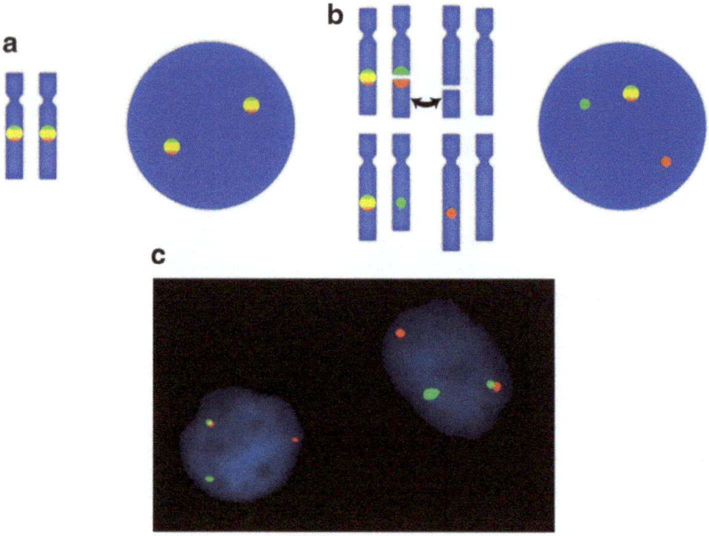

FIGURE 2.8. FISH with break-apart probes to determine the presence of a translocation involving a specific region. (**a**, **b**) Schematic representation with normal (**a**) and abnormal (**b**) results of FISH. (**c**) FISH result in a case of anaplastic large cell lymphoma (ALCL) with t(2;5) translocation. The normal (nontranslocated) 2p23 ALK region is seen as two immediately adjacent *orange–red/green* signals or as a fused *yellow* signal; the 2p23 ALK region that has suffered a t(2;5) (or another translocation) is seen as one *orange–red* and one *green* signal (courtesy of Michelle Dolan, M.D., Cytogenetics Laboratory, and Jonathan Henriksen, Department of Laboratory Medicine and Pathology, University of Minnesota).

each of the partner chromosomes involved in the translocation) (Fig. 2.9a–c).

In contrast to a conventional G-banded cytogenetic analysis in which all chromosomal abnormalities can be identified, FISH can identify only the translocation specifically targeted by the probe set used. Therefore, FISH tests should be ordered based on the differential diagnosis generated by the cytomorphologic or immunophenotypic data, especially if the entities considered in the differential (e.g., FL vs. MZL, FL vs. MCL, etc.) are characterized by different translocations. Because of considerable cytomorphologic and immunophenotypic overlap, one of the most difficult differential diagnoses is between DLBCL and Burkitt lymphoma.

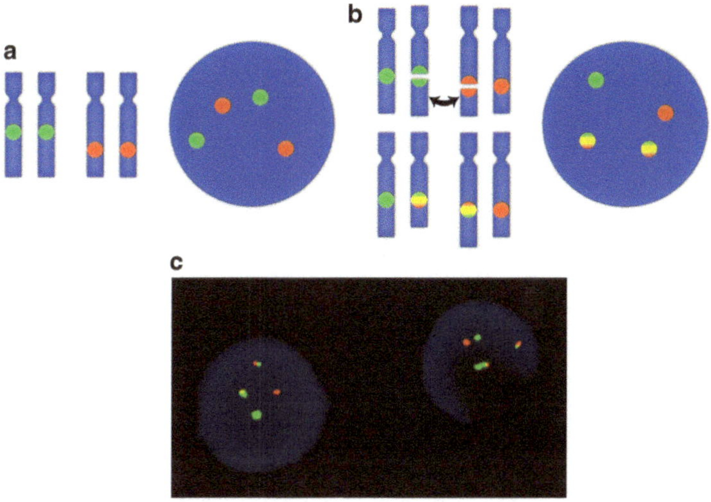

FIGURE 2.9. FISH with dual color, dual fusion probes to determine the presence of a specific translocation. (**a**, **b**) Schematic representation with normal (**a**) and abnormal (**b**) results of FISH. (**c**) FISH result in a case of follicular lymphoma (FL) with t(14;18) IGH/BCL2 translocation. The nuclei show one *orange–red* signal and one *green* signal representing the normal (nontranslocated) chromosomes and two *orange–red/green* or *yellow* fusion signals representing the two chromosomes resulting from the reciprocal translocation (courtesy of Michelle Dolan, M.D., Cytogenetics Laboratory, and Jonathan Henriksen, Department of Laboratory Medicine and Pathology, University of Minnesota).

In this situation, determining the presence of a translocation involving MYC using a break-apart probe may be diagnostically useful.

FISH studies can also be helpful in determining prognosis. For example, in CLL/SLL, a FISH panel test for B-CLL may include, among others, probes for the demonstration of the deletion of markers with prognostic implications such as *MYB* (6q23), *ATM* (11q22.3), 13q14.3, and *TP53* (17p13.1) (Fig. 2.10a–c).

Molecular Studies

Molecular studies are rarely used in the work-up of lymph node fine needle aspirates, but may be helpful in cases where other

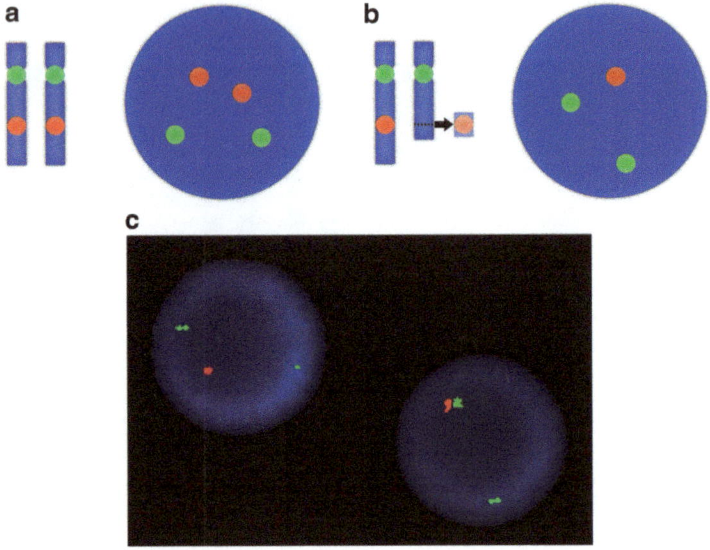

FIGURE 2.10. FISH with locus-specific probes to determine the presence of a specific deletion. (**a**, **b**) Schematic representation with normal (**a**) and abnormal (**b**) results of FISH. (**c**) FISH result in a case of small lymphocytic lymphoma (CLL/SLL) with del 17p13.1 (TP53), associated with worse prognosis. Only one *orange–red* signal is present, while the two *green* signals signify the presence of both centromeres (courtesy of Michelle Dolan, M.D., Cytogenetics Laboratory, and Jonathan Henriksen, Department of Laboratory Medicine and Pathology, University of Minnesota).

ancillary studies could not be performed, were nondiagnostic, or yielded ambiguous results. Molecular studies are helpful in determining the clonality of lymphoid proliferations through DNA-based antigen receptors assays (Southern blot or PCR based) and in aiding the correct classification of lymphomas by demonstrating translocations characteristic for certain lymphomas by PCR, as in the case of t(14;18) of follicular lymphomas, or their fusion gene transcript by RT-PCR, as in the case of the t(2;5) of ALCL.

Antigen Receptor Assays by Southern Blot Analysis or PCR

Southern blot analysis is the most specific of the molecular methods used but it is not commonly used because of the need for fresh samples, large amounts of high quality DNA, slow turn-around time, and high cost. PCR-based techniques, on the contrary, are fast, require very small amounts of cellular sample, and can be performed on material from cell blocks or from cells scraped from smears.

B-cells and T-cells recognize antigens by structurally similar heterodimer proteins composed of both variable and constant regions linked by disulfide bonds, the B-cell surface immunoglobulin receptor (*IG*), and the *TCR*. These are encoded by the *IG* and *TCR* genes, which belong to the same antigen receptor supergene family. Both *IG* and *TCR* genes undergo somatic rearrangements in the earliest stages of lymphoid differentiation and are, therefore, present in the vast majority of immature and mature lymphoid cells.

The *IGH* gene at chromosome 14q32 contains multiple *V*, *J*, *D*, and *C* gene segments that rearrange by somatic recombination to achieve the enormous diversity of antigen receptors. Rearrangements occur sequentially in an orderly fashion; *D* is first rearranged to *J* and then *V* is rearranged to *DJ*. These rearrangements occur with deletion of the intervening DNA and, therefore, result in variably sized DNA segments that are different from the initial nonrearranged DNA referred to as *germline configuration* and between different rearranged cells.

Similar rearrangements occur in the *TCR* genes. The *TCR* is composed of either one alpha and one beta polypeptide chain (αβ *TCR*) or one gamma and one delta polypeptide chain (γδ *TCR*). The corresponding four *TCR* genes are rearranged sequentially: First *TCR*δ (14q11), then *TCR*γ (7p15), *TCR*β (7q34), and finally *TCR*α (14q11). The *TCR*γ gene is usually targeted for clonality studies because it is less complex than *TCR*β. *TCR*γ rearrangements are present in both αβ and γδ T-cells and the vast majority of T-cell neoplasms.

The diversity of sizes of the rearranged *IG* or *TCR* genes is diagnostically useful in determining clonality, as DNA amplified from reactive, polyclonal lymphoid populations shows a wide range of gene sizes, whereas neoplastic lymphoid cells, which are in principle all derived from a common clone, show identically rearranged *IG* or *TCR* genes.

Southern blot analysis uses restriction endonuclease enzyme digestion of the DNA extracted from the lymphocyte population. The fragments are then separated by electrophoresis and immobilized on a nylon membrane, and then hybridized to a radiolabeled fragment of the gene of interest (*IGH* or *TCR*β). A band is detected if the sample contains more than about 5–10% clonal, presumably neoplastic cells admixed with polyclonal cells. Polyclonal cells appear as a background smear because of the variable size of the fragments resulting from endonuclease digestion.

PCR-based assays for B-cell clonality use a variety of V and J specific or consensus primers that amplify the *IGH* V-(D)-J region, also known as the CDR3 (complementarity determining region 3) or N region; the amplimer is then detected using conventional electrophoresis in agarose, nondenaturing polyacrylamide gel electrophoresis with ethidium bromide staining, or the more sensitive capillary electrophoresis. If a polyclonal lymphoid population is present, each lymphocyte will have an N region of a different size, and no bands or peaks will be seen on gel electrophoresis and capillary electrophoresis, respectively. In contrast, clonal populations will show a definite band or peak (Fig. 2.11a–c).

FIGURE 2.11. *IGH* rearrangement studies. (**a**) Schematic representation of the *IGH* rearrangements, location of PCR framework 2 (FR2) and framework 3 (FR3) primers and the common antisense primer that anneals in the J region of the *IGH* gene and possible results of the PCR reaction on capillary electrophoresis. Expected size range for FR2 PCR products is 220–250 bp and that of FR3 products is 70–150 bp. Polyclonal lymphoid populations show a Gaussian distribution of sizes of the PCR products while clonal B-cell populations show a discrete peak. Our laboratory defines a peak as clonal if it meets the following requirements: an electropherogram peak height of >1,500 fluorescent units; and a peak height three times the height of the polyclonal background. (**b**) Results of PCR using FR2 and FR3 primers for determination of *IGH* gene rearrangement in a case of reactive lymphadenopathy. This is an example of a negative B-cell gene rearrangement test that shows multiple small bands in the FR2 reaction between 220 and 250 bp (*top panel*) and a polyclonal bell shaped curve in FR3 reaction between 70 and 150 bp (*bottom panel*). Note the absence of a discrete peak. (**c**) Results of PCR using FR2 and FR3 primers for determination of *IGH* gene rearrangement in a case of B-cell lymphoma. This is an example of a positive B-cell gene rearrangement test that shows positive clonal peaks in the FR2 (*top panel*) and FR3 (*bottom panel*) regions. Both these clonal peaks are >1,500 RFU and the peak heights are three times the height of the polyclonal background (courtesy of Bharat Thyagarajan, M.D., Molecular Diagnostics Laboratory, Department of Laboratory Medicine and Pathology, University of Minnesota).

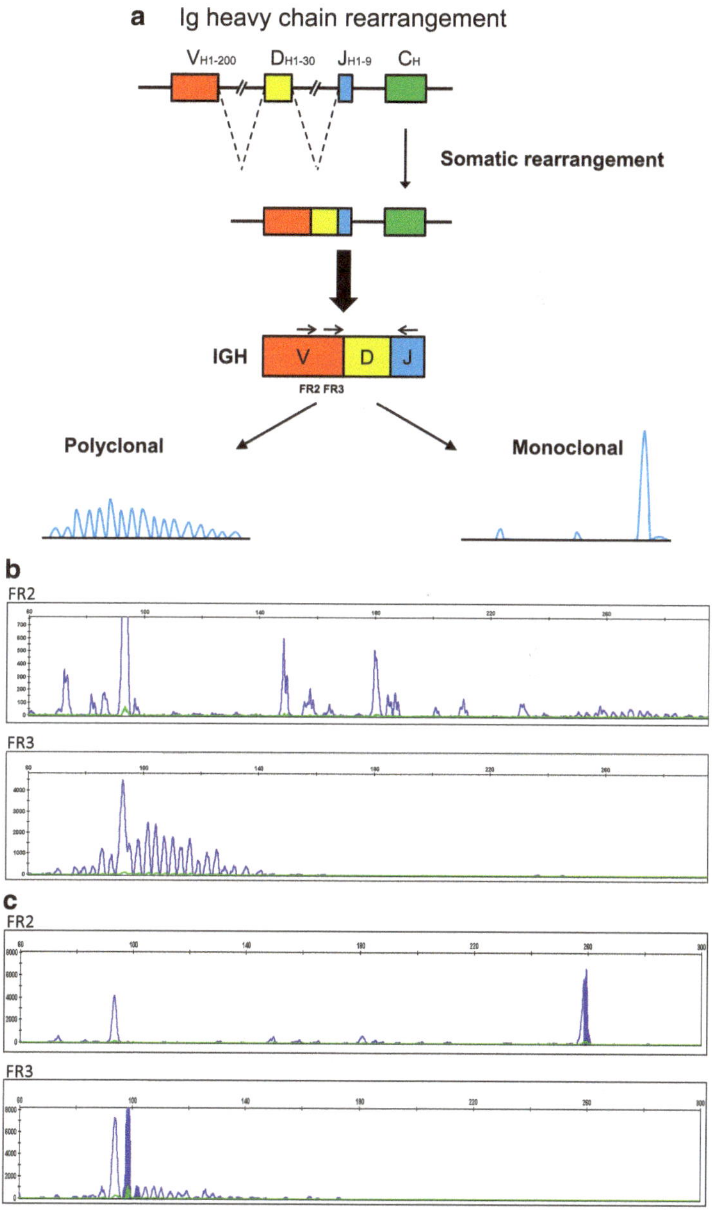
a
Ig heavy chain rearrangement
VH1-200
DH1-30
JH1-9
CH
Somatic rearrangement
IGH
V
D
J
FR2 FR3
Polyclonal
Monoclonal
b
FR2
FR3
c
FR2
FR3

PCR-based assays to determine T-cell clonality employ various combinations of V family and J region primers on the *TCRγ* with amplimer detection and results interpretation similar to those described above. A clone can be detected if there are about 5% of clonal T-cells in a background of polyclonal cells in nondenaturing polyacrylamide gels, with higher sensitivities for capillary electrophoresis (Fig. 2.12a–c).

The sensitivity of PCR-based methods for determining B-cell or T-cell clonality is significantly lower in cell populations obtained from fixed and paraffin-embedded specimens compared to that in fresh specimens.

For detection of *IGH* rearrangements in B-cell lymphoid proliferations, the false negative rate may be as high as 30% in germinal center/postgerminal center lymphomas, such as follicular lymphoma and DLBCL. This occurs due to the fact that B-cells undergo somatic hypermutation in the *IGH* V region in response to antigen exposure in the germinal center, and lymphomas occurring beyond this stage of B-cell development may show high degrees of somatic hypermutation which may modify the PCR primer-binding sites. No equivalent somatic hypermutation process occurs in rearranged *TCR* genes and mispriming is therefore not a problem in T-cell lymphoma clonality determination.

If only a small number of lymphocytes are available for the test, PCR-based antigen receptor assays may give false-positive results due to pseudoclonality caused by the presence of different rearrangements of identical length.

It should be stressed again that detection of clonality is not in and for itself equivalent with malignancy (lymphoma). Apart from technical problems such as contamination or pseudoclonality, real clonal expansions of lymphoid populations may occur in benign disorders such as immunodeficiency states, autoimmune diseases (Sjögren syndrome and Hashimoto thyroiditis), and viral infections (HIV, EBV, and HHV8).

Antigen receptor rearrangements are not entirely lineage specific, as the clonal *IGH*, or *TCR* gene rearrangement detected may be discordant with the B-cell or T-cell lymphoma immunophenotype, i.e., *TCR* rearrangements may be detected in B-cell lymphomas and *IGH* rearrangements in B-cell lymphomas. This occurs especially in lymphoblastic lymphomas but can rarely occur in other lymphomas.

DNA-Based Tests for Identifying Translocations

In addition to conventional cytogenetics and FISH, translocations and their products can also be identified by various molecular techniques including Southern blot, PCR, and RT-PCR.

However, FISH is more commonly used to identify translocations. The very high sensitivity, with capabilities of detection of less than 1 in 1,000 cells showing the translocation makes some of these molecular methods suitable for detection of minimal residual disease.

Differentiating Lymphoid from Nonlymphoid Neoplasms and Establishing the Nature and Potential Site of Origin of a Metastatic Malignancy

Lymph nodes are the most common site of metastasis and metastatic malignancies outnumber primary lymphoid neoplasms in most lymph node locations. When the primary malignancy is known, metastases are frequently diagnosed by the cytomorphologic features of the lymph node aspirate and comparison with the morphology of the primary tumor. However, about 10–15% of all malignancies first present with metastases and the primary site may be difficult to determine even after a thorough clinical evaluation. In addition, second nonlymphoid or lymphoid primaries may occur in patients with known malignancies. Even when the primary malignancy is not known, cytomorphologic features usually allow a diagnosis of metastatic carcinomas or of a metastasis from another malignancy. However, in cases of small cell malignancies (small cell carcinoma and small blue cell tumors) that are very poorly differentiated, the differential diagnosis with lymphoid malignancies may be difficult or impossible based on cytomorphologic features alone. Since an accurate diagnosis is crucial in determining the best management of the patient, a panel of immunohistochemical stains will usually allow distinction of lymphomas from metastatic carcinomas, melanomas, and other metastatic malignancies. A first panel of antibodies usually includes CD45RB (LCA) as a marker of hematolymphoid neoplasms, keratins (usually a cocktail of cytokeratins such as cytokeratin AE1/AE3 and cytokeratin 8/18) and epithelial membrane antigen (EMA) as epithelial markers, S100 as

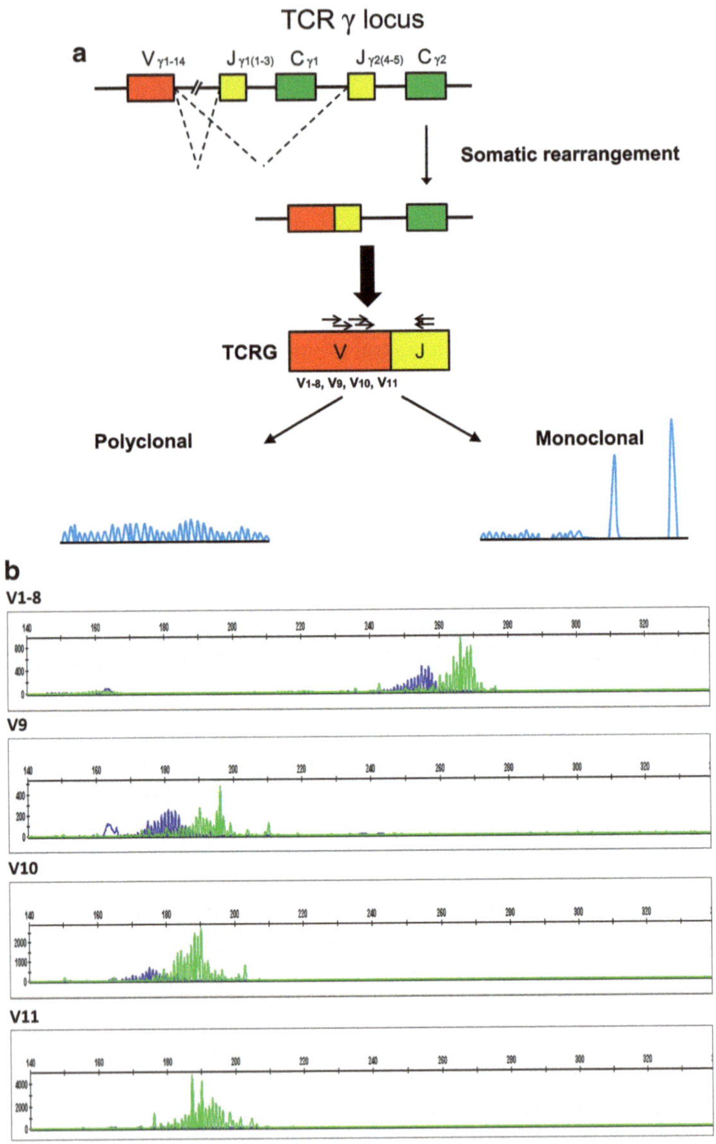

FIGURE 2.12. TCRG rearrangement studies. (**a**) Schematic representation of the TCRG rearrangements, location of PCR primers and results of the PCR reaction on capillary electrophoresis. Primer VG1 binds to regions V1–V8, VG9 binds to V9, VG10 binds to V10 and VG11 binds to V11 paired with two antisense primers JG and JP (labeled with different fluorescent dyes, JG1/2 with blue and JP1/2 with green) that recognize different J regions. The expected size range of PCR products of the VG1/JG1/2 reaction is 250–300 bp, while that of the remaining reactions is 160–210 bp.

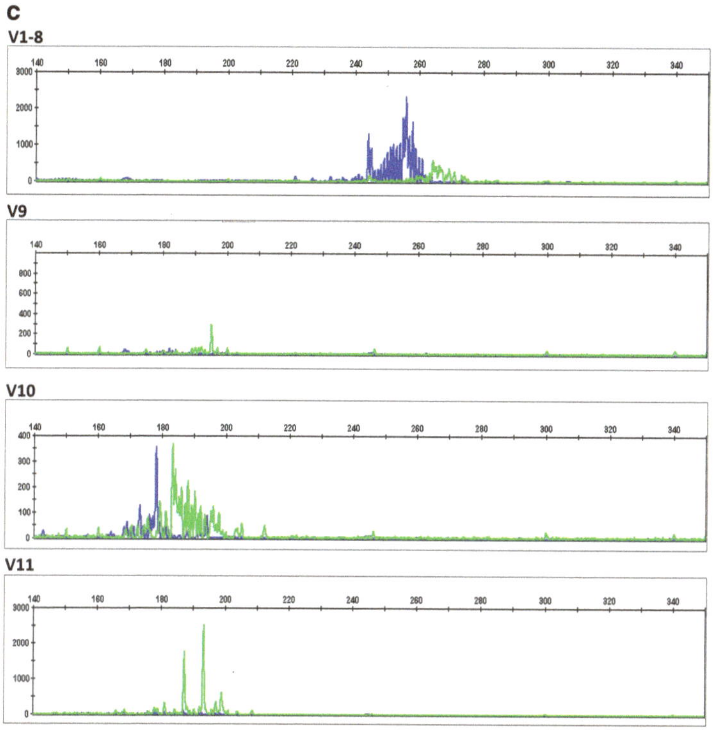

FIGURE 2.12. (continued) Polyclonal lymphoid populations show a Gaussian distribution of sizes of the PCR products while clonal T-cell populations show one or two discrete peaks. Our laboratory defines a peak as clonal if it meets the following requirements: an electropherogram peak height of 1,500 fluorescent units; and a peak height three times the height of the polyclonal background. (**b**) Results of PCR using VG1, VG9, VG10 and VG11 primers for the determination of TCRG gene rearrangement in a case of reactive lymphadenopathy. This is an example of a negative T gene rearrangement test. The VG1 reaction (*top panel*) shows a polyclonal background between 250 and 300 bp. The VG9 (*second panel*), VG10 (*third panel*) and VG11 reactions (*bottom panel*) show a polyclonal background between 160 and 210 bp. Though the VG11 panel shows clonal peak heights that are >1,500 RFUs, none of the peak heights are three times the height of the polyclonal background. (**c**) Results of PCR using VG1, VG9 VG10 and VG11 primers for the determination of TCRG gene rearrangement in a case of T-cell lymphoma. This is an example of a positive T gene rearrangement test. Two positive clonal peaks are detected in the VG11 reaction (*bottom panel*). The height of both peaks is >1,500 RFUs and the peak height three times the height of the polyclonal background. The other three reactions are negative and show a polyclonal background (courtesy of Bharat Thyagarajan, M.D., Molecular Diagnostics Laboratory, Department of Laboratory Medicine and Pathology, University of Minnesota).

a melanocytic marker, and vimentin is frequently used to determine if immunoreactivity of the cells is preserved. Based on the results of this initial panel, additional stains will be selected to confirm the epithelial, hematolymphoid, or melanocytic nature of the metastatic lymphadenopathy, or to rule out less common metastatic malignancies, such as sarcomas and germ cell tumors.

If the immunostains confirm a metastatic carcinoma and the primary site is not known, an attempt is made to determine the primary site by using panels of immunostains that are either "organ specific" such as thyroglobulin, calcitonin, HepPar1, renal cell carcinoma antigen, uroplakin, TTF1, and CDX2, or are differentially expressed by different metastatic carcinomas, such as cytokeratins 7 and 20. It should be noted that no antibody is actually organ specific and that cross-reactivity with other tissues is increasingly reported with the use of these antibodies.

Finally, if a metastasis is suspected but cannot be confirmed by cytomorphology as in the case of cystic or necrotic metastases, chemical determination of thyroglobulin or calcitonin in the lymph node aspirate may be diagnostic of a metastasis from the thyroid. Similarly, the presence of HPV DNA in a cystic lymph node aspirate from the neck usually indicates a cystically degenerated metastasis from a squamous cell carcinoma.

Suggested Reading

Allen TC, Cagle PT (2009) Basic concepts of molecular pathology. Springer, New York

Angelakis E, Roux V, Raoult D, Rolain JM (2009) Real-time PCR strategy and detection of bacterial agents of lymphadenitis. Eur J Clin Microbiol Infect Dis 28(11):1363–1368

Bahrami A, Truong LD, Ro JY (2008) Undifferentiated tumor: true identity by immunohistochemistry. Arch Pathol Lab Med 132(3):326–348

Caraway NP (2005) Strategies to diagnose lymphoproliferative disorders by fine-needle aspiration by using ancillary studies. Cancer 105(6):432–442

Cheng L, Zhang DY (2008) Molecular genetic pathology. Humana, Totowa

Craig FE, Foon KA (2008) Flow cytometric immunophenotyping for hematologic neoplasms. Blood 111(8):3941–3967

Dey P (2006) Role of ancillary techniques in diagnosing and subclassifying non-Hodgkin's lymphomas on fine needle aspiration cytology. Cytopathology 17(5):275–287

Ellis DW, Eaton M, Fox RM, Juneja S, Leong AS, Miliauskas J, Norris DL, Spagnolo D, Turner J (2005) Diagnostic pathology of lymphoproliferative disorders. Pathology 37(6):434–456

Eyzaguirre E, Haque AK (2008) Application of immunohistochemistry to infections. Arch Pathol Lab Med 132(3):424–431

Finn WG, Peterson LC (2004) Hematopathology in oncology. Kluwer, Boston

Fowler LJ, Lachar WA (2008) Application of immunohistochemistry to cytology. Arch Pathol Lab Med 132(3):373–383

Garcia CF, Swerdlow SH (2009) Best practices in contemporary diagnostic immunohistochemistry: panel approach to hematolymphoid proliferations. Arch Pathol Lab Med 133(5):756–765

Gudgin EJ, Erber WN (2005) Immunophenotyping of lymphoproliferative disorders: state of the art. Pathology 37(6):457–478

Higgins RA, Blankenship JE, Kinney MC (2008) Application of immunohistochemistry in the diagnosis of non-Hodgkin and Hodgkin lymphoma. Arch Pathol Lab Med 132(3):441–461

Ioachim HL, Medeiros LJ (2009) Ioachim's lymph node pathology. Wolters Kluwer Health/Lippincott Williams & Wilkins, Philadelphia

Jevremovic D, Viswanatha DS (2009) Molecular diagnosis of hematopoietic and lymphoid neoplasms. Hematol Oncol Clin North Am 23(4):903–933

Jones D (2010) Neoplastic hematopathology: experimental and clinical approaches. Humana, Totowa

Jorgensen JL (2005) State of the Art Symposium: flow cytometry in the diagnosis of lymphoproliferative disorders by fine-needle aspiration. Cancer 105(6):443–451

Nguyen DT, Diamond LW, Braylan RC (2007) Flow cytometry in hematopathology a visual approach to data analysis and interpretation. Humana, Totowa

O'Leary TJ, Abbondanzo SL, Frisman DM (2003) Advanced diagnostic methods in pathology: principles, practice, and protocols. W.B. Saunders, Philadelphia

Pfeifer JD, Arber DA (2006) Molecular genetic testing in surgical pathology. Lippincott Williams & Wilkins, Philadelphia

Spagnolo DV, Ellis DW, Juneja S, Leong AS, Miliauskas J, Norris DL, Turner J (2004) The role of molecular studies in lymphoma diagnosis: a review. Pathology 36(1):19–44

Taylor CR (2009) IHC and the WHO classification of lymphomas: cost effective immunohistochemistry using a deductive reasoning "decision tree" approach. Appl Immunohistochem Mol Morphol 17(5):366–374

Taylor CR (2009) The WHO classification of lymphomas: cost-effective immunohistochemistry using a deductive reasoning "decision tree" approach: part II: the decision tree approach: diffuse patterns of proliferation in lymph nodes. Appl Immunohistochem Mol Morphol 17(6):470–482

3 Lymphadenopathy: Anatomic and Clinical Clues to Fine Needle Aspiration Diagnosis

The cytopathologic evaluation of a lymph node FNA requires knowledge of the patient's clinical history, physical examination, and available laboratory test results.

When possible, the cytopathologist should obtain a rapid clinical history and conduct a brief physical examination. Duration of the lymphadenopathy, local and constitutional symptoms, prior medical history, history of cat scratch, trips to endemic areas, family history, and medication intake, among other factors, must be recorded as well as the location, overlying skin appearance, tenderness, consistency, fixation, size, number, and confluence of lymph nodes. The availability of this information will result in a presumptive clinical diagnosis and determine the handling of the FNA material, i.e., immediate smear interpretation and further sampling for ancillary tests such as cultures, special stains for organisms, immunophenotypic studies, immunocytochemistry, genetic analysis, etc.

Enlarged Lymph Nodes

Lymph nodes are "absent" in newborns and more numerous in children than in adults. In healthy adults, the only palpable lymph nodes may be the inguinal nodes, which are located below the inguinal ligament, measure <1.5 cm, and are oval and soft. In healthy

S.E. Pambuccian and R.H. Bardales, *Lymph Node Cytopathology*, Essentials in Cytopathology 10, DOI 10.1007/978-1-4419-6964-4_3,

children, small lymph nodes may be palpable in the anterior cervical, axillary, and inguinal regions; they measure <1 cm and are also oval and soft. An epitrocheal lymph node larger than 0.5 cm should be considered abnormal in all patients. Lymph node pain may be secondary to inflammation, hemorrhage, or infarction.

Localized or regional lympadenopathy is defined as the enlargement of lymph nodes within contiguous anatomic regions. *Generalized lymphadenopathy* is defined as enlargement of more than two noncontiguous lymph node regions and may also include hepatosplenomegaly.

A round, firm, well-defined lymph node that is present for more than 8 weeks, or a lymph node that is fixed to the skin, deep anatomic planes, or other lymph nodes should be considered for FNA regardless of location, patient age, or symptoms. A regional or generalized lymphadenopathy associated with constitutional symptoms in children or adults should also be considered for FNA.

A palpable regional or generalized lymphadenopathy is commonly the result of nonneoplastic pathologic conditions in children and adults. Viral, bacterial, or mycobaterial infections, depending on the world region, are the most common causes of benign regional lymphadenopathy in children. However, some children with systemic disease such as infectious mononucleosis, viral hepatitis, CMV disease, influenza, rubella, or malignancy may have regional lymphadenopathy, commonly cervical. The most common malignant causes of lymphadenopathy in children are lymphomas and leukemias, followed by solid tumors such as neuroblastoma, rhabdomyosarcoma, Wilms tumor, nasopharyngeal carcinoma, and osteosarcoma.

Regional firm, fixed, and confluent lymph nodes are more common in malignancies other than non-Hodgkin lymphoma. Regional lymphadenopathy in a patient with a history of malignancy may represent a metastatic deposit; however, the cytopathologist should not be influenced by the clinical information in evaluating the smear. In patients with no history of malignancy, the differential diagnosis is based on the clinical scenario, including the age of the patient, the clinical history, physical examination, and the location of the lymph node. In a young patient, regional lymphadenopathy may be seen in Hodgkin lymphoma with or without B symptoms (fever, anorexia, weight loss, or pruritus). Non-Hodgkin lymphoma usually is associated with generalized lymphadenopathy, splenomegaly, and constitutional symptoms.

Lymph Node Groups and Lymphatic Drainage

Localized processes, i.e., infections or malignancies, cause regional lymphadenopathy which is limited to the lymph nodes receiving afferents from that area. Therefore, understanding the pattern of lymphatic drainage is helpful in the evaluation of a patient with lymphadenopathy. Table 3.1 lists the lymph nodes and their areas of afferent lymphatic drainage.

TABLE 3.1. Lymph node chains and their areas of afferent lymphatic drainage.

Lymph node location	Lymphatic drainage
Head	
Occipital	Occipital region of the scalp
Posterior auricular	Posterior part of the external acoustic meatus
Anterior auricular	Lateral region of the ear lobe and adjacent temporal region
Intraparotid	Root of the nose, eyelids, frontotemporal region, external acoustic meatus, and tympanic cavity
Facial infraorbital, buccal, and mandibular	Eyelids, conjunctiva, and skin and mucous membranes of the nose and cheek
Neck	
Submandibular	Medial palpebral commissure, cheek, side of the nose, upper lip, gums, anterior part of the margin of the tongue
Submental	Central portions of the lower lip and floor of the mouth and the apex of the tongue
Superficial cervical: superficial to the sternocleidomastoid muscle	Lower parts of the ear lobe and parotid region
Anterior cervical: ventral to the larynx and trachea	Lower part of the larynx, the thyroid gland, and the cranial part of the trachea
Deep cervical, upper and middle: a chain along the carotid sheath and the internal jugular vein from the base of the skull to the root of the neck under the sternocleiodomastoid muscle	Occipital area of the scalp and ear, back of the neck, part of the tongue, larynx, thyroid gland, trachea, nasopharynx, nasal cavities, palate, and esophagus. The most superior (digastric) is easily palpable in processes affecting the tonsil or pharynx
Deep cervical, lower: beyond the posterior margin of the sternocleidomastoid muscle into the supraclavicular triangle closely related to the brachial plexus and subclavian vein	Back of the scalp and neck, the superficial pectoral region, part of the arm and occasionally, part of the superior surface of the liver. They also receive afferents from the superior deep cervical nodes

(continued)

TABLE 3.1. (continued)

Lymph node location	Lymphatic drainage
Left supraclavicular	
Left subclavian vein and brachial plexus	The right thoracic duct drains in the left subclavian vein and receives lymph from the cisterna chyli (receives the right and left lower intercostal, gastric, superior and inferior mesenteric, right and left lumbar, and right and left internal and external iliac lymphatics), left deep cervical, left supraclavicular, and left mediastinal lymphatics
Right supraclavicular	
Right subclavian vein and brachial plexus	The right lymphatic duct drains in the right subclavian vein and receives lymph from the right mediastinal, right deep cervical, and right supraclavicular lymphatics and no drainage from the abdomen or pelvis
Upper limb	
Epitrochlear	The middle, ring, and little fingers, and the superficial medial aspect of the hand and forearm
Deltopectoral: immediately below the clavicle	Superficial afferents from the arm
Axillary: lateral, anterior, posterior, central, and medial groups	Breast, upper limb, dorsal part of the neck, and trunk above the umbilicus
Thorax: visceral	
Anterior mediastinal	Thymus and pericardium and the sternal nodes
Posterior mediastinal	Esophagus, dorsal part of the pericardium, diaphragm, and convex surface of the liver
Tracheobronchial: tracheal, bronchial, bronchopulmonary, and pulmonary groups	Lungs, bronchi, and thoracic part of the trachea
Parietal abdomen and pelvis	
External iliac	The adductor region of the thigh, glans penis, clitoris, membranous urethra, prostate, fundus of the bladder, uterine cervix, and upper part of the vagina
Common iliac	Internal and external iliac nodes
Internal iliac	Pelvic viscera, the deeper parts of the perineum, including the membranous and cavernous portions of the urethra, and the buttock and dorsum of the thigh

(continued)

TABLE 3.1. (continued)

Lymph node location	Lymphatic drainage
Lumbar periaortic: celiac, superior mesenteric, inferior mesenteric, right and left lateral, and retro-aortic groups	Abdominal viscera, kidney and adrenal, testis, ovary, fallopian tube, uterine body, and the lateral abdominal muscles
Visceral abdomen and pelvis	
Celiac: gastric, hepatic, and pancreatosplenic groups	Stomach, duodenum, liver, gallbladder, pancreas, and spleen
Superior mesenteric: mesenteric, ileocolic, and mesocolic groups	Jejunum, ileum, cecum, vermiform appendix, and ascending and transverse colon
Inferior mesenteric	Descending and sigmoid colon and the upper part of the rectum
Lower limb	
Popliteal	The deep areas of the leg and the superficial fibular side of the foot and lateral area of the leg
Inguinal: superficial (distal to the inguinal ligament), and subinguinal: superficial and deep	The skin of the penis, scrotum, perineum, buttock, and abdominal wall below the umbilicus, the dorsum of the foot and medial areas of the leg, and the deep region around the femoral vessels, the glans penis, and clitoris

Cervical Lymphadenopathy

The following are causes of lymphadenopathy by age groups.

Children

- Bilateral cervical lymphadenopathy:
  - Viruses that affect the upper respiratory tract (respiratory syncytial virus, adenovirus, measles, and influenza).
  - Sinus histiocytosis with massive lymphadenopathy (Rosai-Dorfman disease), seen more often in males. Other regions may be involved.
  - Sarcoidosis. Uncommon in children. Commonly associated with symmetric hilar lymphadenopathy.

- Unilateral cervical:
  - Frequently acute suppurative lymphadenitis, often preceded by upper respiratory infection, pharyngitis, or otitis.
- Chronic lymphadenopathy offers a broader differential diagnosis:
  - Viral or bacterial upper respiratory tract infections, atypical mycobacterial infection (*Mycobacterium avium intracellulare*, *Mycobacterium scrofulaceum*), *Mycobacterium tuberculosis*, EBV or CMV infection, toxoplasmosis (frequently posterior cervical), or less commonly histoplasmosis, actinomycosis, or HIV.
  - Cat scratch disease (when the scratch is on the face) may cause significant cervical lymphadenopathy and may persist for months. Epitrochlear or axillary lymphadenopathy may also be found.
  - Rare causes include tularemia, brucellosis, and anthrax.
- Noninfectious causes of regional cervical lymphadenopathy:
  - Collagen vascular diseases, metabolic storage diseases, and less frequently medications such as phenytoin (can elicit generalized lymphadenopathy).
  - Kikuchi disease.
  - Kawasaki disease, associated with vasculitis. Generalized lymphadenopathy does not occur.
  - Rarely, immunization with live attenuated measles, DPT, Salk vaccine, and typhoid fever vaccination.
  - Langerhans cell histiocytosis. In one third of patients is often a manifestation of a systemic process with generalized lymphadenopathy.
  - Castleman disease. Rare in the pediatric population. The cervical lymphadenopathy commonly is associated with mediastinal or hilar lymphadenopathy.

Adolescents and Young Adults

- Kimura lymphadenopathy. Affects the salivary glands and subcutaneous tissue of the neck, with regional cervical lymphadenopathy most frequent in oriental male patients.

- Sinus histiocytosis with massive lympadenopathy (Rosai-Dorfman disease). Regions other than the neck may be involved.
- Sarcoidosis. Typically affects adults who usually have bilateral cervical lymphadenopathy and commonly symmetric hilar lymphadenopathy.
- Systemic lupus erythematosus. Patients commonly have cervical lymphadenopathy, although mesenteric, axillary, or inguinal lymphadenopathy may occur.
- Castleman disease. The cervical lymphadenopathy commonly is associated with mediastinal or hilar lymphadenopathy, particularly in the hyaline vascular variant.
- Hodgkin lymphoma. Commonly shows cervical and mediastinal lymph node involvement.
- Sporadic Burkitt lymphoma in the appropriate clinical and geographic settings.
- Metastatic germ cell tumor, papillary thyroid carcinoma, and nasopharyngeal carcinoma (30% show bilateral adenopathy). Not uncommonly, metastatic nasopharyngeal, oropharyngeal, and papillary carcinomas may be the first manifestation of the malignancy in any age group. Other malignancies are very uncommon.

Adults and the Elderly

- Toxoplasmosis may occur with cervical lymphadenitis without local or systemic symptoms.
- Kimura lymphadenopathy can also be seen in Orientals of these age groups.
- Castleman disease occurs in a broad age range. Patients with the plasma cell variant tend to be older, and the mediastinum is involved less frequently than in the hyaline vascular variant.
- Metastatic carcinoma increases in incidence parallel to the patient's age and is by far a more common cause of regional lymphadenopathy than are malignant lymphomas, especially in patients more than 50 years old. Metastatic squamous cell carcinoma of the head and neck is frequent after the age of 40 and is the single most important consideration after the age of 60, particularly when there is a history of alcohol and tobacco use, even a remote one.
- Myeloid sarcoma occasionally can be seen concurrently or may be the first manifestation of the disease and can involve cervical lymph nodes.

Axillary Lymphadenopathy

- Dermatopathic lymphadenopathy, measles, and cat scratch disease.
- Leishmaniasis. Axillary and inguinal lymph nodes may be involved second and third to the epitrochlear nodes in endemic areas.
- Hodgkin and non-Hodgkin lymphomas.
- Metastatic deposits, particularly from breast carcinoma, melanoma, and squamous cell carcinoma in decreasing order of frequency.

Supraclavicular Lympadenopathy

- Left and right supraclavicular lymphadenopathy should be considered pathologic in any age group.
- In children, it often reflects associated mediastinal pathology, including Hodgkin lymphoma and neuroblastoma arising from the high thoracic or cervical sympathetic ganglion. It can be found as extension of the primary pulmonary focus in pulmonary tuberculosis.
- In adults, supraclavicular lymphadenopathy is a metastasis of malignancies located below the clavicle in more than 70% of cases. However, less than 1% of carcinomas in the thorax and abdomen lead to malignant supraclavicular lymphadenopathy. Abdominal and pelvic malignancies are more likely to metastasize to the left supraclavicular lymph nodes (Virchow's node). Lung, breast, and head and neck malignancies show no differences in metastatic patterns to the left or right supraclavicular lymph nodes, and the metastasis is usually ipsilateral to the primary tumor.
- Most patients have known primary malignancies or strong clinical evidence of the primary tumor. Occasionally, a left supraclavicular lymphadenopathy may be the first manifestation of an unknown malignancy, as seen in aggressive prostatic adenocarcinoma.

Mediastinal Lymphadenopathy

- Mediastinal adenopathy occurs as a mediastinal mass and may be found in the anterior, middle, and posterior mediastinum. The differential diagnosis is based on imaging studies, laboratory tests, and clinical presentation. The following is a list of pathologic processes occurring in these anatomic locations.

  - Anterior mediastinum: Substernal goiter, thymoma, thymic cyst, germ cell tumor, mesenchymal tumors.
  - Middle mediastinum: Unilateral: tuberculosis, metastatic carcinoma (lung, esophagus), bronchogenic cyst, sarcoma. Bilateral: lymphoma, sarcoidosis, histoplasmosis, Castleman disease.
  - Posterior mediastinum: benign and malignant neurogenic tumors, primary neuroectodermal tumor, germ cell tumor, duplication cyst.

- In cases of mediastinal lymphadenopathy in patients with extrathoracic malignancy, metastasis from such a source is likely. On the contrary, when there is no history of malignancy, malignant and benign diagnoses are seen in equal proportion; however, if malignant, a lung primary is the source in >80% of cases.
- In children, and in contrast to the fact that most common causes of lymphadenopathy are benign, most mediastinal masses are malignant. Hodgkin lymphoma is most common in children, whereas non-Hodgkin lymphoma is more common in adults. Mediastinal large B-cell lymphoma has a slight predilection for young women.
- Histoplasmosis and cryptococcosis are the most common fungal lymphadenitis, usually in the presence of pulmonary involvement or disseminated disease.

Inguinal Lymphadenopathy

- Unilateral: dermatopathic lymphadenopathy, leg infections, herpes simplex, syphilis, lymphogranuloma venereum, tuberculosis. Malignancies of the skin of the lower extremities, cervix, vulva, skin of the trunk, anus/rectum, ovary, and penis occur in decreasing order. Sarcoma, melanoma, and metastatic carcinoma (prostate, testis, bladder, breast, lung, and kidney) have also been described.
- Bilateral: measles, venereal disease, non-Hodgkin lymphoma.
- Cat scratch disease may cause tender chronic inguinal lymphadenitis.

Intra-abdominal and Retroperitoneal Lymphadenopathy

- Whipple disease can involve mesenteric lymph nodes.
- Tuberculosis may affect the upper para-aortic nodes and cause large necrotic and calcified masses.
- Malignancies of the lower extremities, male and female pelvic and genital organs, lymphoma, and germ cell tumors particularly if lower para-aortic.

Generalized Lymphadenopathy

- The principal consideration is non-Hodgkin lymphoma that may be accompanied by constitutional symptoms; however, infectious mononucleosis and other viral processes, sarcoidosis, and autoimmune disorders may produce a similar clinical picture.
- Castleman disease in adults commonly occurs with generalized lymphadenopathy and organomegaly.
- Collagen vascular diseases: 75% of rheumatoid arthritis and 12% of systemic lupus erythematosus have generalized lymphadenopathy.
- Sarcoidosis typically affects adults, who have generalized lymphadenopathy commonly involving bilateral neck and hilar regions (symmetric lymphadenopathy).
- Whipple disease. Peripheral lymphadenopathy is seen in half of the patients.
- Epstein-Barr virus, CMV, and herpes simplex.
- AIDS with coexisting reactive nonspecific lymphoid hyperplasia, infectious processes, and non-Hodgkin lymphoma.
- In children: systemic infections (viral, bacterial, fungal, or protozoal), autoimmune diseases, storage diseases, drug reactions, histiocytic disorders, and malignant processes, including leukemia and lymphoma (lymphoblastic and rarely Burkitt). Kikuchi disease may occur with generalized lymphadenopathy and systemic symptoms, including hepatosplenomegaly.
- Bilateral epitrochlear node involvement may be part of a generalized lymphadenopathy in malignant and benign conditions as seen in areas of endemic Leishmaniasis.

Lymph Node Mimics

In evaluating a patient with suspected regional lymphadenopathy, one must be certain that the mass is indeed a lymph node. The clinical differential diagnosis of a mass includes lymph nodes as well as tumors mimicking lymph nodes, particularly when the mass is in the neck.

Location of the mass in the various regions of the neck is helpful for the preliminary diagnosis. A mass in the posterior neck usually is a lymph node. The lateral and anterior neck harbors lymph nodes and tumors that mimic lymph nodes, including cysts. A fluctuant mass may indicate the presence of fluid, i.e., abscess, cyst or a primary or metastatic tumor with cystic degeneration.

- Congenital malformations have consistent locations in the neck region.
  - *Cystic hygromas* are often found at birth or soon thereafter, commonly develop in the posterior triangle, and are soft and multiloculated.
  - *Branchial cleft anomalies* are usually located in the lateral mid- or superior neck below the angle of the jaw along the anterior border of the sternocleidomastoid muscle. They may be behind the muscle, and 10% are bilateral.
  - *Thyroglossal duct cysts* are the most common congenital neck masses in children, are usually located in the anterior midline near the hyoid bone, and move vertically with swallowing and tongue protrusion. Some cysts may occur in the paratracheal region.
  - *Dermoid cysts* are superficial, smooth, and are commonly located in the midline near the suprasternal area in children.
  - *Neonatal torticollis* typically occurs in the first 2 months of life as a benign fibrous mass within the sternocleidomastoid muscle. The infant's head may be tilted to the side of the lesion.
- A hard dermal or subcutaneous nodule may resemble a lymph node and usually corresponds to a *pilomatrixoma* in the first decade of life, a *sebaceous cyst* in adults, or, less commonly, a *skin metastasis*, which are usually multiple.
- *Lipomas* and other *mesenchymal lesions* may resemble lymph nodes.

- A pulsatile mass in the lateral superior neck may represent a prominent carotid arch or a *carotid-body tumor*. If ultrasound is available, a color Doppler examination is helpful.
- Occasionally, a prominent transverse process of the lower cervical vertebra or a "*cervical rib*" may mimic a firm lower lateral cervical lymph node.

Ultrasound Evaluation of Lymph Nodes

High-frequency real-time transcutaneous, endoscopic, or endobronchial ultrasound is used in the evaluation of superficial, mediastinal, abdominal, and pelvic lymph nodes. A lymph node, when discrete, is sonographically distinguishable from the adjacent soft tissue and vessels. For all lymph nodes, gray-scale and color Doppler ultrasound are used for the evaluation of the ultrasound features, which include size, shape (oval, round, or irregular), echogenicity (hypoechoic, hyperechoic, or anechoic), composition (cystic, solid, or mixed), the presence or absence of calcifications, irregular borders, and internal blood flow.

Clinical and ultrasound features may be predictive of malignant involvement with palpable and nonpalpable cervical, mediastinal, or peri-intestinal lymph nodes. Ultrasound features considered abnormal in the lymph nodes include size greater than 1 cm, hypoechogenicity, sharp, distinct margins, and round shape. When all four features are present in one lymph node, the accuracy of predicting malignancy is 80%. However, all four features are present in only 25% of malignant lymph nodes. The ultrasound features may be less reliable predictors of malignant involvement in pulmonary malignancies when compared with GI cancers.

Ultrasound evaluation and color Doppler are also helpful for differentiating well-defined round lymph nodes from blood vessels, cysts, and complex cystic/solid lesions. A cyst shows no vascular blood flow; a lymph node shows internal speckled, predominantly hilar and/or peripheral blood flow; and a blood vessel will show intense uniform vascular blood flow. A complex solid/cystic mass may represent a metastatic lymph node or a soft-tissue tumor with cystic degeneration such as a Schwannoma.

When the FNA of a complex lymph node is performed under ultrasound guidance, once the fluid is evacuated, a careful ultrasound evaluation of the lesion should be performed for detection of a residual solid mass. If a mass is present, a repeat aspiration with a 27- or a 25-gauge needle should be conducted under ultrasound guidance.

Suggested Reading

Azarow KS, Pearl RH et al (1993) Primary mediastinal masses. A comparison of adult and pediatric populations. J Thorac Cardiovasc Surg 106(1):67–72

Brown RL, Azizkhan RG (1998) Pediatric head and neck lesions. Pediatr Clin North Am 45(4):889–905

Bhutani MS, Hawes RH et al (1997) A comparison of the accuracy of echo features during endoscopic ultrasound (EUS) and EUS-guided fine-needle aspiration for diagnosis of malignant lymph node invasion. Gastrointest Endosc 45(6):474–479

Chang DB, Yang PC et al (1992) Ultrasonography and ultrasonographically guided fine-needle aspiration biopsy of impalpable cervical lymph nodes in patients with non-small cell lung cancer. Cancer 70(5):1111–1114

Cervin JR, Silverman JF et al (1995) Virchow's node revisited. Analysis with clinicopathologic correlation of 152 fine-needle aspiration biopsies of supraclavicular lymph nodes. Arch Pathol Lab Med 119(8):727–730

Dangore-Khasbage S, Degwekar SS et al (2009) Utility of color Doppler ultrasound in evaluating the status of cervical lymph nodes in oral cancer. Oral Surg Oral Med Oral Pathol Oral Radiol Endod 108(2): 255–263

Ferry JA, Harris NL (1997) Atlas of lymphoid hyperplasia and lymphoma. WB Saunders, Philadelphia

Gupta RK, Naran S et al (2003) The diagnostic value of fine needle aspiration cytology (FNAC) in the assessment of palpable supraclavicular lymph nodes: a study of 218 cases. Cytopathology 14(4):201–207

Gupta RK, Naran S et al (2003) Diagnostic value of needle aspiration cytology in the assessment of palpable axillary lymph nodes. A study of 336 cases. Acta Cytol 47(4):550–554

Ioachim HL, Medeiros LJ (2009) The normal lymph node. In: Ioachim H, Medeiros LJ (eds) Ioachim's lymph node pathology, 4th edn. Lippincott Williams & Wilkins, Philadelphia, pp 2–14

Standring S (2008) Gray's anatomy. The anatomical basis of clinical practice, 40th edn. Elsevier London, UK
Twist CJ, Link MP (2002) Assessment of lymphadenopathy in children. Pediatr Clin North Am 49(5):1009–1025
Wright CD, Mathisen DJ (2001) Mediastinal tumors: diagnosis and treatment. World J Surg 25(2):204–209
Zaren HA, Copeland EM 3rd (1978) Inguinal node metastases. Cancer 41(3):919–923

4 Cytology of Normal/Reactive Lymph Nodes

The goal of a lymph node FNA is essentially to distinguish benign from malignant lymphoid processes. Non-neoplastic disorders that can manifest in lymph nodes include those with specific diagnoses and nonspecific reactive hyperplasia (the most common diagnosis). The role of FNA is paramount in determining the etiology of non-neoplastic disorders so that appropriate management can be instituted.

Origin, Functions, and Dynamics of the Lymph Node

All lymphoid cells originate in the bone marrow. The B cells mature in the bone marrow, and the T cells migrate to the thymus, where they differentiate further. From the bone marrow and thymus, the cells colonize the secondary lymphoid organs, which include the lymph nodes, spleen, and mucosa-associated lymphoid tissue (MALT); the immune response takes place in these organs (Fig. 4.1).

In an early B-cell reaction, the naïve B cells from the primary lymphoid follicle in the cortex are transformed into IgM+ blasts in the paracortex. These cells may enter the follicles to initiate the formation of the germinal center, or they may differentiate into the IgM-secreting plasma cells of the primary immune response in the medulla.

S.E. Pambuccian and R.H. Bardales, *Lymph Node Cytopathology*, Essentials in Cytopathology 10, DOI 10.1007/978-1-4419-6964-4_4,

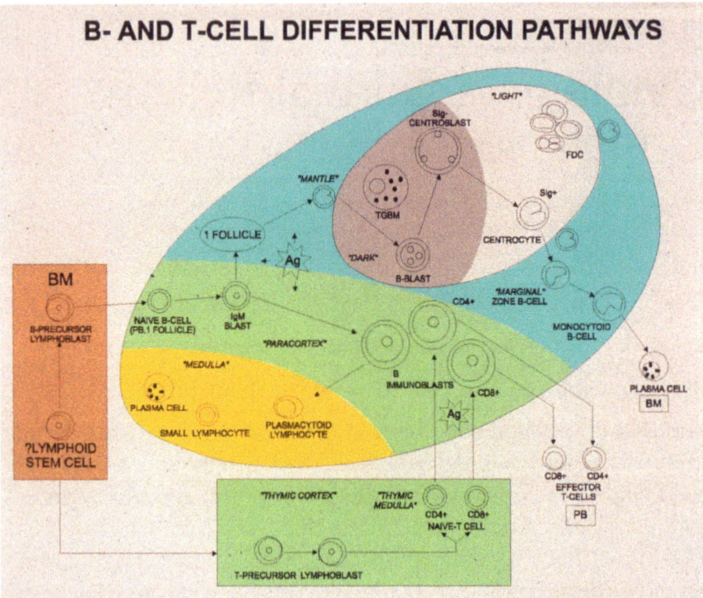

FIGURE 4.1. Diagram of B- and T-cell differentiation pathways.

The germinal center formation begins with the entry of IgM+ blasts into the primary follicle to form centroblasts. As proliferation continues, centroblasts migrate to a more peripheral zone of the germinal center to become immunoglobulin-secreting centrocytes.

The centrocytes may become memory cells and reside in the mantle zone (around the germinal center), which contains B lymphocytes identical to those of the primary follicle. The B cells also leave the germinal center to form the marginal zone around the periphery of the mantle zone. The centrocytes may also differentiate further into plasmablasts and plasma cells that migrate into the medullary area.

All naïve cells, centroblasts, centrocytes, mantle zone, marginal zone, and memory cells express pan-B-cell markers: CD19, CD20, CD22, and CD79a. In addition, centroblasts and centrocytes express CD10. Primary follicles and mantle zone lymphocytes express CD5+ and sIgM+.

The T cells enter a lymph node via the endothelial venule and, if not activated, leave the lymph node via the efferent lymphatic system. Most T cells are found in the paracortex, where they become T immunoblasts. Few T cells are present in the follicles.

T lymphocytes express pan-T-cell markers: CD2, CD3, CD5, and CD7. Depending on the membrane glycoprotein, they belong to the CD4 (helper), CD8 (suppressor), or NK cells.

Histologic Basis of a Normal/Reactive Lymph Node

Cortical or B-Cell Area

The main components of the cortical area are the primary and secondary lymphoid follicles. The primary lymphoid follicles (not stimulated) are perpendicular to the capsule, measure approximately 1 mm, and are composed of small and dark lymphocytes (naïve B cells). The secondary lymphoid follicles (stimulated or reactive) are composed of the germinal center, mantle zone, and marginal zone.

- The *germinal center* is composed of centroblasts, centrocytes, small lymphocytes, supporting reticulum cells, follicular dendritic cells (FDCs), and macrophages. Histologically, the germinal center shows a dark centroblast-rich central and a light centrocyte-rich peripheral zone. The cell composition changes with the antigenic stimulus and as the reactive process evolves in time; but in general, the cells are heterogeneous (small, large, cleaved, and noncleaved) and paler than those in the mantle and marginal zones.
- The *mantle zone* is composed of small B lymphocytes.
- The *marginal zone* cells are less tightly packed and have slightly more cytoplasm than the mantle zone cells. Histologically, this zone is prominent in the spleen and mesenteric lymph nodes, but inconspicuous in the peripheral lymph nodes.

Paracortical or T-Cell Area

This area is located in the deep cortex between the follicles and the medulla. It is the thymus-dependent area, which is composed predominantly of T lymphocytes.

The cells are of variable size and include small lymphocytes, T and B immunoblasts, IgM+ blasts, and interdigitating dendritic cells (IDCs) that are the antigen-presenting cells of the paracortex.

Medullary Area

This area is located toward the hilus of the lymph node and is the main area for antibody production. The medullary cords contain lymphocytes, plasmacytoid lymphocytes, plasmablasts, and large numbers of mature plasma cells. The medullary sinuses contain the lymph, monocytes, macrophages, mast cells, and a few small lymphocytes.

Lymph Node Cells and Their Diagnostic Significance

Because a normal lymph node is usually not sampled by FNA, the lymph node cells considered as "normal" are those aspirated from reactive and variably enlarged lymph nodes. The FNA of a normal/reactive lymph node shows lymphocytes and plasma cells in various stages of maturation and activation as well as accessory cells such as dendritic cells, histiocytes, and mast cells.

A *small lymphocyte* measures between 6 and 12 μm. In general, the nuclear size must be up to two times the size of a red blood cell or equal to or smaller than a histiocyte nucleus or a neutrophil. The small "mature" or "circulating" lymphocytes (naïve cells of the primary follicle and mantle zone cells) measure 6 μm. If a small "mature" lymphocyte becomes activated, it penetrates the germinal center and can measure 10–12 μm.

A *large lymphocyte* measures >20 μm. The nucleus is >3 times the size of a red blood cell or small lymphocyte, or larger than 1.5–2 times a histiocyte nucleus or neutrophil. Immunoblasts and some centroblasts fall in this category (Figs. 4.2 and 4.3).

The *intermediate-sized lymphocyte* measurements are between those of small and large lymphocytes. Centrocytes and most centroblasts fall in this category.

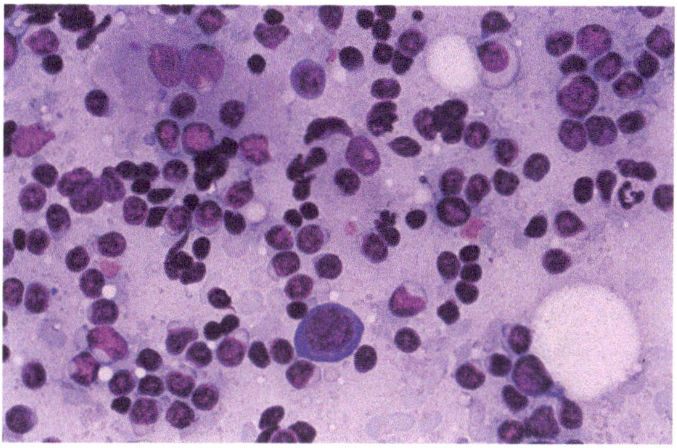

FIGURE 4.2. Normal lymphoid cells. Small lymphocytes, centrocytes, centroblasts, one immunoblast, and two histiocytes (*left upper corner*) are seen as examples of small-, medium-, and large-sized lymphocytes. Red blood cells and one neutrophil can be used as size guidelines (DiffQuik stain, high power).

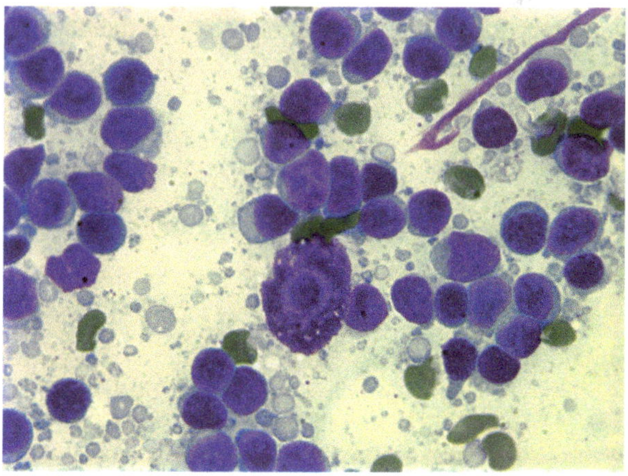

FIGURE 4.3. Early phase of reactive lymphoid hyperplasia. A mixed population of lymphocytes of various sizes, few small lymphocytes, and one mast cell in the center of the frame is seen (Giemsa stain, high power).

Small- and Intermediate-Sized Round Lymphocytes

Small round lymphocytes show regular nuclear contours, dense, coarse chromatin, nonvisible nucleoli, and a narrow rim of cytoplasm. They are found in the medullary cords and sinuses and in the paracortex (T cells). A few round, small T CD4+ cells are also found in the germinal center.

The naïve cells from the primary follicle and the mantle zone cells exhibit round or slightly irregular nuclei and slightly more open chromatin; otherwise, they are almost indistinguishable from small round lymphocytes.

The cells of the marginal zone are small B cells with slightly irregular nuclei and moderate amounts of pale cytoplasm.

The following entities show small round lymphocytes on FNA cytology:

- The resolving phase of reactive lymphoid hyperplasia.
- The hyaline-vascular variant of Castleman disease: mantle zone lymphocytes are cytologically similar to those of Hassal corpuscles of thymoma.
- Hodgkin lymphoma, lymphocyte predominant (a particular type of B-cell lymphoma that originates in the germinal centers) and classical (lymphocyte-rich, nodular sclerosis, mixed cellularity, and lymphocyte depletion) types.
- T-cell/histiocyte-rich diffuse large B-cell lymphoma.
- B-chronic lymphocytic leukemia/small lymphocytic lymphoma (B-CLL/SLL)
- T-CLL/SLL (REAL classification).
- Lymphoplasmacytic lymphoma that also shows plasmacytoid lymphocytes and plasma cells.

Intermediate-sized lymphoid cells predominate in:

- Mantle cell lymphoma.
- Marginal zone B-cell lymphoma. Monocytoid B-cell lymphoma and MALT lymphoma have been grouped as nodal and extranodal types of marginal-zone B-cell lymphoma, respectively, and except for the clinical setting, they are indistinguishable on FNA cytology.

- Precursor B- and T-cell lymphomas.
- Burkitt lymphoma in the appropriate clinical and geographic setting.
- Peripheral T-cell lymphoma.

Monocytoid B Cells

The cells are located within or adjacent to the subcapsular and cortical sinuses. They are believed to be related to marginal zone cells and are of intermediate size with oval, indented, bean-shaped nuclei and abundant pale cytoplasm.

Monocytoid B cells are seen in cytology smears from:

- Toxoplasmosis, CMV, early cat scratch disease, and early HIV-related lymphadenopathy.
- Monocytoid B-cell lymphoma (nodal form of marginal zone B-cell lymphoma).
- Rare cases of classical Hodgkin lymphoma.

Centrocytes and Centroblasts

Most follicular center cells have irregular nuclear contours. The "small cleaved" cells (small centrocytes) and "large cleaved" cells (large centrocytes) lack nucleoli, and the "large noncleaved" cells (large centroblasts) have nucleoli. The "small noncleaved" cells are blastic, of intermediate size, and comprise the minority of cells in the germinal center.

Centrocytes are sIg+ IgA+ or IgG+ cells with finely granular chromatin. Centroblasts are sIg-cells with finely dispersed chromatin, 1–3 peripheral nucleoli, and deeply basophilic narrow cytoplasm.

Follicular center cells (Figs. 4.4 and 4.5) are seen in cytology smears from:

- Reactive lymphoid hyperplasia, dermatopathic lymphadenopathy (early stages), early bacterial infection, early cat scratch disease, primary and secondary syphilis, early HIV, toxoplasmosis, rheumatoid arthritis, Kimura lymphadenopathy, and Castleman disease (plasma cell variant).

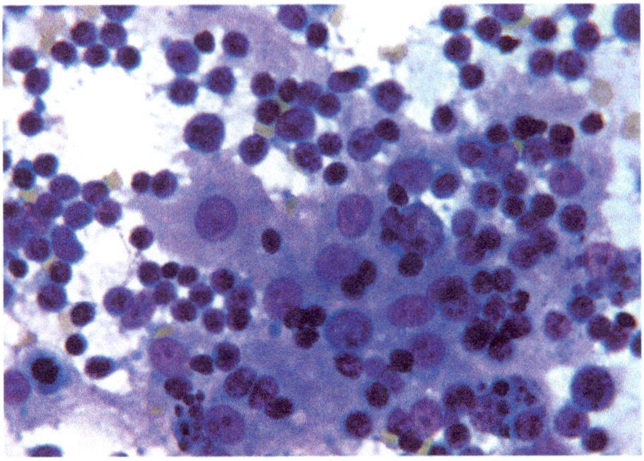

FIGURE 4.4. Lymphohistiocytic aggregate. Lymphocytes of various sizes are present admixed with histiocytes (DiffQuik stain, high power).

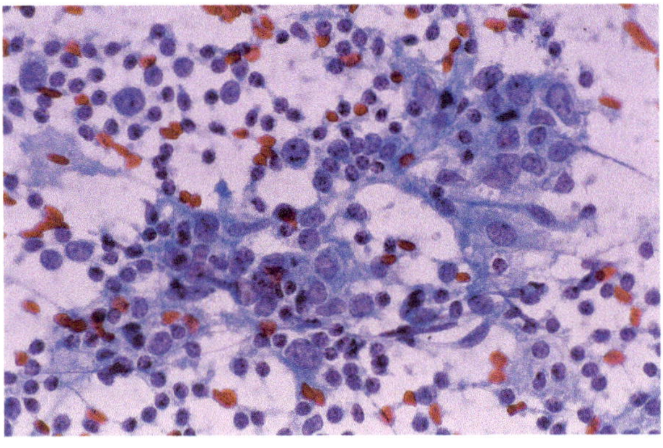

FIGURE 4.5. Lymphohistiocytic aggregate. Lymphocytes of various sizes admixed with follicular dendritic cells with characteristic elongated cytoplasm and bland nuclei are present (Papanicolaou stain, high power).

- Hodgkin lymphoma with partial lymph node involvement. Fifteen percent of lymphocyte predominant Hodgkin lymphoma may have reactive germinal centers.
- Lymph node involvement of cutaneous T-cell lymphoma (Sezary syndrome).

- Lymph node metastases.
- Follicular lymphoma, centroblastic diffuse large B-cell lymphoma, diffuse follicle center cell lymphoma, and peripheral T-cell lymphoma.

Plasmacytoid Monocytes

These are located in the junction of the paracortex and medullary cords and show ill-defined cell borders, pale cytoplasm, and round, pale nuclei slightly larger than those of small lymphocytes. They are found in Kikuchi disease and Castleman disease (hyaline-vascular variant).

Immunoblasts

T and B immunoblasts resemble each other and are located predominantly in the paracortex and scattered in the medullary cords. They are the largest lymphoid cells in the lymph node and have large, deeply basophilic cytoplasm, one round nucleus with a single nucleolus, or an irregular nucleus with 2 or 3 marginal nucleoli Fig. 4.2.

Immunoblasts are seen in cytology smears from:

- Infectious mononucleosis, herpes simplex, and CMV lymphadenitis.
- Kikuchi disease, Lyme disease, juvenile rheumatoid arthritis, Castleman disease (plasma cell variant in early stages), reactions to vaccination (smallpox vaccine, no longer given), and drug-induced (specially anticonvulsants such as Dilantin) lymphadenopathy.
- The mesenteric lymph nodes draining a suppurative appendicitis or intestinal perforation.
- Immunoblastic lymphoma and some peripheral T-cell lymphomas.

Follicular Dendritic Cells (FDCs)

It is difficult to recognize FDCs by light microscopy. FDCs show elongated cytoplasm and a large and irregular or elongated pale nucleus with a small nucleolus. They can be bi-, tri-, or multinucleated with nuclear molding. They are located in the germinal centers, interact with B lymphocytes, and are CD21+, CD15+, C3b+, HLA-DR+, CD1a+, and S100 protein+ (Fig. 4.5).

FDCs are seen in smears from:

- Hodgkin lymphoma, angioimmunoblastic T-cell lymphoma, and the hyaline-vascular variant of Castleman disease (shows lymphocyte-depleted germinal centers with preserved FDCs).
- FDC sarcoma/tumor.

Interdigitating Dendritic Cells (IDCs)

The IDCs are large with abundant pale and ill-defined cytoplasm, a markedly irregular nucleus, and inconspicuous nucleoli. They are located in the paracortex, interact with T lymphocytes, and are HLA-DR+, CD1a+, and S100 protein+.

Various numbers of IDCs are seen in smears from dermatopathic lymphadenopathy. The malignant counterpart is interdigitating dendritic-cell sarcoma/tumor.

Histiocytes

Along with FDCs and IDCs, the monocytic/histiocytic cells are part of the mononuclear phagocyte system and are found in the subcapsular, cortical, and medullary sinuses. They originate in the bone marrow, migrate to the peripheral tissues, and reach the lymph nodes. The cells are large with indistinct cytoplasmic borders and are positive for the histiocytic markers CD68, lysozyme, α1-antitripsine, α1-antichymotrypsin, and S100 protein. They phagocytose apoptotic nuclear debris and form the tingible-body macrophages of the germinal centers Figs. 4.2 and 4.4. Under specific stimulation, they may transform into epithelioid cells and form granulomas.

Histiocytes are seen in smears from:

- Hereditary storage disease and dermatopathic (containing hemosiderin, melanin, or lipid) lymphadenopathy.
- T-cell/histiocyte-rich diffuse large B-cell lymphoma and peripheral T-cell lymphoma.
- Rosai–Dorfman disease. Histiocytes have abundant, pale, vacuolated cytoplasm and engulfed cells (usually lymphocytes or “emperipolesis”).

- Toxoplasma, leishmania, and rheumatoid arthritis lymphadenitis. Histiocytes with rare or no granulomas.
- Herpes simplex and varicella zoster, SLE (hematoxylin bodies in the necrosis), Kikuchi disease ("crescentic," "signet-ring," and with foamy histiocytes). Histiocytes with necrosis, but no granulomas.
- Mycobacteria (particularly in children), fungi (commonly histoplasmosis and cryptococcosis), brucellosis, leishmaniasis, yersinia, Chlamydia, and the late stage of cat scratch disease lymphadenitis show histiocytes with necrotizing granulomas. Lymphogranuloma venereum, tularemia, chancroid, pseudotuberculous mesenteric lymphadenitis, listeriosis, glanders, and melioidosis show necrotizing granulomas that mimic cat scratch disease.
- Primary and secondary syphilis. Non-necrotizing granulomas.
- Whipple disease (PAS+ intracytoplasmic bodies), foreign body (lipid, proteinaceous, silicone, etc.), sarcoidosis, Crohn's disease, *mycobacterium avium intracellulare*, and lepromatous leprosy lymphadenitis. Lipogranulomas with clusters of foamy histiocytes and epitheliod cells.
- Sarcoidosis and rarely rheumatoid arthritis. Hyaline PAS+ material or amyloid can be seen in long-standing rheumatoid arthritis. Tight granulomas with little or no necrosis.
- Hodgkin lymphoma and metastatic carcinoma lymphadenitis with or without lymph node metastasis. Granulomas and necrosis.
- Histiocyte rich T-cell angioimmunoblastic large-cell lymphoma and angioimmunoblastic T-cell lymphoma. Histiocytes.
- High-grade non-Hodgkin lymphomas. Tingible-body macrophages.
- Langerhans cell histiocytosis (histiocytosis X) and Langerhans cell sarcoma that are the neoplastic proliferations of Langerhans cells without or with malignant cytologic features.

Plasma Cells

Plasma cells along with plasmacytoid lymphocytes are present in the medullary cords and produce the lymph node immunoglobulin. Plasma cells react with CD138 (syndecan 1).

Variable numbers of plasma cells are seen in the cytology smears from:

- Primary and secondary syphilis, the plasma cell variant of Castleman disease, and rheumatoid arthritis lymphadenitis (numerous plasma cells).
- Dermatopathic lymphadenopathy, SLE, Rosai–Dorfman disease, Kimura lymphadenopathy, late and chronic HIV lymphadenitis, lymph node involvement of cutaneous T-cell lymphoma (Sezary syndrome), angioimmunoblastic T-cell lymphoma, and some cases of Hodgkin lymphoma.
- Plasma cell myeloma/plasmacytoma, lymphoplasmacytic lymphoma, and nodal marginal zone lymphoma.

Mast Cells

Mast cells are present in the medullary sinus and are seen in smears from Kimura lymphadenopathy, mast cell disease involving lymph nodes, and mastocytoma. Scattered mast cells may be seen in reactive lymphoid hyperplasia, B-CLL/SLL, and lymphoplasmacytic lymphoma (Fig. 4.3).

Eosinophils

Variable numbers are seen in cytology smears from:

- Dermatopathic lymphadenopathy, infectious mononucleosis, allergic reactions, including drugs such as Dilantin, Kimura lymphadenopathy, Rosai–Dorfman disease, Castleman disease (hyaline vascular variant), and foreign-body lymphadenitis.
- Hodgkin lymphoma, precursor B- and T-cell lymphoma, peripheral T-cell lymphoma, angioimmunoblastic T-cell lymphoma, cutaneous T-cell lymphoma with lymph node involvement (Sezary syndrome), Langerhans cell histiocytosis, and rare cases of mast cell disease involving lymph nodes.

Neutrophils

Variable numbers are seen in smears from:

- Acute bacterial lymphadenitis.
- Necrotizing granulomatous lymphadenitis, particularly in cat scratch disease as the disease progresses.

- Herpes simplex and varicella zoster lymphadenitis (neutrophils and necrosis).
- Yersinia, lymphogranuloma venereum, Kikuchi disease, early HIV lymphadenitis, and some cases of Hodgkin lymphoma.
- Rheumatoid arthritis, but absent in SLE lymphadenitis.

The cell composition in a normal/reactive lymph node also depends on the body location. Mesenteric lymph nodes have wide medullary cords and sinuses, and the smears have a predominance of plasma cells, monocytes, macrophages, and mast cells. Cervical lymph nodes have numerous secondary lymphoid follicles, and the smears show germinal center cells.

Lymphoglandular Bodies and Their Diagnostic Significance

The lymphoglandular bodies (LGBs) seen in cytologic smears from lymph nodes are small (2–10 μm), usually round, homogeneous, or vacuolated cytoplasmic fragments. Their presence implies a lymphoid origin for the disease process, either benign or malignant. However, LGBs in various proportions (>1 to <10 LGBs/high-power field) have been described in <10% of nonlymphoid

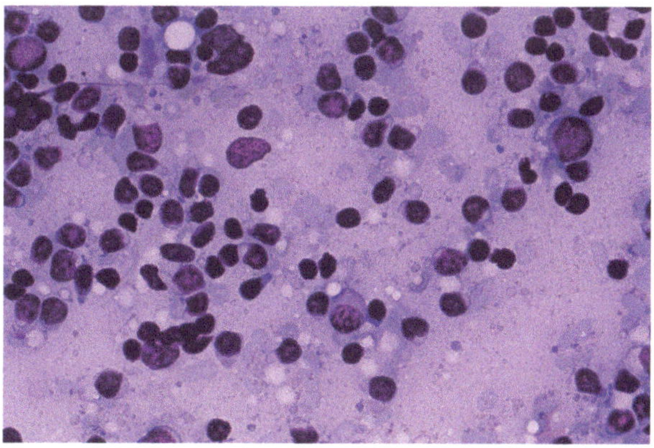

Figure 4.6. Lymphoglandular bodies (LGBs). This reactive lymphoid cell pattern shows numerous LGBs as result of cytoplasmic fragmentation (DiffQuik stain, high power).

malignancies such as small and nonsmall carcinomas, Wilms tumor, seminoma, and ganglioneuroblastoma. Thus, with rare exceptions, only the presence of large numbers of LGBs is characteristic of lymphoid tissue (Fig. 4.6).

The presence of numerous LGBs is particularly useful in the differentiation of non-Hodgkin lymphoma from poorly differentiated carcinoma. However, 14% of non-Hodgkin lymphomas have few or no LGBs. Certainly, the overall FNA pattern and cytomorphology must be correlated with the appropriate clinical setting for a final cytologic diagnosis.

Suggested Reading

Flanders E, Kornstein MJ et al (1993) Lymphoglandular bodies in fine-needle aspiration cytology smears. Am J Clin Pathol 99(5):566–569

Harris NL (2001) Mature B-cell neoplasms. Introduction, pathology and genetics. In: Jaffe ES, Harris NL, Stein H, Vardiman JW (eds) WHO classification of tumors of the haematopoietic and lymphoid tissues. IARC Press, Lyon, pp 121–126

Ioachim HL, Medeiros LJ (2009) The normal lymph node. In: Ioachim H, Medeiros LJ (eds) Ioachim's lymph node pathology, 4th edn. Lippincott Williams & Wilkins, Philadelphia, pp 2–14

Jaffe ES, Harris NL, Stein H, Vardiman JW (2001) Tumors of haematopoietic and lymphoid tissue. WHO-IARC Press, Lyon

Kurtin PJ (2000) Marginal zone B cells, monocytoid B cells, and the follicular microenvironment. Determinants of morphologic features in a subset of low-grade B-cell lymphomas. Am J Clin Pathol 114(4):505–508

Stein H (1999) Lymphocyte differentiation. In: Mason DY, Harris NL (eds) Human lymphoma: clinical implications of the REAL classification. Springer, New York

5 Overall Assessment of the Aspirate: Diagnostic Clues

The questions that the pathologist tries to sequentially answer when evaluating fine needle aspiration biopsies of lymph nodes are:

1. Is the aspirate adequate?
2. Is the nodule clinically considered to be a lymph node really a lymph node?
3. Is the lymphadenopathy caused by a benign or malignant process?
4. If it is a benign process, is it infectious? Can the infectious agent be identified?
5. If it is malignant, is it a metastasis or lymphoma?
6. If it is a metastasis what is the type (carcinoma, melanoma, sarcoma)? Where did it most likely originate?
7. If it is lymphoma, is it non-Hodgkin or Hodgkin lymphoma?
8. If it is non-Hodgkin lymphoma, is it of B or T cell type? What is the subtype? Is it possible to grade it?
9. If it is Hodgkin lymphoma, is it possible to determine the subtype?

These questions are answered by a thorough morphologic examination which begins with a low power assessment of the aspirate. The initial low-power examination can frequently answer the questions:

1. Is the aspirate adequate for examination?
2. Is it representative of a lymph node?

S.E. Pambuccian and R.H. Bardales, *Lymph Node Cytopathology*, Essentials in Cytopathology 10, DOI 10.1007/978-1-4419-6964-4_5,

3. What is the overall pattern of the aspirate based on the cohesion (or lack thereof) of the cells, size of cells and variation in size of the cells.

   (a) Is the aspirate composed of an evenly dispersed population of cells or are there aggregates of cells?
   (b) Are the majority of cells small or large? Is the aspirate monomorphic (i.e., most cells are either small or large) or polymorphic (i.e., there a more or less even admixture of small and large cells)?
   (c) Are there very large pleomorphic (very large, atypical, anaplastic) cells admixed with lymphoid cells?

A differential diagnosis can be formulated according to the pattern of the aspirate and ancillary studies can be ordered to narrow down the differential diagnostic possibilities to a definitive diagnosis.

The low power examination is best made on both air-dried smears stained with Romanovsky-type stains (Diff-Quik, Wright stain or May-Grunwald-Giemsa stain) and fixed smears stained with Papanicolaou or hematoxylin and eosin stains. The two types of cytologic preparations are complementary to each other. Air-dried smears allow a better low-power assessment of cell size because they exaggerate the size differences between cells and allow a better assessment of the background elements. Fixed smears, on the other hand, allow a better assessment of cell aggregates and allow a better visualization of the nuclear chromatin and the differences between the very compact chromatin of small lymphocytes and the more open chromatin of larger cells. Wright-stained cytospin preparations are frequently made from the cell suspension submitted for flow cytometry and are useful as a quality assurance measure since they allow the assessment of the overall quality of the sample, the intactness and viability of the cells and of the predominant cell size. Liquid-based ("monolayer") preparations may be made from needle rinses and show very good cytologic detail (Fig. 5.1). However, we caution against the exclusive use of liquid-based preparations for lymph node fine needle aspirates as background elements are more difficult to identify, cells appear smaller, their nucleoli more prominent, aggregates of cells may become fragmented and lymphocytes may become artificially aggregated in tight clusters. All of these differences from the cytologic features seen in smears to which pathologists

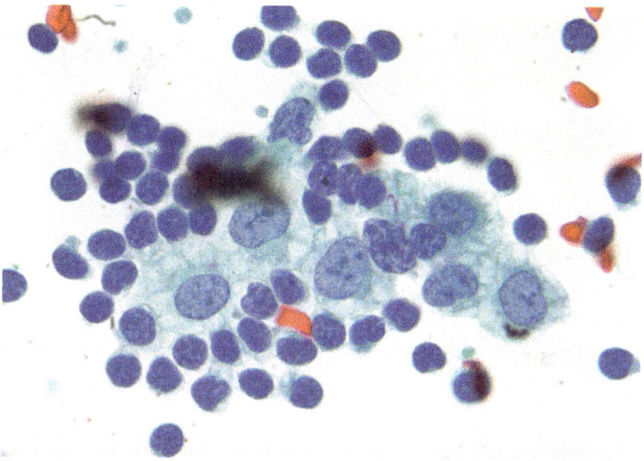

FIGURE 5.1. Liquid-based (Surepath®) preparation of a reactive lymph node aspirate showing a "lymphohistiocytic aggregate" composed of small lymphocytes, centrocytes, and follicular dendritic cells. Note the crisp nuclear and cytoplasmic detail (Papanicolaou stain, ×1,000).

have become accustomed, may cause diagnostic difficulties or even cause misdiagnoses.

Assessment of Sample Adequacy

Adequacy of a lymph node aspirate depends on the presence of:

(a) Sufficient cellularity on smears, cell block sections and samples submitted for flow cytometry or other ancillary tests.
(b) Smears and cell block sections of good quality, devoid of extensive artifacts.

Gross examination of a well-prepared fine needle aspiration smear from a lymph node usually shows an ovoid purple colored cellular area (Fig. 5.2). The presence of a trailing "feather edge" is important to accurately evaluate cellular morphology and cell size. Smears in which the whole surface of the slide is covered by cellular material are usually suboptimal, since they do not allow uniform, thin smearing. When air-dried Romanovsky-stained smears are grossly examined, they have an intensely purple color due to the abundance of lymphoid cells present.

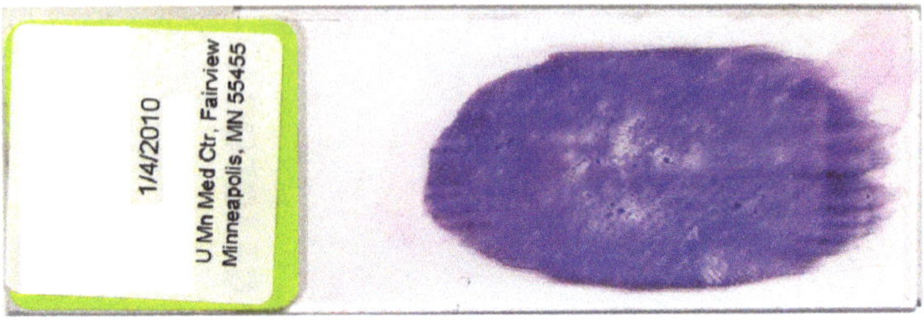

FIGURE 5.2. Gross picture of a Diff-Quik-stained smear of a lymph node fine needle aspirate showing the characteristic "bullet shape" and a feather edge.

Cellularity

Smears from well-performed fine needle aspirates of lymph nodes are usually extremely cellular with variable numbers of admixed red blood cells, depending on the needle size and aspiration technique. Larger needle size tends to be associated with hemodilution of the aspirate. Imaging-guided aspirates, such as ultrasound-guided FNA, endoscopic ultrasound-guided FNA (EUS-FNA) and endobronchial ultrasound guided transbronchial needle aspiration (EBUS-TBNA) of lymph nodes also tend to be more hemodiluted, most likely due to the unavoidable movement of the target during the aspiration procedure, with resulting increase in needling trauma. For such imaging-guided aspirates, we have recently proposed that 40 lymphoid cells per high power field (40×) in the area of highest cellularity should be considered the minimum number of lymphoid cells to consider an aspirate not showing granulomas or metastatic malignancy as adequate.

Scant cellularity is unusual in lymph node aspirates, but may be related to the underlying pathology. It is most often caused by fibrosis/sclerosis of the lymph node, as seen in Hodgkin lymphoma (particularly the nodular sclerosis type), some large B-cell lymphomas and metastatic desmoplastic carcinomas.

Another potential cause of scant cellularity is the partial replacement of the lymph node by acellular material (mucin, colloid, amyloid, chondroid material, or other types of matrix material).

Artifacts

Smears that are too thickly smeared, show extensive crush artifact or are very hemodiluted are not optimal for cytologic evaluation. A definitive diagnosis is usually not possible and any interpretation rendered on such smears should include the statement that the material is suboptimal for the evaluation because suboptimal or unsatisfactory smears are frequently the cause of cytologic misdiagnoses.

Optimal smearing technique, which can be learned and mastered with experience, is essential to obtain relatively thin smears without prominent crush artifact (Fig. 5.3). Some crush artifact is unavoidable, especially when follicular germinal cell fragments are present (Fig. 5.4). *Lymphoid tangles*, which are spider-like structures formed of strings of purple-staining (hematoxylinophilic) material, are the result of a similar crush artifact. They occur as the result of crushing the more fragile nuclei of lymphoid cells, when the aspirate also contains a population of more resilient cells such as benign or malignant epithelial cells (lymphocytic thyroiditis, Warthin tumor or metastatic lymphadenopathy) or epithelioid histiocytes (granulomatous lymphadenitis).

Neoplastic lymphoid cells tend to crush more easily, and high grade lymphomas may at times exhibit a tendency to crush similar

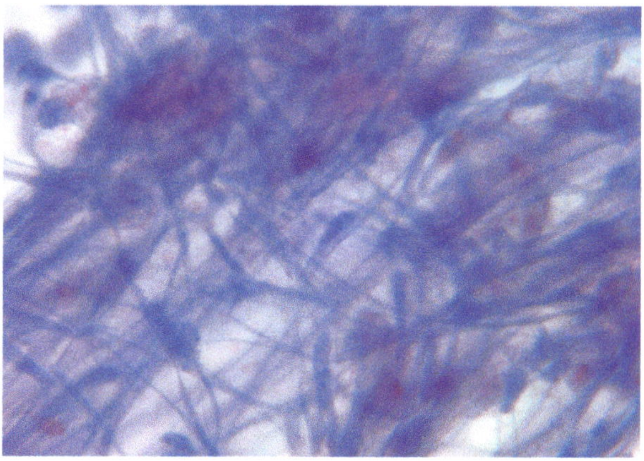

FIGURE 5.3. Lymph node fine needle aspirate showing extensive crush artifact precluding morphologic interpretation (Papanicolaou stain, ×1,000).

to that seen in small-cell carcinomas. One of the more characteristic smearing artifacts is the presence of *smudge cells* also referred to as *basket cells* (Fig. 5.5) or *shadow cells* of Gumprecht, in honor of the German internist who described them in 1896. Smudge cells represent lymphoid cells stripped of their cytoplasm, where the

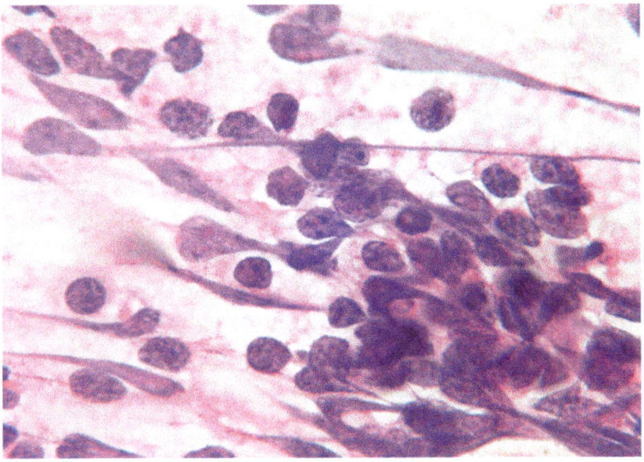

FIGURE 5.4. Minor degrees of crush artifact are common in lymph node fine needle aspirates and have no diagnostic significance (Hematoxylin and eosin, ×1,000).

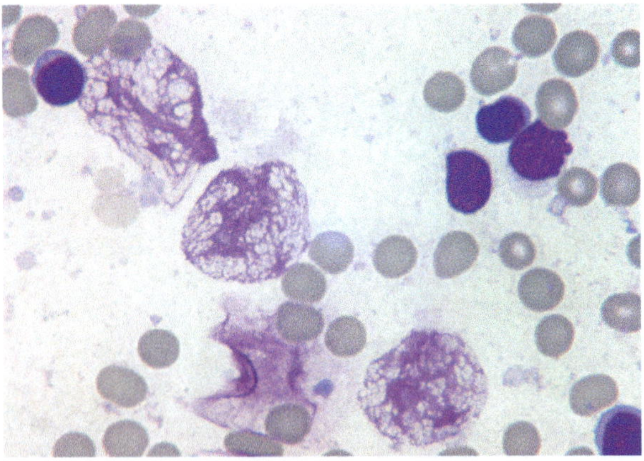

FIGURE 5.5. Fine needle aspiration smear of a lymph node with small lymphocytic lymphoma (CLL/SLL) showing numerous *smudge cells* or *basket cells* (Diff-Quik, ×1,000).

basophilic nuclear material becomes dispersed after the disruption of the nuclear membrane. The resulting thin strands of interwoven pale staining basophilic material are larger and more irregularly shaped than the nuclei of surrounding lymphocytes. Such cells are more common in aspirates of small lymphocytic lymphoma, where they can represent a large proportion of the neoplastic cells. Occasional smudge cells, however, can be seen in aspirates from other lymphoid neoplasms and even in aspirates from benign lymphadenopathies.

Background Elements

After the aspirate smears are determined to be adequate for diagnosis, the next step is to assess the background of the smears. The background usually shows blood and lymphoglandular bodies (LGBs) but may show a variety of noncellular elements that may be diagnostically useful:

- Necrotic debris in necrotizing granulomatous lymphadenitis (Fig. 5.6), other infectious lymphadenitides, aggressive lymphomas, metastatic lymphadenopathies, and lymph node necrosis/ infarction (Fig. 5.7).

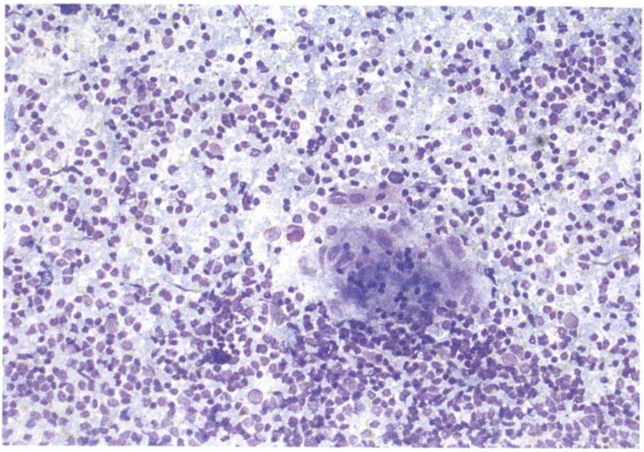

FIGURE 5.6. Fine powdery necrotic debris, the cytologic equivalent of caseous necrosis, seen in the background of the upper part of the image of a fine needle aspirate from an atypical mycobacterial necrotizing granulomatous lymphadenitis in a 3-year-old boy. Note the epithelioid granuloma in the center of the image (Diff-Quik, ×200).

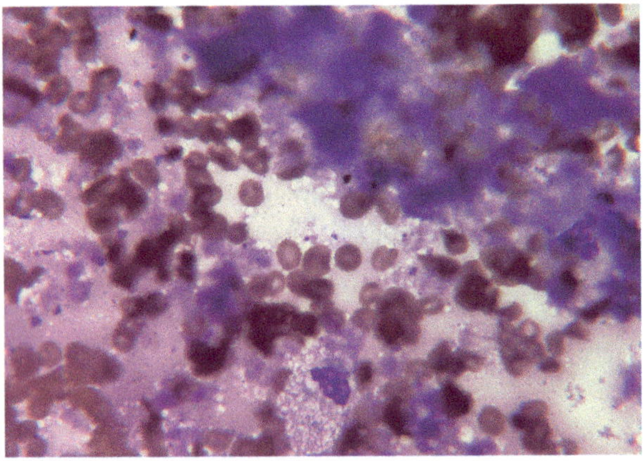

FIGURE 5.7. Coarse clumps of necrosis in an aspirate from a totally necrotic/infarcted lymph node. An occasional foamy histiocyte is present, but no lymphocytes are seen. Such aspirates should be carefully scrutinized for the presence of malignant cells (Diff-Quik, ×1,000).

- Fat vacuoles in fatty replacement of the lymph node.
- Foreign refractile material in silicone lymphadenopathy and postarthroplasty lymphadenopathy.
- Keratin debris in metastatic squamous cell carcinoma.
- Pigment such as melanin in metastatic melanoma (Fig. 5.8).
- Amyloid in metastatic medullary carcinoma and plasma cell disorders (Fig. 5.9).
- Colloid in metastatic thyroid carcinomas.
- Mucin in metastatic mucinous adenocarcinomas.
- Chondroid or myxoid matrix in metastatic sarcomatoid carcinomas or sarcomas.
- Fibrillary material (neuropil) in metastatic neuroblastoma (Fig. 5.10).
- "Tigroid background" in metastatic seminoma (Fig. 5.11).

Because structures other than lymph nodes can be clinically misidentified as lymph nodes, a determination should be made if the aspirate is representative of a lymph node. This may not be possible if no morphologically preserved cellular elements are present, as is the case with aspirates from cystic or necrotic structures or when the fine needle aspirate is composed exclusively of metastatic malignant cells.

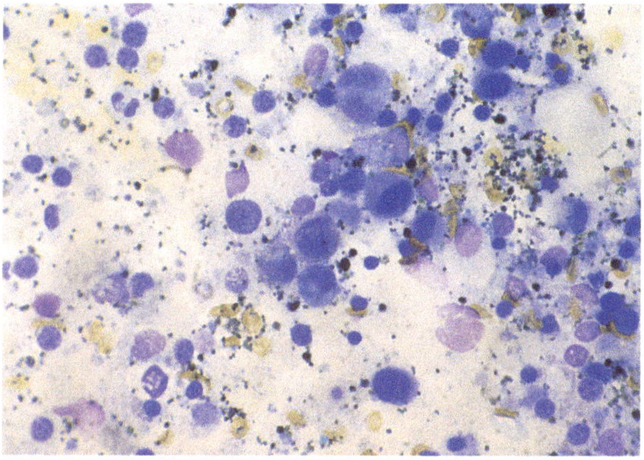

FIGURE 5.8. Coarse melanin pigment in the background of a lymph node aspirate showing metastatic melanoma (Diff-Quik, ×400).

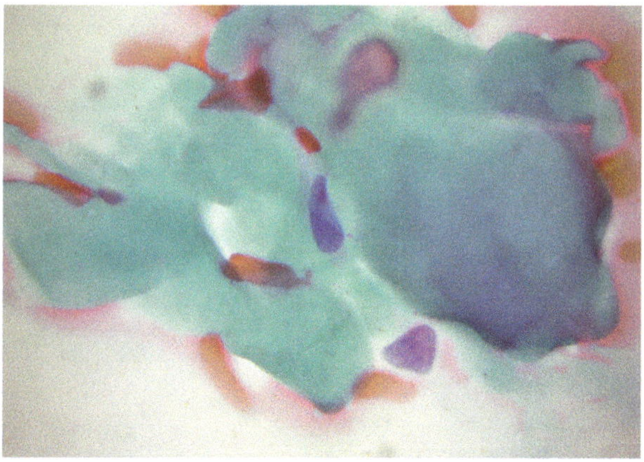

FIGURE 5.9. Amyloid clumps in an aspirate of a lymph node involved by localized amyloidosis ("amyloid tumor") (Papanicolaou stain, ×1,000).

However, most fine needle aspirates from lymph nodes can be readily identified as such due to the presence of a dispersed population of lymphoid cells with numerous LGBs in the background (Fig. 5.12).

LGBs are also referred to as Söderstrom bodies in honor of Nils Söderstrom, the Swedish pioneer of fine needle aspiration who drew

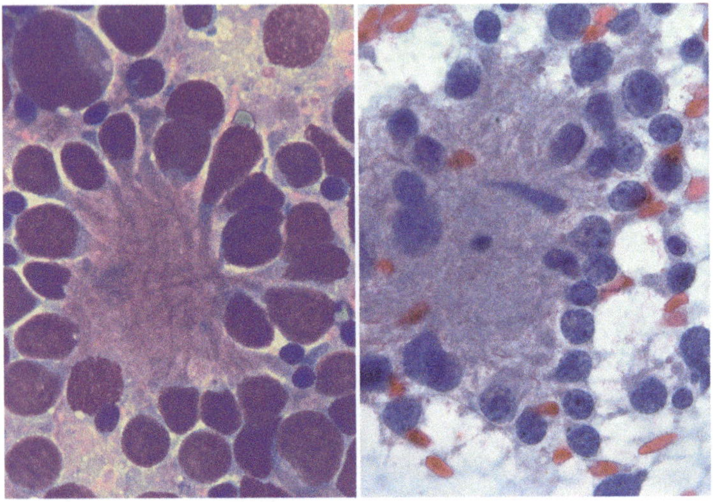

FIGURE 5.10. Neuropil and rosette formation in an aspirate from a lymph node metastasis of neuroblastoma (*left* Diff-Quik, ×400, *right* Papanicolaou ×400).

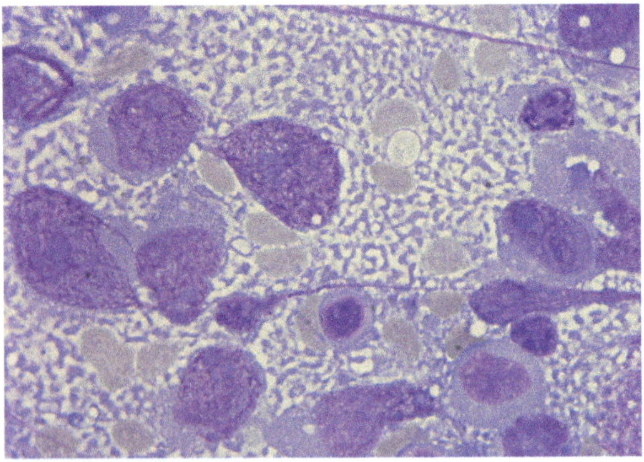

FIGURE 5.11. Tigroid background in an aspirate of a seminoma metastatic to a retroperitoneal lymph node. The strands comprising the "tigroid" background have staining characteristics similar to the cytoplasm of the neoplastic cells. Note the very large size of the tumor cells as compared to the lymphocytes (Diff-Quik, ×1,000).

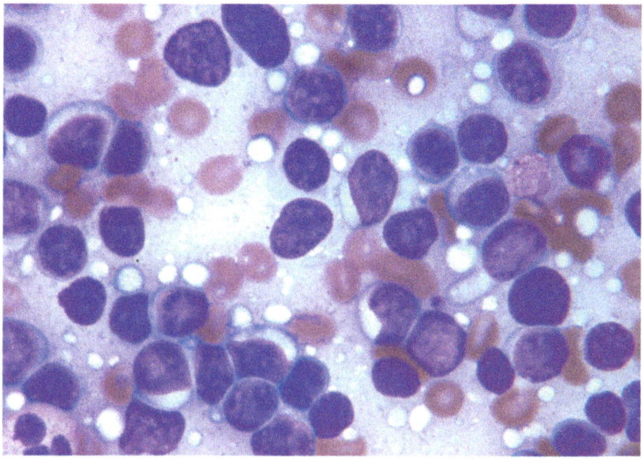

FIGURE 5.12. Numerous lymphoglandular bodies (LGBs) are present in this lymph node aspirate from a reactive lymphadenopathy. Note that LGBs have similar staining characteristics to the cytoplasm of the lymphocytes (Diff-Quik, ×1,000).

attention to their significance in 1968. The term lymphoglandular does not imply that they are of glandular origin but rather that they are characteristic of lymph nodes ("lymph glands") and other lymphoid tissues such as spleen, tonsils, and thymus. LGBs are seen in the background of almost all aspirates from lymph nodes and are more abundant in lymphomas than in aspirates from benign lymph nodes. Aspirates from aggressive lymphomas, which are composed of more fragile cells tend to show more numerous LGBs than low-grade lymphomas. As already mentioned, LGBs are not entirely specific for lymphoid tissue or lymphomas since they are also seen in malignant melanoma, small cell carcinoma of the lung, undifferentiated carcinoma, seminoma, and small blue cell tumors of childhood. However, in all of these situations their number is smaller than in aspirates of lymphoid proliferations and the presence of over 20 LGBs per high power field is virtually diagnostic of an aspirate from a lymphoid organ or extranodal lymphoid proliferation.

The presence of even abundant LGBs does not imply that the neoplastic cells identified in the aspirate are lymphoid (i.e., represent a lymphoma) since they may be derived from benign lymphocytes present in metastatic lymphadenopathies.

Cellular Aggregates

The next step in the examination of lymph node aspirates is to scan for the presence of cellular aggregates.

Since lymphocytes do not adhere to each other and are actually in a constant state of flow within the lymph node, no cohesion is expected in lymph node aspirates. However, dendritic cells, which form the support for lymphocytes, are cohesive and FNA results in so-called lymphohistiocytic aggregates that are actually follicular germinal center fragments formed of follicular dendritic cells, macrophages and lymphocytes (centrocytes and centroblasts) (Fig. 5.13). Clusters of pigmented histiocytes may be seen in mediastinal anthracotic lymph nodes (Fig. 5.14).

The presence of other cellular aggregates is abnormal and any aggregates present in the aspirate should be examined at high power. The presence of abundant follicular fragments confers a vaguely nodular appearance at low power examination of the aspirates of follicular lymphomas (Figs. 5.15 and 5.16). The aggregates of follicular lymphoma are composed predominantly of centrocytes and tend to be less polymorphous in composition than lymphohistiocytic aggregates of reactive lymphadenopathies (Fig. 5.17).

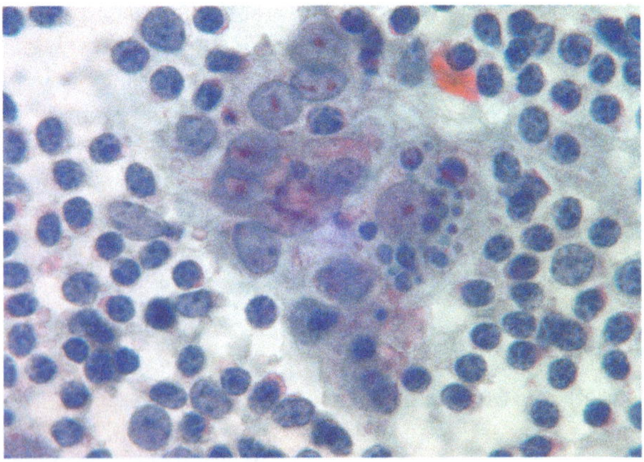

FIGURE 5.13. High power appearance of a lymphohistiocytic aggregate in a lymph node aspirate from a reactive lymphadenopathy. The aggregate is composed of a tingible body macrophage, several follicular dendritic cells and small lymphocytes (Papanicolaou stain, ×1,000).

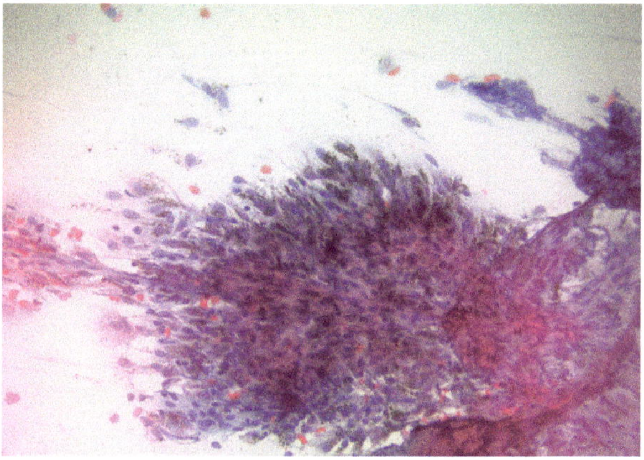

FIGURE 5.14. Low power appearance of an aggregate of pigmented sinus histiocytes from a endobronchial ultrasound-guided transbronchial aspirate of an anthracotic mediastinal lymph node (Papanicolaou stain, ×200).

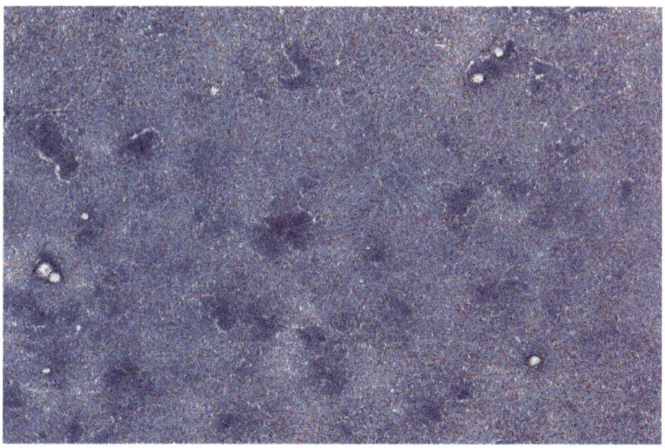

FIGURE 5.15. Scanning magnification appearance of nodularity in an aspirate from a follicular lymphoma (Papanicolaou stain, ×40).

Abnormal cell aggregates are seen in granulomatous lymphadenitides, where the epithelioid or spindle cell histiocytes show a haphazard orientation of nuclei ("fish-in-the-net" appearance) (Fig. 5.18), and metastatic malignancies. Metastatic carcinomas,

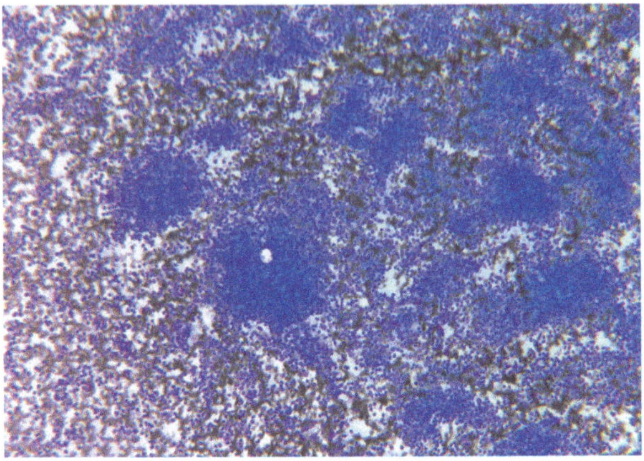

FIGURE 5.16. Low power appearance of the nodular cell aggregates in an aspirate from a grade 1 follicular lymphoma (Diff-Quik, ×100).

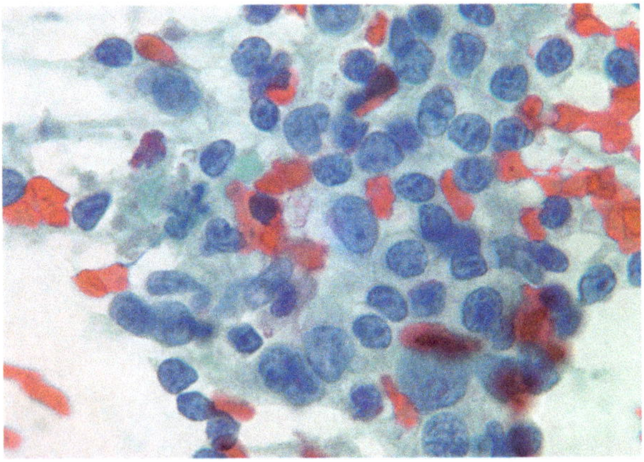

FIGURE 5.17. High power appearance of a nodular cell aggregate in an aspirate from a grade 1 follicular lymphoma. The aggregate is composed of centroblasts, small lymphocytes, follicular dendritic cells and a centroblast (Papanicolaou stain, ×1,000).

melanomas, and sarcomas frequently show aggregates of malignant cells, the identification of which establishes the diagnosis. Lymphomas, particularly anaplastic large cell lymphomas can rarely show cellular cohesion and form aggregates.

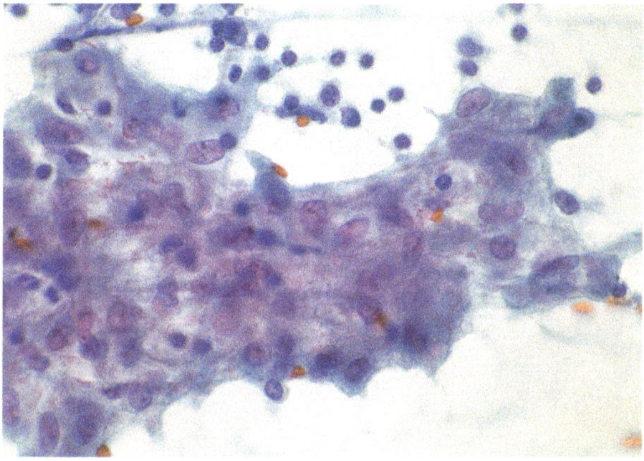

FIGURE 5.18. Loose aggregate of epithelioid histiocytes forming a granuloma in an aspirate of a lymph node involved by sarcoidosis. Note the poorly defined cytoplasmic borders, the spindle-shaped and twisted nuclei of the histiocytes and their open chromatin with distinct small nucleoli (Papanicolaou stain, ×600).

Cell Size and Monotony

The next step in the overall evaluation of the aspirate consists of the assessment of the cell size of the predominant cells present in the smears and of the degree of variability in cell sizes that characterizes the smears. Cell size is best determined in thin areas of the smear, especially in the feather edge of the smear by comparison of the size of the nuclei with red blood cells and nuclei of histiocytes or endothelial cells. Cells and their nuclei appear larger in Diff-Quik-stained smears than in fixed smears, but also in thinner peripheral areas of the smear as compared to thicker central areas of the smear. Cell size should not be estimated in areas where it is exaggerated by air drying artifacts that may occur at the edges of the smear or in damaged cells and naked nuclei. Large cells are by definition cells that have nuclei that are similar in size or larger than the nuclei of histiocytes (Fig. 5.19). They are also characterized by their paler-staining (vesicular) nucleus in fixed smears and the presence of visible to prominent nucleoli. Such cells are normally present in lymph node aspirates (centroblasts and immunoblasts)

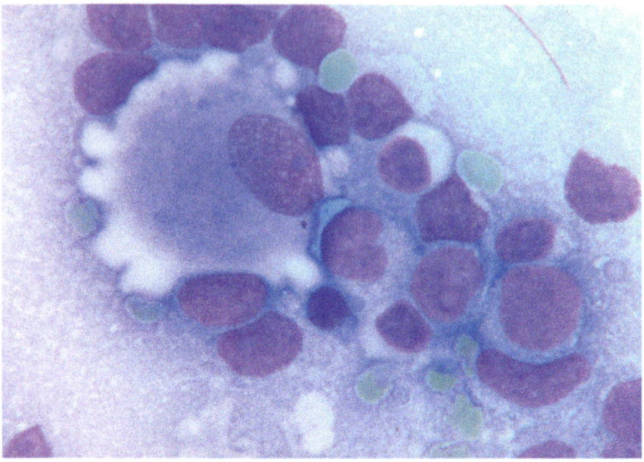

FIGURE 5.19. Histiocyte with abundant pale cytoplasm surrounded by small lymphocytes and occasional large lymphocytes (Diff-Quik, ×1000).

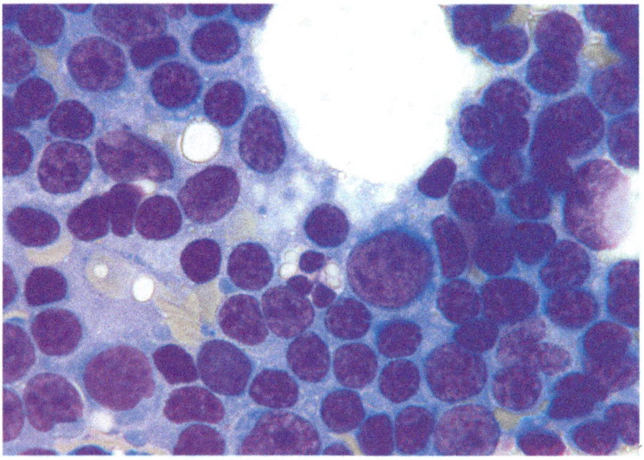

FIGURE 5.20. Polymorphous lymphoid population in an aspirate from reactive lymphadenopathy Note the accentuation of cell size differences in air-dried smears. (Diff-Quik, ×1,000).

but constitute a minority of lymphoid cells present. Their presence contributes to the polymorphous appearance of the smears of reactive lymphadenopathies (Figs. 5.20 and 5.21).

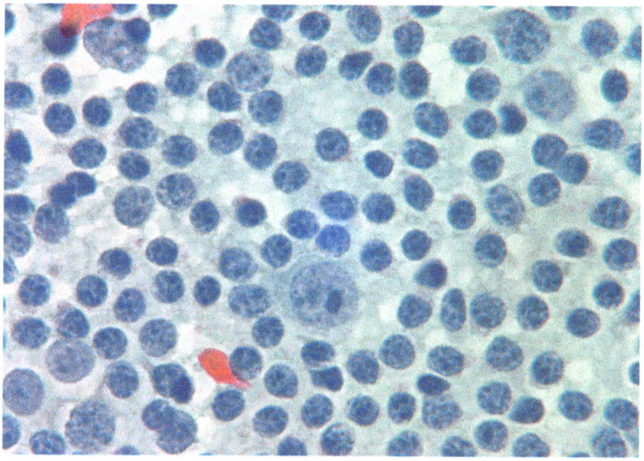

FIGURE 5.21. Polymorphous lymphoid population in an aspirate from reactive lymphadenopathy Note the immunoblast in the center of the image (Papanicolaou stain, ×1,000).

Typical benign aspirates from lymph nodes show evenly dispersed predominantly small lymphoid cells with occasional large lymphocytes, histiocytes, and follicular dendritic cells. On low power, they have a polymorphous appearance due to the difference in cell sizes and the difference in nuclear chromaticity. They may show lymphohistiocytic aggregates or partially crushed tissue fragments that have not completely disaggregated during smearing.

Smears showing monotonous small or large cells or the presence of very large pleomorphic large cells are distinctively abnormal and have to be scrutinized for the presence of malignancy.

A diagnostic algorithm based on the predominant cell size is presented in the next chapter.

Suggested Reading

Bangerter M, Herrmann F, Griesshammer M, Gruss HJ, Hafner M, Heimpel H, Binder T (1997) The abundant presence of Soderstrom bodies in cytology smears of fine-needle aspirates contributes to distinguishing high-grade non-Hodgkin's lymphoma from carcinoma and sarcoma. Ann Hematol 74(4):175–178

Feldman PS, Covell JL, Kardos TF (1989) Fine needle aspiration cytology: lymph node, thyroid, and salivary gland. American Society of Clinical Pathologists Press, Chicago

Flanders E, Kornstein MJ, Wakely PE Jr, Kardos TF, Frable WJ (1993) Lymphoglandular bodies in fine-needle aspiration cytology smears. Am J Clin Pathol 99(5):566–569

Francis IM, Das DK, al-Rubah NA, Gupta SK (1994) Lymphoglandular bodies in lymphoid lesions and non-lymphoid round cell tumours: a quantitative assessment. Diagn Cytopathol 11(1):23–27

Michael CW, Hunter B (2000) Interpretation of fine-needle aspirates processed by the ThinPrep technique: cytologic artifacts and diagnostic pitfalls. Diagn Cytopathol 23(1):6–13

Moriarty AT (2005) Lymph node. In: Renshaw AA (ed) Aspiration cytology: a pattern recognition approach. ElsevierSaunders, Philadelphia, pp 477–533

Murakami T, Kayano H, Itoh T, Shimizu Y, Ban S, Ogawa F, Sannohe S, Kondo S, Shimizu M (2008) Lymphoglandular bodies in malignant tumors: with special reference to histologic specimens. Ann Diagn Pathol 12(4):249–251

O'Dowd GJ, Frable WJ, Behm FG (1985) Fine needle aspiration cytology of benign lymph node hyperplasias. Diagnostic significance of lymphohistiocytic aggregates. Acta Cytol 29(4):554–558

Soderstrom N (1968) The free cytoplasmic fragments of lymphoglandular tissue (lymphoglandular bodies). A preliminary presentation. Scand J Haematol, 5(2):138–152

Suh YK, Shabaik A, Meurer WT, Shin SS (1997) Lymphoid cell aggregates: a useful clue in the fine-needle aspiration diagnosis of follicular lymphomas. Diagn Cytopathol 17(6):467–471

Thunnissen FB, Kroese AH, Ambergen AW, Peterse JL, Jansen JW, Ladde BE, van Pel R, Tiebosch AT, Schaafsma W (1997) Which cytological criteria are the most discriminative to distinguish carcinoma, lymphoma, and soft-tissue sarcoma? A probabilistic approach. Diagn Cytopathol 17(5):333–338

van Heerde P, Go D, Koolman-Schellekens MA, Peterse JL (1984) Cytodiagnosis of non-Hodgkin's lymphoma. A morphological analysis of 215 biopsy proven cases. Virchows Arch A Pathol Anat Histopathol 403(3):213–233

6
Overview of the Algorithmic Pattern-Based Approach to Lymph Node FNA

After exclusion of inadequate aspirates, lymph node FNAs can be broadly divided into those that are dominated by neutrophils, necrosis, and/or granulomas, smears showing cellular aggregates and smears with a dispersed single cell pattern. This broad classification can be made at the initial on-site assessment of the aspirate and will guide the differential diagnostic considerations, and the choice of ancillary studies as outlined in Algorithms 1, 2, and 3. The first algorithm is useful in the diagnosis of lymph node aspirates with a predominance of necrosis, neutrophils, or granulomas, where the most important ancillary tests are microbiologic cultures. The second algorithm is useful in the diagnosis of lymph node aspirates that show predominantly cellular aggregates, where the most important ancillary tests are immunohistochemical stains performed on cell block preparations. The third algorithm is useful in the diagnosis of the most commonly encountered lymph node aspirates, those where dispersed cells predominate; in these aspirates the most useful ancillary test is flow cytometry.

S.E. Pambuccian and R.H. Bardales, *Lymph Node Cytopathology*,
Essentials in Cytopathology 10, DOI 10.1007/978-1-4419-6964-4_6,

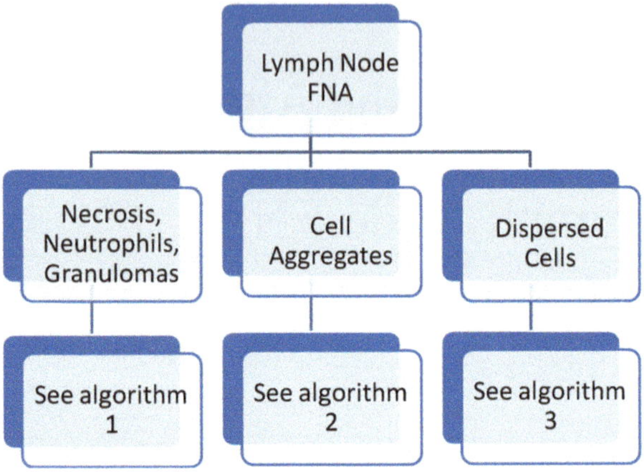

Algorithm 1:

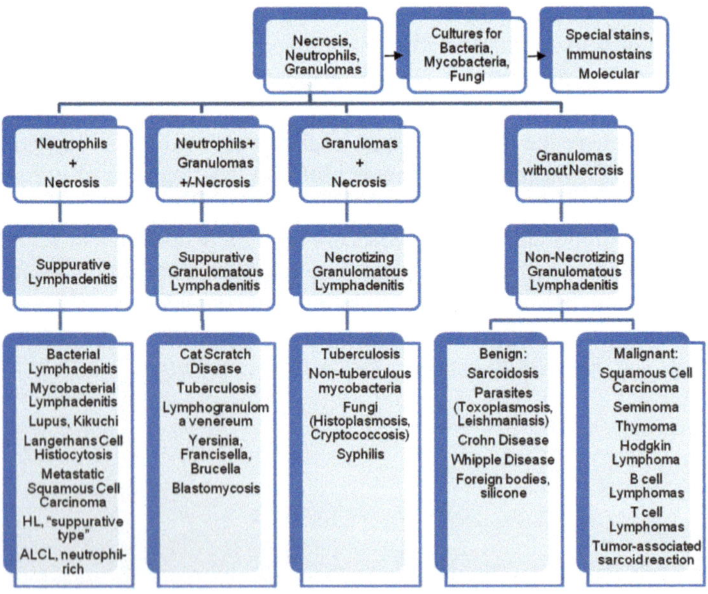

HL Hodgkin lymphoma, *ALCL* Anaplastic large cell lymphoma

Algorithm 2:

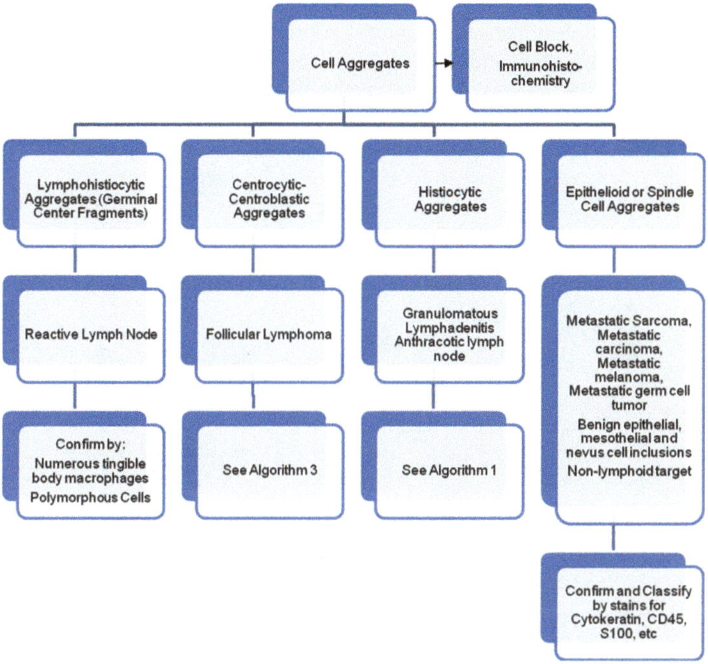

Algorithm 3:

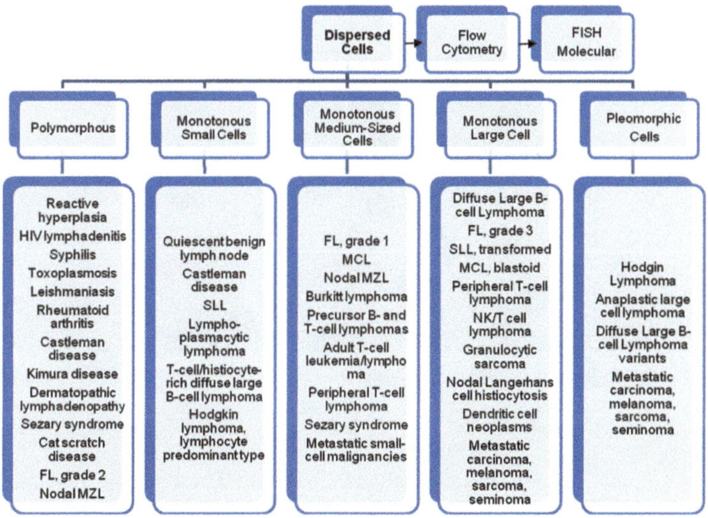

FL Follicular lymphoma, *SLL* small lymphocytic lymphoma, *MCL* Mantle cell lymphoma, *MZL* Marginal zone lymphoma

Figures 6.1–6.5 show schematic representations of the dispersed cell patterns. The following chapters include a discussion of these patterns.

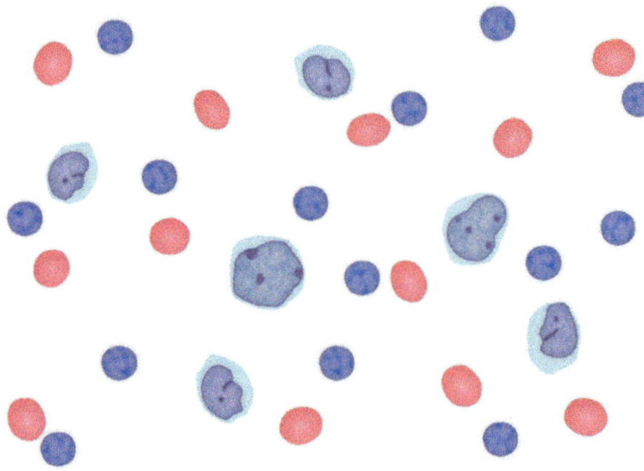

FIGURE 6.1. Polymorphous cell pattern. (Drawing by Jonathan Henriksen, Department of Laboratory Medicine and Pathology, University of Minnesota).

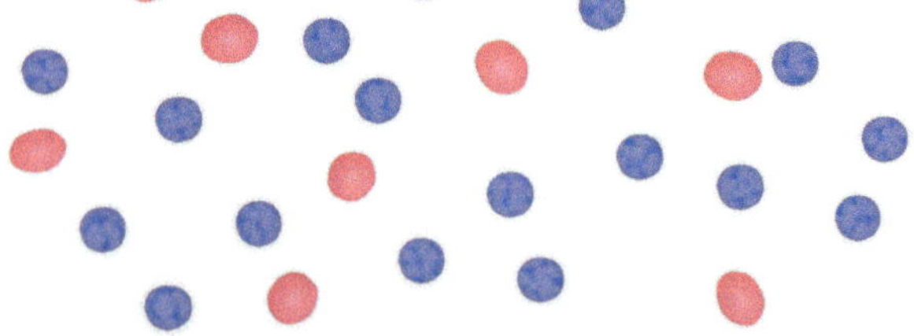

FIGURE 6.2. Monotonous small cell pattern. (Drawing by Jonathan Henriksen, Department of Laboratory Medicine and Pathology, University of Minnesota).

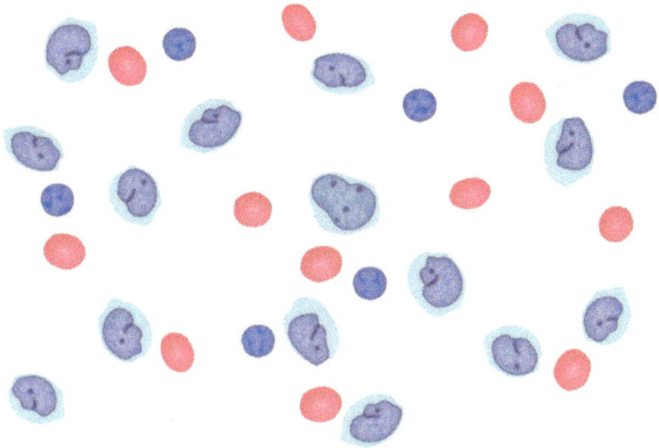

FIGURE 6.3. Monotonous medium-sized cell pattern. (Drawing by Jonathan Henriksen, Department of Laboratory Medicine and Pathology, University of Minnesota).

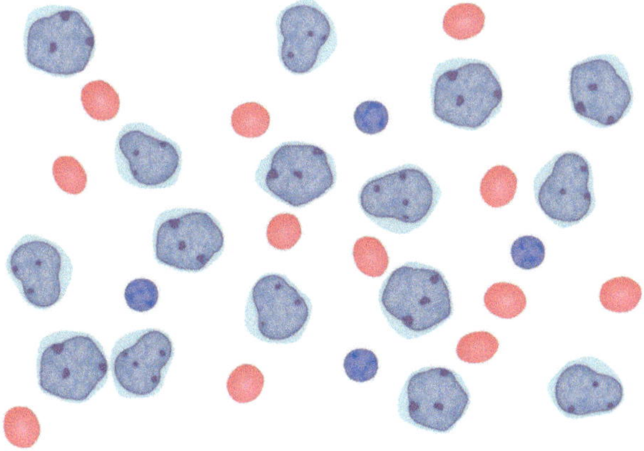

FIGURE 6.4. Monotonous large cell pattern. (Drawing by Jonathan Henriksen, Department of Laboratory Medicine and Pathology, University of Minnesota).

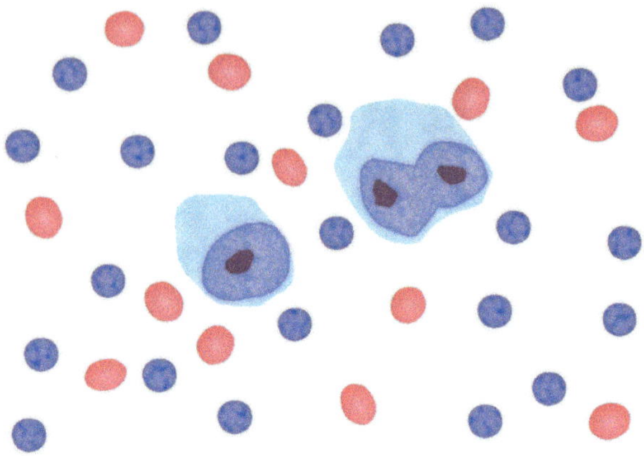

FIGURE 6.5. Pleomorphic (anaplastic) cell pattern. (Drawing by Jonathan Henriksen, Department of Laboratory Medicine and Pathology, University of Minnesota).

7 The Polymorphous Lymphoid Cell Pattern

The following is a list of entities showing this pattern. The cytologic description is based on Romanovsky-stained, air-dried smears. We use the WHO classification and nomenclature for lymphoid neoplasms, unless otherwise is noted.

- Nonspecific reactive lymphoid hyperplasia
- Early human immunodeficiency virus lymphadenitis
- Primary and secondary syphilis lymphadenitis
- Toxoplasma lymphadenitis
- Leishmania lymphadenitis
- Rheumatoid arthritis (RA) lymphadenopathy
- Castleman lymphadenopathy – plasma-cell variant
- Kimura lymphadenopathy
- Early dermatopathic lymphadenopathy
- Sezary syndrome (SS)
- Early cat scratch lymphadenitis
- Follicular lymphoma, grade 2
- Diffuse follicular center cell lymphoma
- Nodal marginal-zone B-cell lymphoma (NMZL)

Reactive lymphoid hyperplasia is the prototype of a cytologic polymorphous lymphoid cell pattern commonly associated with a benign, reactive and reversible lymphadenopathy. Bacteria, viruses, chemicals, and iatrogenic drugs are identified in approximately 10% of cases. The etiology remains unknown in most cases.

S.E. Pambuccian and R.H. Bardales, *Lymph Node Cytopathology*, Essentials in Cytopathology 10, DOI 10.1007/978-1-4419-6964-4_7,

The expansion of a particular lymph node area(s) (follicular, paracortical, medullary, or sinusoidal) depends on the antigenic stimulus and is reflected in the cytologic pattern. Follicular hyperplasia and plasma cells represent a B-cell immune response. The cytology shows small, round lymphocytes, centroblasts, centrocytes, immunoblasts, plasmacytoid lymphocytes, plasma cells, and histiocytes/tingible body macrophages in various numbers. Paracortical hyperplasia with predominance of immunoblasts represents a T-cell response.

The cytologic pattern of a lymph node reaction may suggest a specific etiology that should be addressed in the cytology report, so that appropriate clinical tests are conducted for reaching the specific diagnosis. An inflammatory pattern is frequently associated with bacteria and fungi. An immune pattern is often the effect of drugs and viruses. Occasionally, distinction from non-Hodgkin lymphoma, particularly follicular lymphoma grades 2 and 3, is difficult, and the use of ancillary tests on cytology material may be necessary for diagnosis.

Nonspecific Reactive Lymphoid Hyperplasia

Etiology. Diverse, mostly unknown.

Clinical Findings. This process affects children, adults, and less commonly the elderly. A local disease process may be found in the area of afferent lymphatic drainage. Lymph nodes are soft, usually small, oval, and single or regional (often cervical in children and inguinal in all age groups). Commonly, the lymphadenopathy resolves in 6–8 weeks; however, the nodes may remain enlarged for a longer time, even months.

Cytology. The smears are cellular and show isolated lymphoid cells and scattered small, loose lymphohistiocytic aggregates (LHAs), best identified at scanning power. The LHAs are fragments of germinal centers composed of centrocytes, centroblasts, dendritic cells, small round lymphocytes, and tingible body macrophages (Fig. 7.1, Fig. 4.5 and Fig. 5.13). In the first 3–4 weeks, the smears show predominantly small round lymphocytes and numerous centrocytes, with variable numbers of centroblasts and immunoblasts. Smears from the next 3–4 weeks show predominantly small round lymphocytes and centrocytes with a few large cells. Scattered histiocytes and numerous lymphoglandular bodies are usually found in the background. Plasmacytoid lymphocytes and plasma cells may be present (see Figs. 7.2–7.4, Figs. 4.2–4.3, Figs. 5.2–5.4, Fig. 5.20 and Table 7.1).

Immunophenotype. Positive pan-B-cell markers are CD19, CD20, CD22, and CD79a. In contrast to follicular lymphomas,

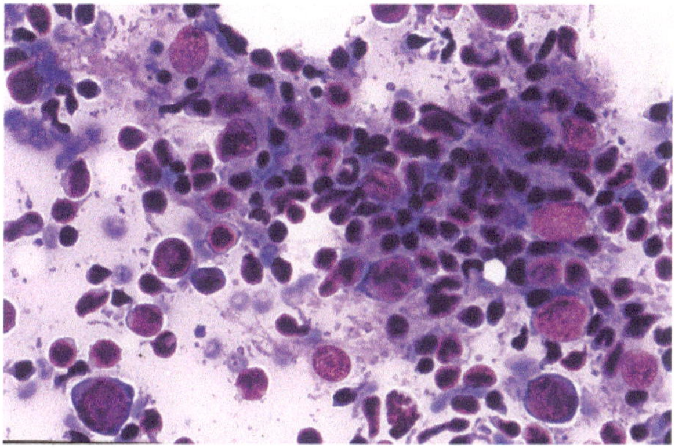

FIGURE 7.1. Characteristic lymphohistiocytic aggregate (LHA) composed of lymphocytes of various sizes and tingible body macrophages (DiffQuik, high magnification).

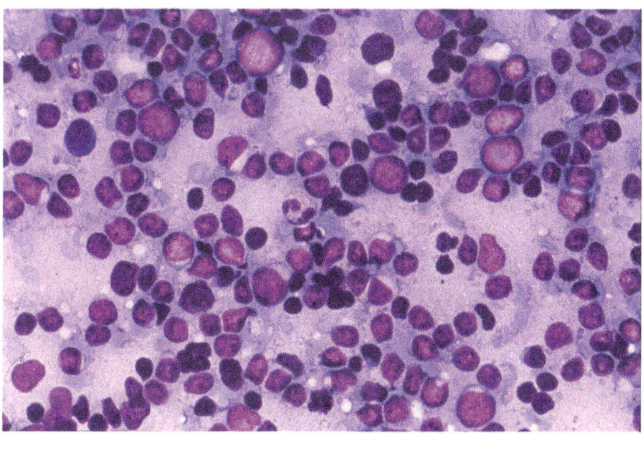

FIGURE 7.2. Reactive lymphoid hyperplasia. Early stage (DiffQuik, high magnification).

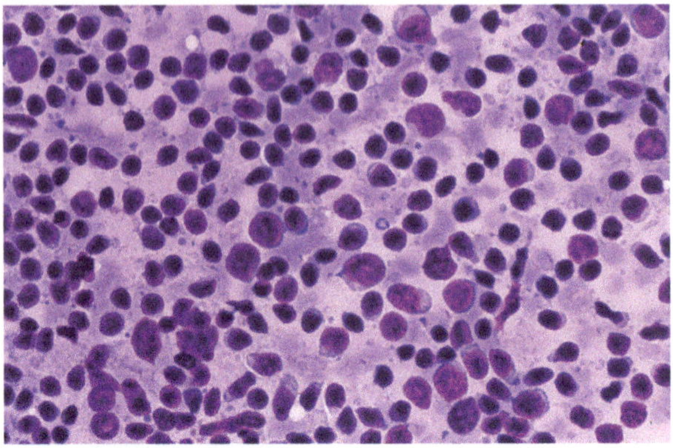

FIGURE 7.3. Reactive lymphoid hyperplasia. Mid-late stage (DiffQuik, high magnification).

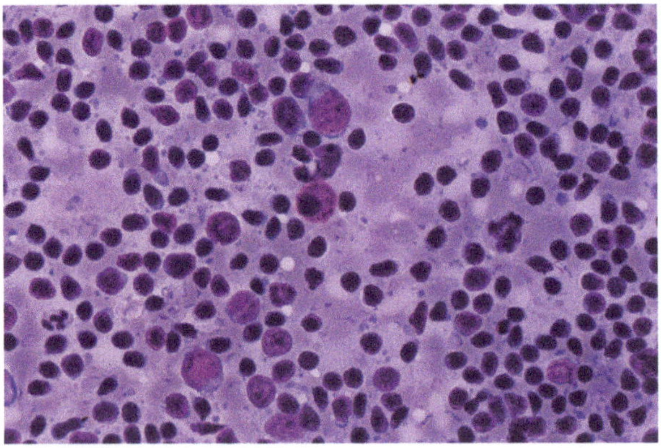

FIGURE 7.4. Reactive lymphoid hyperplasia. Late stage (DiffQuik, high magnification).

only rare BCL-2+ and CD10+ cells are present. The κ/λ ratio is 3–5 to 1. Scattered T-cells are positive for CD3, CD5, CD4, and CD8. Histiocytes are CD68+, and follicular dendritic cells are CD21+. Ki-67 is positive, indicating a high proliferating fraction.

Cytogenetics. In contrast to the finding in follicular lymphoma, no *bcl-2* gene rearrangement is found.

TABLE 7.1. Reactive lymphoid hyperplasia versus follicular lymphoma.

	RLH	FL-2
Age	Children > adults > elderly	Rare in children
Cytology		
LHAs	Present	Absent
Pseudo LHAs	Absent	Present
Centrocytes and centroblasts	Variable numbers	Centrocytes > centroblasts
Cytologic atypia	Absent or mild	Present
Mitosis	Present	Rare
Small round lymphocytes	Present	Rare/absent
Immunoblasts	Present	Rare/absent
Plasma cells	Present	Rare/absent
TGBs	Present	Rare/absent
Eosinophils	May be present	Rare/absent
Markers		
Light chain	Both κ and λ	Monotypic κ or λ
BCL-2 and BCL-6	Negative	Positive
CD10	Negative	Positive
MIB-1/Ki-67	High proliferation	Low proliferation

RLH reactive lymphoid hyperplasia, *FL-2* follicular lymphoma grade 2, *LHAs* lymphohistiocytic aggregates, *TBMs* tingible body macrophages

Key Points. The cytologic diagnosis of reactive lymphoid hyperplasia should be made with caution in the elderly. A prominent histiocytic response may be seen in lymph nodes draining the lymphatic afferents of a malignant process, regardless of the presence or absence of an actual nodal metastasis. The smear background of Hodgkin lymphoma shows follicular hyperplasia.

Early Human Immunodeficiency Virus Lymphadenitis

Etiology. HIV-1 is an RNA lentivirus, of the family of retroviruses.

Clinical Findings. See Chap. 12. In the acute phase of HIV infection, the patients have influenza-like symptoms that include fever and generalized lymphadenopathy that last a few weeks.

The lymphadenopathy may persist in the chronic phase and last for several years.

Cytology. In the acute phase, there are prominent reactive lymphoid hyperplasia, numerous tingible body macrophages, and high mitotic activity. Lymphocytes of intermediate and large size are predominant, with a paucity of small round lymphocytes. Scattered monocytoid cells and multinucleated cells with clustered grape-like nuclei and neutrophils are seen.

The germinal centers involute, follicular hyperplasia decreases, and plasma cells predominate in the chronic and late phase. Endothelial and fibrous stromal fragments with a paucity of lymphocytes and plasma cells are seen in the late burned-out phase.

Immunophenotype. Positive pan-B and pan-T-cell markers. Lack of monoclonal light chain restriction. Multinucleated cells are positive for dendritic cell markers CD21 and CD35.

Key Points. The cytology of the acute phase may be difficult to distinguish from follicular lymphoma. Similar acute-phase cytologic patterns may be seen in measles, CMV, varicella, and EBV lymphadenitis, and serology is necessary for confirming the diagnosis. The incidence of non-Hodgkin lymphoma is increasing in AIDS patients undergoing antiretroviral therapy.

Primary and Secondary Syphilis Lymphadenitis

Etiology. Treponema pallidum, a bacterial spirochete 5–15 μm long and <1 μm thick, is acquired through sexual contact or transmitted from mother to fetus.

Clinical Findings. See Chap. 12. Regional inguinal and less commonly cervical lymphadenitis (draining the site of entry) is present in primary syphilis or generalized in secondary syphilis. The lymph nodes are large, firm, and painless. Whereas chancre is seen in primary syphilis and may last up to 4 weeks, skin and mucosal rash/eruptions and condylomata lata accompany the secondary stage, which may last up to 2 years. Tertiary syphilis with visceral involvement develops thereafter.

Cytology. Florid follicular hyperplasia with small round lymphocytes, scattered immunoblasts, and numerous plasma cells is the characteristic pattern. Noncaseating granulomas are occasionally seen.

Key Points. Visualization of the *T. pallidum* by dark-field preparation, immunofluorescence, and Warthin–Starry stain or amplification by PCR is used for diagnosis along with serologic tests.

Toxoplasma Lymphadenitis

Etiology. See Chap. 12. The responsible organism is *Toxoplasma gondii*, a protozoan that is prevalent in warm and humid climates. Cats (definitive hosts) eliminate oocysts in their stools, and humans (intermediary hosts) are infected, usually by ingestion of oocysts. Other routes of infestation include transplacental transmission to the fetus and renal or bone marrow transplantation.

Clinical Findings. A posterior cervical lymphadenopathy is common in immunocompetent individuals who may be asymptomatic or have mild nonspecific symptoms. Lymph nodes are of variable size, firm, tender or painless, and they may persist for months. The disseminated form occurs in immunosuppressed hosts, is symptomatic, and is often fatal.

Cytology. Smears show a polymorphous lymphoid cell population, plasma cells, and tingible body macrophages. Immunoblasts, scattered monocytoid cells, and epithelioid cells, both single and in small aggregates, are also present. Microgranulomas may be present, but necrosis or giant cells are not a feature. The background may show crescent-shaped trophozoites and/or cysts (Fig. 7.5).

Key Point. When organisms are not identified, the diagnosis of *Toxoplasma* lymphadenitis must be confirmed by serology.

Leishmania Lymphadenitis

Etiology. See Chap. 12. The *Leishmania donovani* in Asia, South America, and Africa or *L. infantum* in Mediterranean regions is transmitted by sand flies (*Phlebotomus* sp.) to mammals, including humans.

Clinical Findings. Regional lymphadenitis is commonly seen in visceral and cutaneous leishmaniasis. The lymph nodes are moderately enlarged, firm, mobile, and nontender.

Cytology. The smear pattern may be similar to that of *Toxoplasma* lymphadenitis. Giant cells, necrosis, and atypical plasma cells may be identified particularly in immunosuppressed patients.

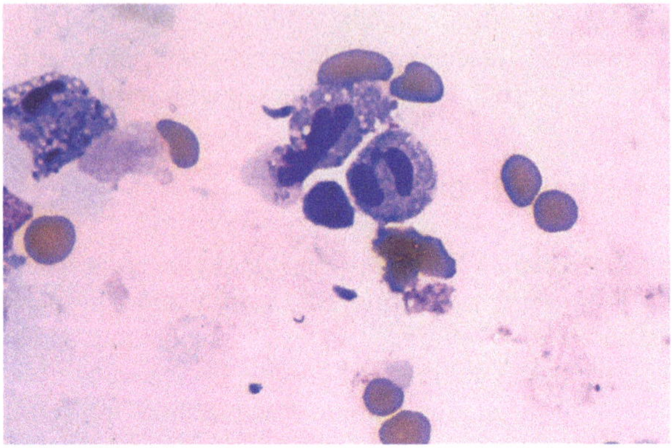

FIGURE 7.5. Toxoplasma. Trophozoites, red blood cells and neutrophils (DiffQuik, high magnification).

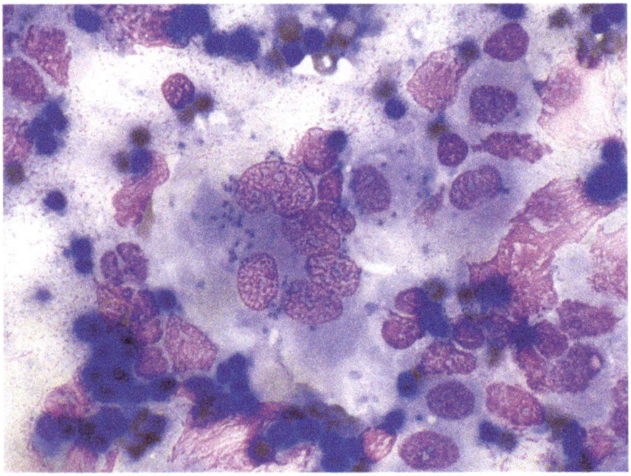

FIGURE 7.6. Leishmania. Leishman–Donovan bodies within histiocytes (DiffQuik, high magnification). Courtesy of Dr. Yahya Daneshbod, Hematopathologist, Department of Pathology, Dr Daneshbod Laboratory, Shiraz, Iran.

Small, ovoid or round organisms (Leishman–Donovan bodies) are present in the histiocytes and giant cells, and are scattered in the background, showing the characteristic rod-shaped kinetoplast (Fig. 7.6).

Rheumatoid Arthritis Lymphadenopathy

Etiology. See Chap. 12. The etiology is unknown. Patients with RA frequently express HLA-DR1or HLA-DR4.

Clinical Findings. RA is most prevalent in females aged 35–50 years and affects proximal small joints (hands and feet) symmetrically and preferentially. Regional or systemic lymphadenopathy occurs in more than 50% of patients, and axillary and cervical, including supraclavicular, lymph nodes are the most commonly involved.

Cytology. A polymorphous lymphoid population and plasma cells are characteristic and reflect the marked follicular hyperplasia and interfollicular lymph node plasmacytosis seen histologically (Fig. 7.7). Scattered immunoblasts, tingible body macrophages, and neutrophils are also identified. Small granulomas and minimal necrosis are seen in rare cases.

Immunophenotype. Pan-B- and pan-T-cell markers are positive. Monoclonal light-chain restriction is lacking.

Key Points. The risk of Hodgkin and non-Hodgkin lymphoma in patients with RA is twice that of the general population. The cytology pattern in both juvenile (Still disease) RA and adult-onset Still disease is similar.

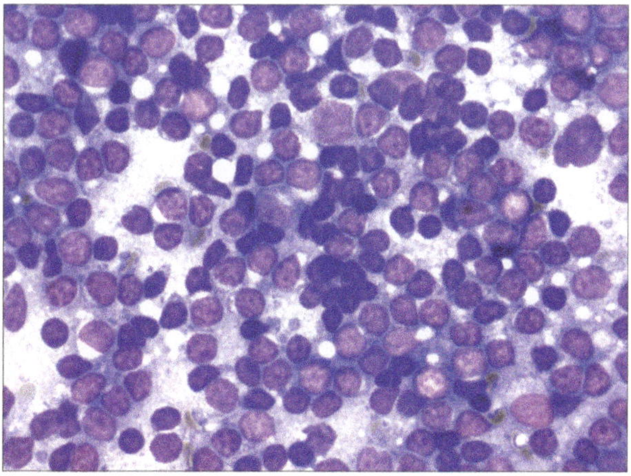

FIGURE 7.7. Rheumatoid arthritis. Reactive lymphocytes are seen. Plasma cells are seen in other cases (Giemsa stain, high magnification).

Castleman Lymphadenopathy: Plasma-Cell Variant

The plasma cell variant of Castleman disease shows a polymorphous lymphoid cell population with numerous small round lymphocytes and plasma cells. Scattered LHAs, histiocytes/tingible body macrophages, and small numbers of immunoblasts are also present.

Staining for human herpesvirus-8 (HHV-8) supports the diagnosis.

Kimura Lymphadenopathy

Etiology. Unknown.

Clinical Findings. See Chap. 12. This is a chronic inflammatory disorder that is prevalent in young adult Asian males. It affects mainly the deep subcutaneous tissue of the head and neck (commonly retroauricular) or the salivary glands and is associated with lymphadenopathy. The lymph nodes are confluent and enlarged. Patients have peripheral eosinophilia and high serum IgE levels.

Cytology. A polymorphous lymphoid cell population is present and reflects the marked follicular hyperplasia. Varying numbers of eosinophils and mast cells are also present. Fragments of collagenous tissue and multinucleated cells with nuclei in a grapevine-like arrangement (polykaryocytes) along with a fibroblastic-vascular stroma lined by endothelial cells are occasionally seen, particularly in cell-block slides.

Immunophenotype. IgE+ dendritic cells.

Early Stages of Dermatopathic Lymphadenopathy

See Chap. 12. Patients have regional (usually axillary or inguinal) or generalized lymphadenopathy and have a coexisting benign or malignant skin disorder.

Follicular lymphoid hyperplasia is present in the early stages of dermatopathic lymphadenopathy, and smears show LHAs, a polymorphous lymphocyte population, and variable numbers of

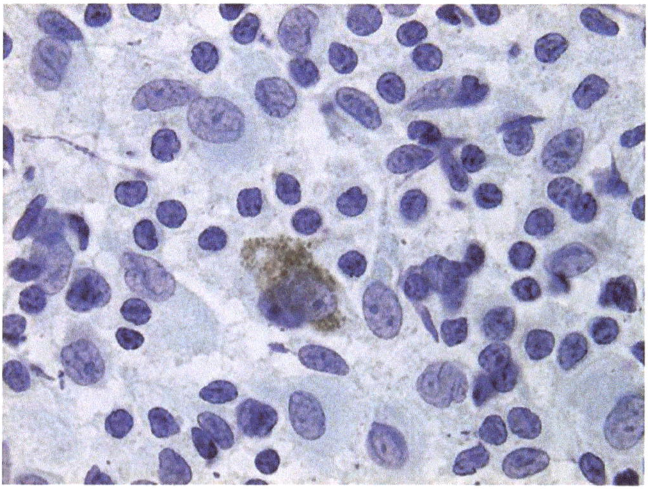

FIGURE 7.8. Dermatopathic lymphadenopathy. A melanin-laden histiocyte is surrounded by histiocytes and cerebriform lymphocytes corresponding to Sezary syndrome (Papanicolaou stain, high magnification). Courtesy of Dr. Javier Saenz de Santamaria, Pathologist, Department of Pathology, Complejo Universitario de Badajoz, Spain.

immunoblasts, plasma cells, and eosinophils. Lipid-, hemosiderin-, or melanin-laden histiocytes and interfollicular dendritic cells are also present (Fig. 7.8). In late stages, the follicles become atrophic, and there is paracortical (immunoblastic) proliferation.

Sezary Syndrome

Three percent of patients with mycosis fungoides (a type of cutaneous T-cell lymphoma) develop SS and have erythroderma and lymphadenopathy. Small and large SS cells with convoluted nuclei are present in the peripheral blood, commonly associated with eosinophilia.

The lymph node cytology shows scattered monomorphic small to intermediate-size SS cells. A pattern of dermatopathic lymphadenopathy with melanin-laden histiocytes may be seen in the background (Fig. 7.8).

Early Cat Scratch Lymphadenitis

In the first week, there is reactive follicular hyperplasia with LHAs, lymphocytes, immunoblasts, histiocytes, rare eosinophils, and neutrophils. The cytologic pattern becomes more characteristic, with prominent necrosis, granulomas, and neutrophils, as the disease process progresses.

Follicular Lymphoma, Grade 2

Follicular lymphomas are the most common non-Hodgkin lymphomas of adults in America and Europe, but are rare in Asia. They originate from the germinal centers, exhibit a nodular histologic pattern, are composed of centrocytes (cleaved) and centroblasts (noncleaved), and have a B-cell immunophenotype. In contrast to reactive lymphoid hyperplasia that is common in children, follicular lymphoma is exceedingly rare in the pediatric population and, when it occurs, usually is localized and follows an indolent clinical course.

Clinical Findings. The patients have regional or generalized lymphadenopathy. The cervical and inguinal lymph nodes are most often involved, show rapid enlargement, are well defined, soft or rubbery, and may be confluent. The texture of the lymph node is not as firm or hard as in metastatic carcinoma, but less firm than in Hodgkin lymphoma. Constitutional symptoms are seen in 20% of patients.

Cytology. The cellularity is usually high, and the smears show a dimorphous or polymorphous cell population with small and large centrocytes (cleaved) and centroblasts (large noncleaved) in equal proportion or with centrocyte predominance. The chromatin is coarse, slightly open, and shows a similar texture in all centrocytes or centroblasts. Occasional small aggregates of neoplastic cells resemble LHAs; however, they consist of centrocytes and follicular dendritic cells; histiocytes/tingible body macrophages are not seen. Mitotic figures are sparse, but may be numerous when the centroblasts outnumber the centrocytes. Rare small lymphocytes, plasmacytoid cells, and plasma cells originating in the interfollicular regions

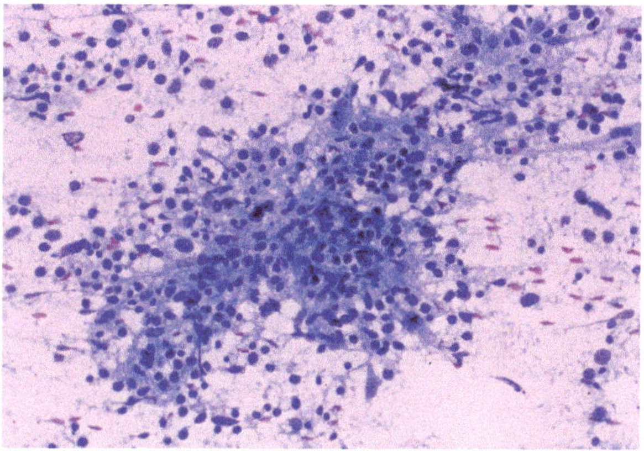

FIGURE 7.9. Follicular lymphoma, grade II. Pseudo LHA (Papanicolaou stain, medium magnification).

may be seen and may be especially conspicuous in partially involved lymph nodes. Necrosis is absent. (Table 7.1 and Figs. 7.9–7.12)

Transformation of follicular lymphoma to diffuse large cell lymphoma, immunoblastic lymphoma, and Burkitt lymphoma can be accurately diagnosed by FNA cytology. Likewise, the signet ring cell variant and floral variants of follicular lymphoma can be diagnosed by aspiration cytology; however, they need histologic evaluation, particularly the former, because it can be nodular or diffuse.

The histologic grading of follicular lymphoma is based on the number of centroblasts per high-power field (HPF) counted in ten neoplastic follicles. Grades 1, 2, and 3 have <6, 6–15, and >15 centroblasts per HPF, respectively. Although similar grading can be used in FNA or liquid-based cytology smears, it has not been fully accepted. Evaluation of the Ki-67 proliferating fraction has been suggested to correlate with the grading system. A major disadvantage of FNA cytology in evaluating follicular lymphomas is the inability to quantify the nodular architecture, a prognostic indicator that can only be evaluated histologically. Similarly, the diffuse follicle center cell lymphoma of mixed cell type, considered by the WHO as a variant of follicular lymphoma, must be evaluated histologically.

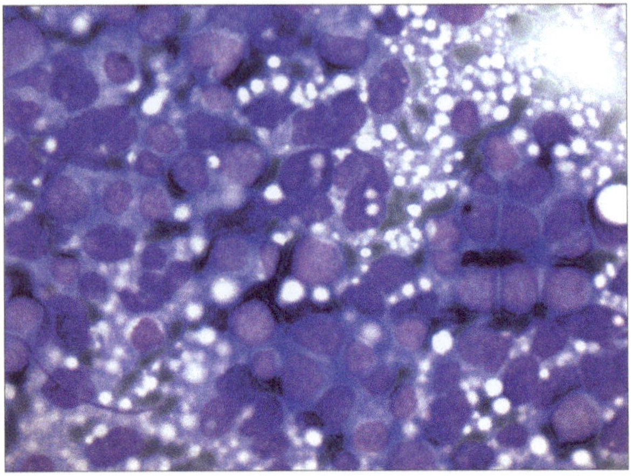

FIGURE 7.10. Follicular lymphoma, grade II. Small aggregates of large and small cells all with irregular nuclear contours are seen along with rare small non-neoplastic lymphocytes (Giemsa stain, high magnification).

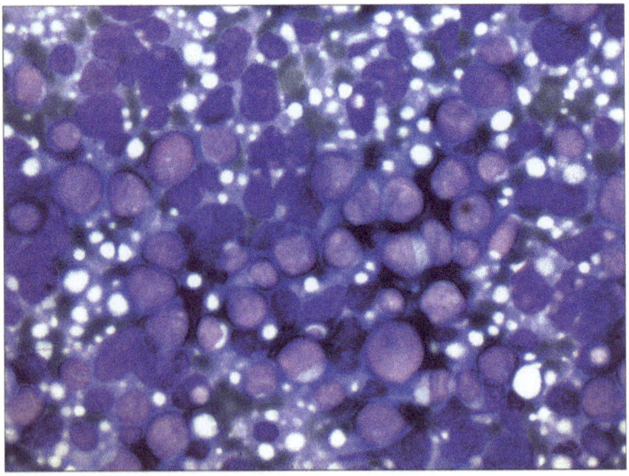

FIGURE 7.11. Follicular lymphoma, grade II. Neoplastic cells with irregular and cleaved nuclei (DiffQuik stain, high magnification).

Immunophenotype. Pan-B-cell markers are CD19+, CD20+, CD22+, CD79a+, and CD10+ (60% of cases). T-markers are CD3–, CD5–, CD23–, and CD43–. Surface κ or λ light chain monoclonality is found. sIgM+ and sIgG+ are less common.

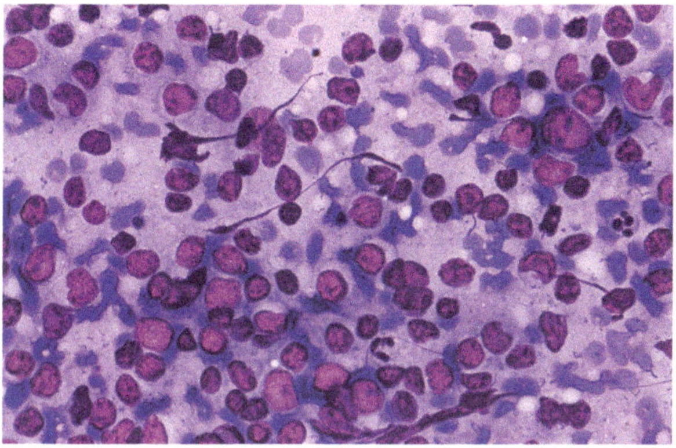

FIGURE 7.12. Follicular lymphoma, grade II. The chromatin pattern is similar in large and smaller neoplastic cells (DiffQuik stain, high magnification).

Positive BCL-2 and BCL-6 protein expression is seen in most cases. The proliferation marker Ki-67 is low.

Cytogenetics. FISH and PCR (on tissue and cytologic material) detect the aberrant *bcl-2* gene rearrangement. This t(14;18) (q32;q21) chromosomal translocation is present in 85% of follicular lymphomas and results in overexpression of the BCL-2 protein, an apoptosis inhibitor.

Diffuse Follicle Center Cell Lymphoma

This variant of follicular lymphoma (as considered by the WHO) is a germinal-center-derived B-cell lymphoma that shows a diffuse histologic pattern and is the diffuse counterpart of nodular follicular lymphoma. In most cases, it represents a transformation of a nodular follicular lymphoma; it rarely arises as a primary diffuse lymphoma.

Cytology. Most cases show predominantly small centrocytes and less frequently a mixed centrocyte and centroblast pattern similar to that of grade 2 follicular lymphoma, and they have the same differential cytologic diagnosis. Similar to the finding in follicular lymphomas, a higher mitotic activity is seen as the proportion of large cells (centroblasts) grows.

Immunophenotype. The immunophenotype is similar to that of follicular lymphoma, including CD10+ and BCL-6+. There is less expression of Ki-67.

Cytogenetics. The *bcl-2* gene is rearranged in <30% of cases of diffuse follicle center cell lymphoma. Remarkably, patients with this type of lymphoma seem to have a better prognosis.

Nodal Marginal-Zone B-Cell Lymphoma

The rare NMZL represents 1.8% of non-Hodgkin lymphomas and, by definition, lacks visceral or splenic involvement. The pathogenesis and cell of origin are unknown. Monocytoid B-cells from the paracortical area that may be related to marginal-zone B-cells are postulated to be the cells of origin (see Chap. 9).

Clinical Findings. Nodal MZL affects predominantly middle-aged and elderly females, although the age varies widely. Patients have regional lymphadenopathy, commonly cervical, axillary, and inguinal in decreasing order of frequency. Abdominal lymphadenopathy is present in 50% of patients and constitutional symptoms are present in 35% of patients. The disease usually follows an indolent course. However, transformation into a diffuse large B-cell lymphoma occurs in a subset of patients and correlates with a worse prognosis.

Cytology. Nodal MZL may involve the various areas of the lymph node (marginal/perifollicular, follicular, sinusoidal) or efface the architecture completely. Neoplastic cells may be seen in a background of a nonspecific reactive lymphoid hyperplasia in partly involved lymph nodes, or they may predominate as a monotonous intermediate-sized cell pattern as described in Chap. 9.

Of note, in most cases of NMZL the neoplastic cells are cytologically polymorphous and show monocytoid cells along with small round lymphocyte- and centrocyte-like cells that require a differential diagnosis with small lymphocytic lymphoma, mantle cell lymphoma, and follicular lymphoma. Centroblast- and immunoblast-like cells are present in various proportions in all cases (Fig. 7.13). Varying degrees of plasmacytoid differentiation, including plasma cells, may be identified.

Immunophenotype. CD19+, CD20+, CD22+, CD79a+; CD5–, CD10–, CD21–, CD23–, CD25–, CD43–, CD68–.

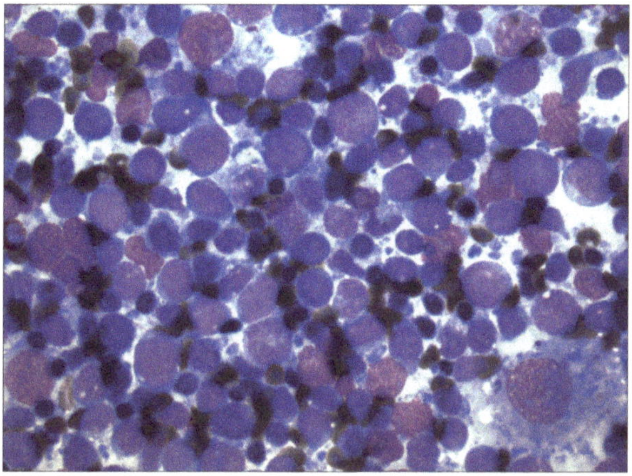

FIGURE 7.13. Nodal marginal-zone B-cell lymphoma. Most cases show a polymorphous lymphoid cell pattern (Giemsa stain, high magnification).

There is surface κ or λ light chain monoclonality. BCL-2 is positive in most cases.

Cytogenetics. Trisomy 3 and t(11;18), which are common in extranodal MZL, are rare in NMZL. Likewise, the 7q21–32 loss found in 40% of splenic MZL is rarely found in NMZL.

Key Points. Because immunophenotypic, cytogenetic, and molecular markers are not well known, the clinical information is important for making the diagnosis. Nodal MZL is a heterogeneous entity with various cytomorphologic patterns.

Suggested Reading

Brandao GD, Rose R et al (2006) Grading follicular lymphomas in fine-needle aspiration biopsies: the role of ThinPrep slides and flow cytometry. Cancer 108(5):319–323

Chow LT, Yuen RW et al (1994) Cytologic features of Kimura's disease in fine-needle aspirates. A study of eight cases. Am J Clin Pathol 102(3):316–321

Das DK (1999) Value and limitations of fine-needle aspiration cytology in diagnosis and classification of lymphomas: a review. Diagn Cytopathol 21(4):240–249

Donnelly A, Hendricks G et al (1995) Cytologic diagnosis of cat scratch disease (CSD) by fine-needle aspiration. Diagn Cytopathol 13(2):103–106

Katzenberger T, Kalla J et al (2009) A distinctive subtype of t(14;18)-negative nodal follicular non-Hodgkin lymphoma characterized by a predominantly diffuse growth pattern and deletions in the chromosomal region 1p36. Blood 113(5):1053–1061

Kishimoto K, Kitamura T et al (2006) Cytologic differential diagnosis of follicular lymphoma grades 1 and 2 from reactive follicular hyperplasia: cytologic features of fine-needle aspiration smears with Pap stain and fluorescence in situ hybridization analysis to detect t(14;18)(q32;q21) chromosomal translocation. Diagn Cytopathol 34(1):11–17

Kondratowicz GM, Symmons DP et al (1990) Rheumatoid lymphadenopathy: a morphological and immunohistochemical study. J Clin Pathol 43(2):106–113

Kumar PV, Moosavi A et al (2001) Subclassification of localized Leishmania lymphadenitis in fine needle aspiration smears. Acta Cytol 45(4):547–554

Laane E, Tani E et al (2005) Flow cytometric immunophenotyping including Bcl-2 detection on fine needle aspirates in the diagnosis of reactive lymphadenopathy and non-Hodgkin's lymphoma. Cytometry B Clin Cytom 64(1):34–42

Matsushima AY, Hamele-Bena D et al (1999) Fine-needle aspiration biopsy findings in marginal zone B cell lymphoma. Diagn Cytopathol 20(4):190–198

Morton LM, Wang SS et al (2006) Lymphoma incidence patterns by WHO subtype in the United States, 1992–2001. Blood 107(1):265–276

O'Dowd GJ, Frable WJ et al (1985) Fine needle aspiration cytology of benign lymph node hyperplasias. Diagnostic significance of lymphohistiocytic aggregates. Acta Cytol 29(4):554–558

Pai RK, Mullins FM et al (2008) Cytologic evaluation of lymphadenopathy associated with mycosis fungoides and Sezary syndrome: role of immunophenotypic and molecular ancillary studies. Cancer 114(5):323–332

Rassidakis GZ, Tani E et al (1999) Diagnosis and subclassification of follicle center and mantle cell lymphomas on fine-needle aspirates: A cytologic and immunocytochemical approach based on the Revised European-American Lymphoma (REAL) classification. Cancer 87(4):216–223

Saikia UN, Dey P et al (2002) Fine-needle aspiration biopsy in diagnosis of follicular lymphoma: cytomorphologic and immunohistochemical analysis. Diagn Cytopathol 26(4):251–256

Shabb N, Katz R et al (1991) Fine-needle aspiration evaluation of lymphoproliferative lesions in human immunodeficiency virus-positive patients. A multiparameter approach. Cancer 67(4):1008–1018

Stani J (1987) Cytologic diagnosis of reactive lymphadenopathy in fine needle aspiration biopsy specimens. Acta Cytol 31(1):8–13

Stewart CJ, Duncan JA et al (1998) Fine needle aspiration cytology diagnosis of malignant lymphoma and reactive lymphoid hyperplasia. J Clin Pathol 51(3):197–203

Suh YK, Shabaik A et al (1997) Lymphoid cell aggregates: a useful clue in the fine-needle aspiration diagnosis of follicular lymphomas. Diagn Cytopathol 17(6):467–471

van Crevel R, Grefte JM et al (2009) Syphilis presenting as isolated cervical lymphadenopathy: two related cases. J Infect 58(1):76–78

Viguer JM, Jimenez-Heffernan JA et al (2005) Fine needle aspiration of toxoplasmic (Piringer-Kuchinka) lymphadenitis: a cytohistologic correlation study. Acta Cytol 49(2):139–143

Yu GH, McGrath CM (2000) Follow-up of morphologically reactive lymphoid proliferations in fine-needle aspirates of elderly patients. Diagn Cytopathol 23(4):249–252

8
The Monotonous Small-Cell Pattern

Small lymphocytes measure <12 μm in diameter, equivalent to the size of a histiocyte nucleus, a segmented neutrophil, or 1.5 to 2 times the size of an erythrocyte. The presence of a monotonous proliferation of small lymphoid cells in an enlarged round and rubbery lymph node is abnormal, and the cytologic findings should be correlated with the clinical scenario. Chronic lymphocytic leukemia/small lymphocytic lymphoma (CLL/SLL) and the resolving or quiescent phase of a reactive lymphoid hyperplasia are the main and most common entities considered in the differential diagnosis and must be distinguished from other neoplastic and non-neoplastic processes. The following is a list of entities showing the monotonous small-cell pattern. The cytologic description is based on Romanovsky-stained, air-dried smears. We use the WHO classification and nomenclature for lymphoid neoplasms unless otherwise is noted.

- Quiescent benign lymph node.
- Castleman disease, hyaline-vascular variant.
- B-cell chronic lymphocytic leukemia/small lymphocytic lymphoma.
- T-cell chronic lymphocytic leukemia (REAL classification).
- Lymphoplasmacytic lymphoma.
- T-cell/histiocyte-rich diffuse large B-cell lymphoma.
- Hodgkin lymphoma, lymphocyte predominant type.

S.E. Pambuccian and R.H. Bardales, *Lymph Node Cytopathology*, Essentials in Cytopathology 10, DOI 10.1007/978-1-4419-6964-4_8,

The Quiescent Benign Lymph Node

The pattern of a quiescent or inactive lymph node is seen in the resolving phase of a reactive lymphoid hyperplasia.

Clinical Findings. Patients are asymptomatic, with isolated or regional, usually cervical or inguinal lymphadenopathy present for more than 8 weeks. The lymph nodes usually measure <1 cm and are oval, firm, movable, and not confluent.

Cytology. The smears are cellular and show mature-appearing lymphocytes. Larger lymphocytes or histiocytes are rare or absent; however, if found, they are helpful for identifying the reactive process (Fig. 8.1).

Immunophenotype. B-cell monoclonality or T-cell gene rearrangement is lacking.

Key Points. The cytology must be interpreted along with the clinical information. The small round lymphocytes are indistinguishable cytologically from those of CLL/SLL, and flow cytometry may be used in selected cases for distinguishing between the two.

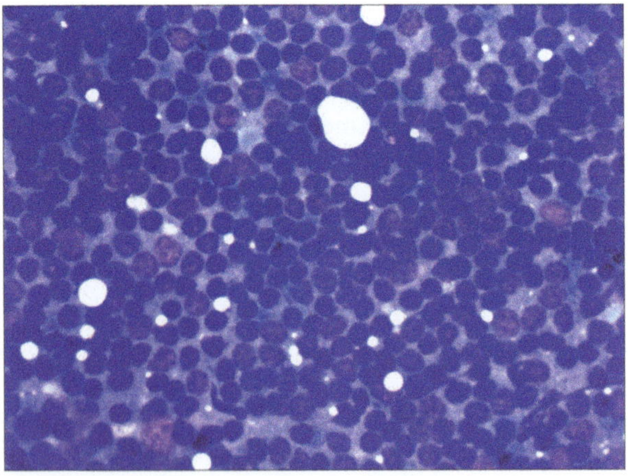

FIGURE 8.1. Quiescent benign lymph node. Characteristic predominant population of small round lymphocytes, rare larger lymphoid cells, and tingible body macrophages (Giemsa stain, high magnification).

Castleman Disease, Hyaline-Vascular Variant

Castleman disease (CD) is a heterogenous group of diseases with variable clinical presentation and prognosis, and most likely multiple etiologies; it is also known as angiofollicular or giant lymph node hyperplasia. Localized hyaline-vascular (HV) and plasma cell (PC) variants as well as the multicentric Castleman disease (MCD) have been described. The latter two have been noted in HIV-positive patients. The human herpes virus type-8, also known as Kaposi sarcoma virus, has been recognized in a subset of patients with PC-CD and MCD. Most cases of MCD show histologic features of PC-CD.

Clinical Findings. HV-CD represents 90% of localized CD and commonly affects the mediastinal and less frequently the cervical and abdominal lymph nodes. Males and females in a broad age range are affected equally; however, patients with HV-CD are usually younger than those with PC-CD. The median size of the lymph nodes is 6 cm (range, 1.5–16 cm). Symptoms are secondary to the compression of local structures, i.e., dysphagia, shortness of breath, or vascular compression. Constitutional symptoms are rare, and patients are frequently asymptomatic.

Cytology. Smears show numerous small lymphocytes representing the hyperplastic mantle zones. Branching hyalinized small blood vessels and germinal center elements have been described in more than 50% of the cases. Rare mitotic figures can be identified. Follicular dendritic cells (FDCs), plasmacytoid monocytes, immunoblasts, and eosinophils are variably present, and rare plasma cells may be seen. Thus, the overall cytomorphology may be described as polymorphous with predominance of small round lymphocytes (Fig. 8.2). The follicular dendritic cells may be atypical.

Immunophenotype. There is no evidence of B-cell monoclonality or T-cell gene rearrangement.

Cytogenetics. Ig heavy-chain and T-cell receptor genes are nearly always germline.

Key Points. Thymoma should be included in the differential diagnosis in the appropriate clinical setting. The mantle-zone lymphocytes are cytologically similar to those of Hassal's corpuscles in thymoma. Follicular dendritic cell sarcoma has been described

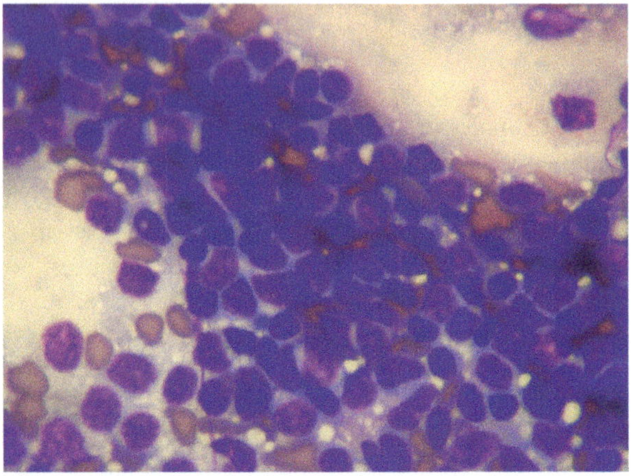

FIGURE 8.2. Castleman disease, hyaline-vascular variant. Predominant small lymphocytes representing the hyperplastic mantle zones (DiffQuik stain, high magnification). Courtesy Dr. Luis de las Casas, Pathologist, Department of Pathology, Texas Tech University, El Paso Texas.

in HV-CD; however, there is no increased risk for developing lymphomas in these patients.

B-Cell Chronic Lymphocytic Leukemia/Small Lymphocytic Lymphoma

The term CLL is used for patients who have lymphocytosis. The term SLL is used when there is lymph node involvement with no leukemia. Patients with B-cell chronic lymphocytic leukemia/small lymphocytic lymphoma (B-CLL/SLL) usually have peripheral-blood and bone marrow involvement at the time of lymph node involvement. FNA of a lymph-node in these patients is usually performed for confirmation of lymph-node leukemic involvement or to exclude a transformation to a large-cell lymphoma (Ritchter's transformation), which occurs in 5% of the patients.

Clinical Findings. This neoplasm is more common in white males than in African-Americans and is least common in Asians. Patients are usually in their fifth decade or older and have generalized lymphadenopathy, hepatosplenomegaly, and asthenia secondary to anemia. The lymph nodes are rounded, firm, and large. The clinical course is indolent except when there is transformation to a large-cell lymphoma and the patients have constitutional symptoms.

Cytology. The smears are cellular, and the pattern is dominated by a monotonous population of small lymphocytes (same size as or slightly larger than a normal lymphocyte) with minimal cytoplasm, a round nucleus, regular or slightly irregular nuclear membrane, coarse clumped and regular chromatin, and an inconspicuous/small nucleolus. The chromatin appears dense and coarse in the Papanicolaou stain. Mitoses are rare, and plasmacytic differentiation is absent (Fig. 8.3). Occasionally larger cells (prolymphocytes and paraimmunoblasts) are seen. The prolymphocytes are of intermediate size and show dispersed chromatin and a visible nucleolus. The larger paraimmunoblasts have broader cytoplasm and a nucleus with vesicular chromatin, a visible large central nucleolus, and they resemble immunoblasts; however, the cytoplasm is pale instead of blue. No histiocytes, tingible-body macrophages, or LHAs are seen in B-CLL/SLL. Mast cells can be observed; however, they are also seen in reactive lymphadenopathy.

Immunophenotype. The cells are positive for CD19, CD20, and CD23. Characteristically, the surface Ig light chain expression is

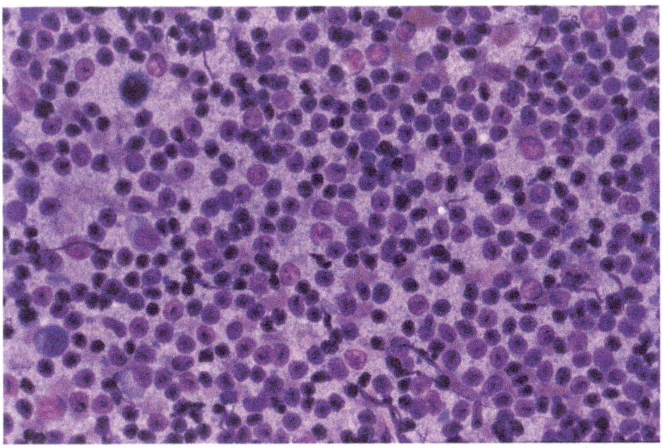

FIGURE 8.3. Chronic lymphocytic leukemia. Monotonous population of small lymphocytes with small inconspicuous nucleolus (DiffQuik stain, high magnification).

dim on flow cytometry. Positivity for CD5 is characteristic. CD10 and FMC7 are negative.

Cytogenetics. Del(13q14) is present in 50% of the patients and is associated with a favorable prognosis. Trisomy 12, t(11;14), and t(14;19) have also been described. Chromosomal aberrations of 17p13.1 and 11q22 are associated with an increased risk of death and can be detected by FISH on FNA material.

Key Points. A polymorphous cell population would indicate a reactive process. A monotonous small/intermediate cell pattern with nuclear irregularities would indicate other neoplasms such as grade 1 follicular, mantle cell, or T-cell lymphoma. Predominance of plasmacytoid lymphocytes would favor a lymphoplasmacytic lymphoma. The prolymphocytic and Ritchter's transformation convey an aggressive clinical course. Cytologically, Ritchter's transformation usually resembles the centroblastic variant of diffuse large B-cell lymphoma, but immunoblastic and T-cell/histiocyte-rich variants can also occur.

T-Cell Chronic Lymphocytic Leukemia

The term T-cell chronic lymphocytic leukemia (T-CLL) used by the REAL classification is not included in the WHO classification, which only considers T-cell prolymphocytic leukemia. However, occasional cases of mature CD4+ T-cell leukemias with nodal involvement and without morphologic features to suggest a prolymphocytic or other T-cell neoplasm have been described.

Clinical Findings. T-CLL is more aggressive than B-CLL, is not curable, and affects the bone marrow, lymph nodes, visceral organs, and skin in adults.

Cytology. The neoplastic cells are small and similar to those of B-CLL in a minority of cases. Most cases show a T-prolymphocytic leukemia cytomorphology, including larger cells with irregular nuclei and broad cytoplasm.

Immunophenotype. Positive T-cell associated antigens are present, and most are CD4+.

Cytogenetics. Inv 14(11q;q32) and trisomy 8q are common.

Key Point. The definitive diagnosis requires immunophenotyping in excised lymph nodes.

Lymphoplasmacytic Lymphoma

Lymphoplasmacytic lymphoma/Walderstrom macroglobulinemia (LPL/WD) is a B-cell neoplasm of small lymphocytes, plasmacytoid lymphocytes, and plasma cells.

Clinical Findings. LPL/WM is especially frequent in elderly white males, who show bone marrow, lymph node, and spleen involvement and commonly serum monoclonal IgM paraprotein, hyperviscosity, and cryoglobulinemia. Lymph nodes are moderately enlarged, and seen in 15% of patients. Fatigue and weakness are common and are usually due to anemia secondary to bone marrow involvement. The hyperviscosisty causes reduced visual acuity and ischemia of the central nervous system. Bleeding diathesis and distal peripheral neuropathy are secondary to the serum IgM paraprotein deposition. Type II cryoglobulins can be associated with Reynaud phenomenon, arthralgias, and vasculitis. Amyloidosis may be seen as a result of monoclonal light-chain deposition.

Cytology. Smears are cellular and show variable numbers of small round lymphocytes, plasmacytoid lymphocytes, and mature plasma cells (Fig. 8.4). Dutcher and Russell bodies can be seen in the plasma cells. Occasional multinucleated cells may be present. Mitoses are rare, and the background shows mast cells.

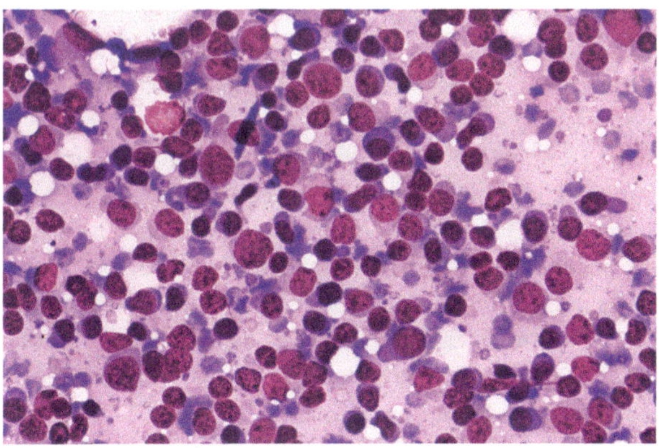

FIGURE 8.4. Lymphoplasmacytic lymphoma. Predominant population of plasmacytoid lymphocytes and rare small lymphocytes (DiffQuik stain, high magnification).

Immunophenotype. B-cell markers CD19, CD20, CD22 are positive. CD23 is negative or dim. CD25, CD27, and FMC7 are positive. Typically, cells are CD5- and CD10-negative. Lymphoplasmacytoid cells are positive for CD38. Plasma cells are positive for CD38 and CD138 and show cytoplasmic IgM, but no surface Ig.

Cytogenetics. Deletions of chromosome 6q are the most frequent genotypic finding.

Key Points. Like any other low-grade small-B cell lymphoma, LPL/WM can undergo transformation to a high-grade lymphoma, particularly centroblastic or immunoblastic diffuse large B-cell lymphoma. The serum IgM paraprotein level can be high in various B-cell lymphomas; thus, it is not a reliable discriminator in the differential diagnosis.

T-Cell/Histiocyte-Rich Diffuse Large B-Cell Lymphoma

Diffuse large B-cell lymphomas (DLBCL) are highly aggressive neoplasms, which are common in Western countries; they comprise five variants: centroblastic, immunoblastic, plasmablastic, anaplastic, and T-cell-rich. DLBCL can develop de novo as a primary tumor or as the transformation of a low-grade small-cell B-cell lymphoma, i.e., CLL/SLL, LPL/WM, follicular, or marginal-zone lymphoma.

Clinical Findings. The T-cell-rich variant is uncommon and is seen mostly in young individuals, with a male predominance. Liver, bone marrow, and spleen involvement is commonly present along with lymphadenopathy and constitutional symptoms. The treatment modality is similar to that for other DLBCLs.

Cytology. The large cell lymphoma cells must be looked for carefully because they comprise <10% of the cellular population and may be centroblastic, immunoblastic, or Reed–Sternberg-like. The mature, small, reactive and non-neoplastic T-lymphocytes comprise 90% of the cell population. Variable numbers of histiocytes are present and may be epithelioid.

Immunophenotype. The lymphoma cells are of B- or T-cell type (see Chapter 10). In addition, the neoplastic cells are CD15-, CD30-, and EBV-negative. The small T lymphocytes show positivity for the pan-T-cell marker CD3.

Key Points. The predominance of small reactive lymphocytes obscures the larger neoplastic cells, and the process can be misdiagnosed as a reactive follicular hyperplasia, lymphocyte-predominance Hodgkin lymphoma (LPHL), or other small-cell lymphomas. In contrast to LPHL, which shows a nodular histologic pattern, the typical T-cell/histiocyte-rich large B-cell lymphoma is diffuse.

Hodgkin Lymphoma, Lymphocyte Predominant Type

The WHO classifies HL into lymphocyte predominance (LP) and classical types. The latter group comprises nodular sclerosis, lymphocyte-rich, mixed cellularity, and lymphocyte-depleted HL. The LP and nodular-sclerosis types have the best prognosis and occur predominantly in young females.

Although the WHO and REAL classifications of lymphoid neoplasms note that LPHL is a particular type of B-cell lymphoma originating in the germinal center, it is temporarily classified in the group of HL.

Clinical Findings. These lymphomas comprise 6% of cases of HL and have a peak in the fourth decade of life. Patients usually have lymphadenopathy and have localized disease with an indolent clinical course and a favorable prognosis. LPHL is commonly associated with stage I (single-lymph node region, usually cervical and supraclavicular) or stage II (two or more lymph node regions on the same side of the diaphragm) disease. The lymph nodes are large, rounded, and firm. Mediastinal and retroperitoneal lymphadenopathy is uncommon. Constitutional symptoms (fever, night sweats, pruritus, anorexia, fatigue, weakness, and weight loss) are rare. In the presence of constitutional symptoms and high-stage disease, the patients are treated with chemotherapy for non-Hodgkin lymphoma.

Cytology. The lymphocytic and/or histiocytic (L&H) cells are the neoplastic cells of LPHL and constitute <10% of the cells in smears. The L&H cells are large, with pale and scant cytoplasm, a convoluted or multilobed nucleus, a thin nuclear membrane, vesicular chromatin, and an inconspicuous nucleolus. The term "popcorn" is used to describe these cells. Such cells can be round, with a more conspicuous nucleolus. Mitoses are rare. In contrast to the finding in lymphocyte-rich classical HL, Reed–Sternberg and Hodgkin cells are not present.

Non-neoplastic cells are the majority and include predominantly small round lymphocytes, scattered histiocytes either singly or in small clusters, and follicular dendritic cells. Approximately 15% of LPHLs show reactive germinal centers, and the smears may show elements of a reactive follicular hyperplasia including centroblasts, centrocytes, and occasional immunoblasts. Eosinophils, neutrophils, and plasma cells are not seen in LPHL; however, they are present in lymphocyte-rich classical HL (Fig. 8.5).

Immunophenotype. Flow-cytometric analysis is usually noncontributory to the diagnosis. Instead, immunohistochemistry is used for diagnosis.

L&H cells are CD20+, CD22+, CD75+, and CD79a+, PAX5/BSAP+, Oct2+, BOB.1+, BCL6+, PU.1+, EMA+/–, CD45+, CD15–, CD30–/+, and negative for EBV or T-cell antigens.

Reactive small round lymphocytes are a mixture of polyclonal B cells and T cells.

Cytogenetics. Ig gene rearrangement has been detected in single L&H cells. Clonal abnormalities have been found in most cases.

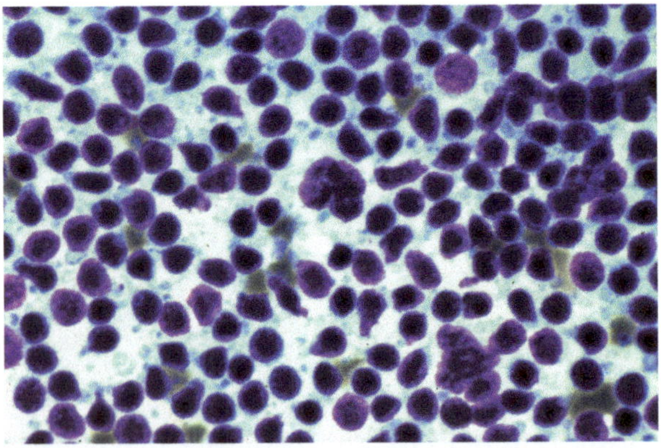

FIGURE 8.5. Hodgkin lymphoma, lymphocyte predominant type. Small round non-neoplastic lymphocytes are predominant. A large cell with convoluted nucleus is seen in the center of the frame (DiffQuik stain, high magnification).

Key Points. Study of cytology and immunophenotype and ultimately lymph node excision are necessary for differentiating among LPHL, lymphocyte-rich classical HL, or T-cell/histiocyte-rich large B-cell lymphoma. Histologically, almost all LPHL have a nodular pattern. Patients with LPHL have an increased risk for developing diffuse large B-cell lymphoma.

Suggested Reading

Bonato M, Pittaluga S et al (1998) Lymph node histology in typical and atypical chronic lymphocytic leukemia. Am J Surg Pathol 22(1):49–56

Caraway N P, Thomas E et al (2008) Chromosomal abnormalities detected by multicolor fluorescence in situ hybridization in fine-needle aspirates from patients with small lymphocytic lymphoma are useful for predicting survival. Cancer 114(5):315–322

Deschenes M, Michel RP et al (2008) Fine-needle aspiration cytology of Castleman disease: case report with review of the literature. Diagn Cytopathol 36(12):904–908

Diehl V, Sextro M et al (1999) Clinical presentation, course, and prognostic factors in lymphocyte-predominant Hodgkin's disease and lymphocyte-rich classical Hodgkin's disease: report from the European Task Force on Lymphoma Project on Lymphocyte-Predominant Hodgkin's Disease. J Clin Oncol 17(3):776–783

Dong HY, Harris NL et al (2001) Fine-needle aspiration biopsy in the diagnosis and classification of primary and recurrent lymphoma: a retrospective analysis of the utility of cytomorphology and flow cytometry. Mod Pathol 14(5):472–481

Fan Z, Natkunam Y et al (2003) Characterization of variant patterns of nodular lymphocyte predominant hodgkin lymphoma with immunohistologic and clinical correlation. Am J Surg Pathol 27(10):1346–1356

Harris NL, Jaffe ES et al (1999) World Health Organization classification of neoplastic diseases of the hematopoietic and lymphoid tissues: report of the Clinical Advisory Committee meeting-Airlie House, Virginia, November 1997. J Clin Oncol 17(12):3835–3849

Hoyer JD, Ross CW et al (1995) True T-cell chronic lymphocytic leukemia: a morphologic and immunophenotypic study of 25 cases. Blood 86(3):1163–1169

Kardos TF, Vinson JH et al (1986) Hodgkins disease: diagnosis by fine-needle aspiration biopsy. Analysis of cytologic criteria from a selected series. Am J Clin Pathol 86(3):286–291

Keller AR, Hochholzer L et al (1972) Hyaline-vascular and plasma-cell types of giant lymph node hyperplasia of the mediastinum and other locations. Cancer 29(3):670–683

Koo CH, Rappaport H et al (1989) Imprint cytology of non-Hodgkin's lymphomas based on a study of 212 immunologically characterized cases: correlation of touch imprints with tissue sections. Hum Pathol 20(12 Suppl 1):1–137

Lim MS, Beaty M et al (2002) T-cell/histiocyte-rich large B-cell lymphoma: a heterogeneous entity with derivation from germinal center B cells. Am J Surg Pathol 26(11):1458–1466

Lin P, Bueso-Ramos C et al (2003) Waldenstrom macroglobulinemia involving extramedullary sites: morphologic and immunophenotypic findings in 44 patients. Am J Surg Pathol 27(8):1104–1113

Meyer L, Gibbons D et al (1999) Fine-needle aspiration findings in Castleman's disease. Diagn Cytopathol 21(1):57–60

Morton LM, Wang SS et al (2006) Lymphoma incidence patterns by WHO subtype in the United States, 1992–2001. Blood 107(1):265–276

Shin HJ, Caraway NP et al (2003) Cytomorphologic spectrum of small lymphocytic lymphoma in patients with an accelerated clinical course. Cancer 99(5):293–300

Stani J (1987) Cytologic diagnosis of reactive lymphadenopathy in fine needle aspiration biopsy specimens. Acta Cytol 31(1):8–13

Stewart CJ, Duncan JA et al (1998) Fine needle aspiration cytology diagnosis of malignant lymphoma and reactive lymphoid hyperplasia. J Clin Pathol 51(3):197–203

Tani E, Johansson B et al (1998) T-cell-rich B-cell lymphoma: fine-needle aspiration cytology and immunocytochemistry. Diagn Cytopathol 18(1):1–4

Tong TR, Lee KC et al (2002) T-cell/histiocyte-rich diffuse large B-cell lymphoma. Report of a case diagnosed by fine needle aspiration biopsy with immunohistochemical and molecular pathologic correlation. Acta Cytol 46(5):893–898

Zhang JR, Raza AS et al (2006) Fine-needle aspiration diagnosis of Hodgkin lymphoma using current WHO classification – re-evaluation of cases from 1999–2004 with new proposals. Diagn Cytopathol 34(6):397–402

9
The Monotonous Intermediate-Sized Cell Pattern

A small lymphocyte measures between 6 and 12 μm, and a large lymphocyte measures >20 μm. The intermediate-sized lymphocyte measurements are between those of small and large lymphocytes.

Once the cytologic diagnosis of an intermediate-sized lymphoid malignancy is made and a metastatic deposit is excluded, the distinction between the various lymphoma types is made with the use of ancillary tests, in particular flow cytometry.

The following is a list of entities showing this pattern, the cytologic description is based on Romanovsky-stained, air-dried smears. We use the WHO classification and nomenclature for lymphoid neoplasms unless otherwise specified.

- Follicular lymphoma, grade 1
- Diffuse follicle center cell lymphoma, grade 1
- Mantle cell lymphoma
- Nodal marginal-zone lymphoma
- Burkitt lymphoma
- Precursor B- and T-cell lymphomas
- Adult T-cell leukemia/lymphoma
- Peripheral T-cell lymphoma
- Sezary syndrome
- Metastatic small-cell malignancies

S.E. Pambuccian and R.H. Bardales, *Lymph Node Cytopathology*, Essentials in Cytopathology 10, DOI 10.1007/978-1-4419-6964-4_9,

Follicular Lymphoma, Grade 1

Most follicular lymphomas are nodular, at least focally, and rare cases are entirely diffuse. Histologically, follicular lymphoma, grade 1 (FL-1) has an average of <6 centroblasts per high-power field counted in ten neoplastic follicles. Although it has not been fully accepted, a similar evaluation can be made on cytology smears.

Clinical Findings. Adults and elderly persons of both genders are affected equally, rarely before the age of 20 years. Patients usually have widespread disease at diagnosis, often with involvement of cervical and inguinal lymph nodes and spleen, but rarely of extranodal sites. The course is indolent, but FL-1 is not curable. Transformation to a large B-cell lymphoma is more frequent than with other low-grade lymphomas.

Cytology. At low magnification, the smears may show aggregates of neoplastic centrocytes in keeping with the nodular histologic counterpart (Fig. 9.1). The monotonous cells have scant or non-visible cytoplasm, clumped chromatin, and inconspicuous nucleoli. The nuclei are variably irregular, angulated, and cleaved but, in general these features are less evident than in tissue sections or Papanicolaou-stained

FIGURE 9.1. Follicular lymphoma, grade I. The nodularity of this lymphoma can also be visualized as cellular aggregates in aspiration biopsy smears (Giemsa stain, low magnification).

smears; deeply cleaved cells may appear to have a bi-lobed nucleus (Fig. 9.2). There are cases in which some cells may be slightly smaller and less irregular, but the chromatin pattern is similar in all neoplastic cells (Fig. 9.3). Larger lymphoma cells or centroblasts are rare and show non-cleaved nuclei, less dense chromatin,

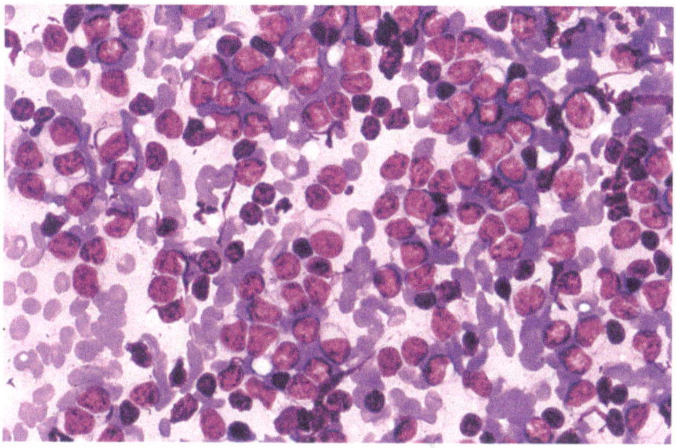

FIGURE 9.2. Follicular lymphoma, grade I. Monotonous intermediate cell pattern and prominent nuclear irregularity and grooving are present (DiffQuik stain, high magnification).

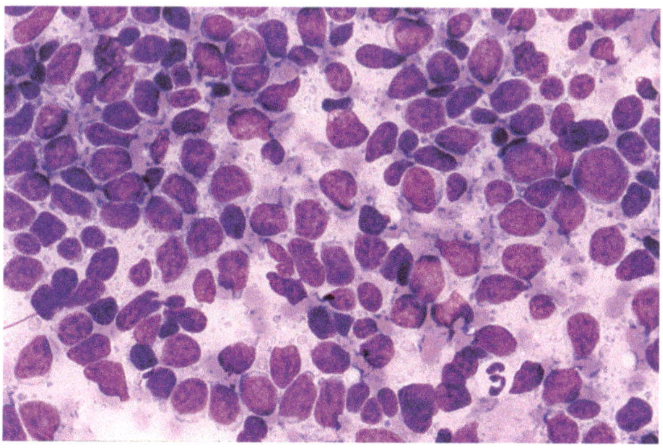

FIGURE 9.3. Follicular lymphoma, grade I. The nuclear chromatin pattern is uniform in the intermediate and in the rare large cells present. The nuclear irregularity is not prominent (Giemsa stain, high magnification).

and a narrow rim of dense cytoplasm; however, larger-cleaved centroblasts may be seen. There are few or no mitoses and rare or absent tingible-body macrophages. Scattered non-neoplastic T cells which may be similar to, although slightly smaller than the neoplastic cells may be seen; they originate in the follicles and interfollicular areas. Signet-ring-cell lymphoma, a rare variant of follicular lymphoma shows intracellular immunoglobulins indenting the nucleus toward the periphery, resembling adenocarcinoma. Numerous lymphoglandular bodies are seen in the background.

Immunophenotype. Briefly, cells express bright, monotypic sIg and B-cell-associated antigens (see Table 9.1). In tissue sections, bcl-2 protein-positive staining is diagnostic of follicular lymphoma. T cells in reactive follicles, which may be numerous, express bcl-2 protein. Thus, bcl-2 positivity should be considered with other markers. The signet-ring-cell lymphoma is keratin- and mucicarmine-negative.

Cytogenetics. There is gene rearrangement of both light and heavy chains and t(14;18)(q32;q21) resulting in a rearrangement of the *bcl-2* gene with subsequent inhibition of apoptosis. FISH seems to be the most sensitive and specific detecting method. Other common

TABLE 9.1. Immunophenotypic profile of small- and intermediate-sized cell lymphomas.

	B-CLL/SLL	MCL	Nodal MZL	FL-1	LPL
Surface κ/λ	+Dim	+Strong	+Strong	+Strong	+Strong
CD5	+	+	+Dim 10%	–	–
CD10	–	–	–	+	–
CD20	+Dim	+	+	+	+
CD23	+90%	+Dim 10%	+10%	–	+Dim/–
FMC7	–	+	+	+	+
BCL-1	–	+	–	–	–
BCL-2	+	+	+Most cases	+	+
BCL-6	–	–	–	+	–
Cyclin D1	–	+	–	–	–

B-CLL/SLL B-chronic lymphocytic leukemia/small lymphocytic lymphoma, *MCL* mantle cell lymphoma, *MZL* marginal-zone lymphoma, *FL* follicular lymphoma, *LPL* lymphoplasmacytic lymphoma

genetic abnormalities include loss of the 1p, 6q, 10q, and 17p chromosome arms and gains of 1, 6p, 7, 8, 12q, X, and 18q/dup.

Key Points. A more polymorphous lymphoid pattern, tingible-body macrophages, and mitoses are seen in reactive lymphoid hyperplasia.

Diffuse Follicle Center Cell Lymphoma, Grade 1

The 2008 WHO classification of mature B-cell neoplasms recommends that lymphomas composed of centrocytes and centroblasts with an entirely diffuse (histologic) pattern may be included in the category of follicular lymphoma. Thus, because the architecture cannot be evaluated in FNA smears, the cytology of grade 1 diffuse follicle center cell lymphoma is similar to that of the follicular lymphoma described above. See diffuse follicle center cell lymphoma in Chapter 7 for more details.

Mantle Cell Lymphoma

Mantle cell lymphoma (MCL) is a B-cell neoplasm that comprises 3–10% of all non-Hodgkin lymphomas. The blastoid and pleomorphic variants are more aggressive.

Clinical Findings. Mantle cell lymphoma occurs in middle-aged to older individuals, with male predominance. Most patients have generalized lymphadenopathy, hepatosplenomegaly, and bone marrow and peripheral blood involvement, and may have GI lymphomatous polyposis.

Cytology. Cytologic preparations show monotonous lymphoid cells with irregular nuclear contours resembling centrocytes (Fig. 9.4). The nuclei show dispersed chromatin and inconspicuous nucleoli; the larger cells may have single small, distinct nucleoli. The cytoplasm is moderate in quantity and is usually mildly basophilic. Rare plasmacytoid lymphocytes may be seen. Neoplastic centroblasts, immunoblasts, or paraimmunoblasts are absent. Scattered epithelioid histiocytes are commonly present. Larger and more pleomorphic cells may be seen in cases of relapse; however, large-cell transformation has not been described. Mitoses can be seen and correlates with a more aggressive course.

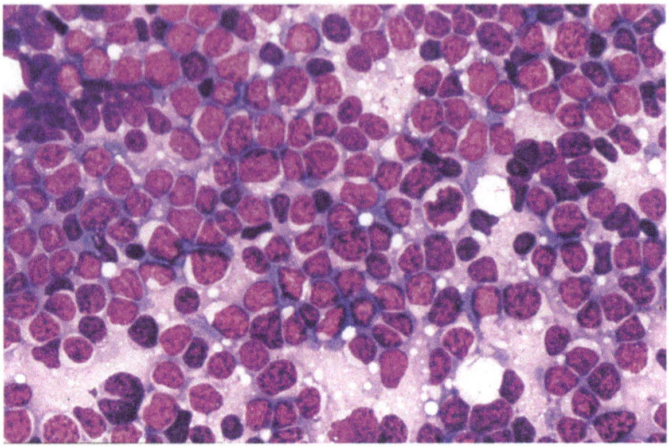

FIGURE 9.4. Mantle cell lymphoma. This lymphoma is cytologically indistinguishable from other intermediate-sized cell lymphomas (DiffQuik stain, high magnification).

Immunophenotype. Monotypic lambda light-chain restriction is more common than kappa. Cells are CD5+, FMC7+, CD43+, BCL2+, BCL6–, and CD10– (Table 9.1). An aberrant phenotype may be seen in the more aggressive variants. Almost all are cyclin D1- and BCL-1-positive.

Cytogenetics. Neoplastic cells show t(11;14)(q13;q32) with *CCND1* translocation in almost all cases. Rare MCLs are negative for both cyclin D1 and the t(11;14), but have the MCL immunophenotype.

Key Points. Most patients cannot be cured. The small-cell variant, which appears to have a more indolent course, shows more clumped chromatin and must be distinguished from small lymphocytic lymphoma. The marginal-zone-like variant exhibits monocytoid cells similar to those in marginal-zone lymphoma.

Nodal Marginal-Zone Lymphoma

Monocytoid B-cell lymphoma and mucosa-associated lymphoid tissue (MALT) lymphoma have been grouped as nodal and extranodal types of MZL, respectively, and have identical histology and cytology (see Chap. 7).

Nodal MZL (NMZL) comprises <2% of all non-Hodgkin lymphomas and is a primary lymph node B-cell neoplasm without splenic or extranodal involvement.

Clinical Findings. Nodal MZL occurs mostly in adults and older individuals, with a similar incidence in males and females. Most patients have asymptomatic regional, often cervical or generalized lymphadenopathy. Some patients have systemic symptoms. Nodal MZL is clinically indolent, and most patients survive longer than 5 years. Some patients may have serologic evidence of hepatitis C infection.

Cytology. Cytology preparations show monocytoid cells, centrocyte-like cells, or cells resembling small/intermediate round lymphocytes, or a combination of the three in various proportions (Fig. 9.5). Monocytoid cells have gray cytoplasm, central nuclei, clumped chromatin, and small nucleoli. Scattered larger transformed cells in various proportions and plasma cells may be seen. Plasma cell differentiation may be prominent in some cases, and scattered eosinophils may be present. A predominance of large cells in a patient with known NMZL may indicate transformation to a large-cell lymphoma.

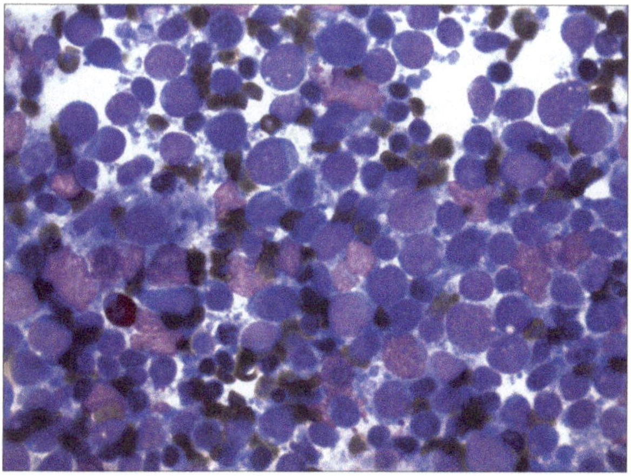

FIGURE 9.5. Nodal marginal-zone lymphoma. This particular example shows a predominance of intermediate-sized lymphocytes (Giemsa stain, high magnification).

Immunophenotype. As seen in Table 9.1, CD5, CD10, BCL6, and cyclin D1 are negative and BCL2 is positive. CD23 may be faintly positive.

Cytogenetics. There is clonal Ig gene rearrangement with predominance of mutated VH3 and VH4 families. The various chromosomal translocations associated with extranodal MZL are not seen in NMZL.

Key Points. One-third of patients with NMZL represent nodal dissemination of MALT lymphoma. Nodal MZL with cytology and immunophenotype similar to that of adult NMZL has been described in children; mostly in males, the prognosis is excellent. In addition to the entities listed in Table 9.1, lymphocyte-rich classical and lymphocyte-predominant Hodgkin lymphoma, T-cell/histiocyte-rich diffuse large B-cell lymphoma, peripheral T-cell lymphoma, and mast cell disease should be considered.

Burkitt Lymphoma

Burkitt lymphoma (BL) is a B-cell lymphoma that often occurs in extranodal sites or as an acute leukemia. The endemic, sporadic, and immunodeficiency-associated variants of BL differ clinically, morphologically, and biologically. Endemic BL occurs in equatorial Africa in areas of endemic malaria and affects predominantly children. Sporadic BL is seen throughout the world, represents <2% of all non-Hodgkin lymphomas in the USA, and affects predominantly children and young adults. Immunodeficiency-associated BL is often associated with HIV infection.

The Epstein–Barr virus (EBV) genome is present in the neoplastic cells in all cases of endemic BL. EBV is detected in approximately 30% of sporadic and immunodeficiency-associated BL.

Clinical Findings. Extranodal sites including the CNS are often involved in all three variants. Lymph node involvement at diagnosis is seen more commonly in adults than in children with sporadic BL. Nodal and bone marrow involvement are frequent in immunodeficiency-associated BL. Patients have bulky disease and signs and symptoms of a few weeks' duration due to the short doubling time of the tumor. Endemic and sporadic BL may be cured with intensive chemotherapy regimens.

Cytology. The tumor cells have nuclei similar to or smaller than those of histiocytes. Nuclei are round with evenly distributed chromatin and with multiple nucleoli of moderate size. The cytoplasm is moderate, non-granular, homogeneous, deeply basophilic, and usually contains a number of clear-lipid-containing vacuoles 1–2 μm in diameter (Fig. 9.6). Numerous mitoses are present as well as numerous macrophages with ingested apoptotic tumor cells. The spectrum of BL is wide, and some cases may show tumor cells with plasmacytoid features, particularly in immunodeficiency-associated BL, or nuclear pleomorphism with more prominent nucleoli.

Immunophenotype. Tumor cells express light-chain restriction and B-cell-associated antigens. BCL2 is negative and BCL6 is positive.

Cytogenetics. *IG;MYC* gene translocation at chromosome segment 8q24 without BCL2 or BCL6 translocation is almost always present.

Key Points. Burkitt lymphoma is a highly aggressive neoplasm and is often extranodal. The three types of BL have identical histology and cytology, but show different epidemiologic, geographic, and molecular findings.

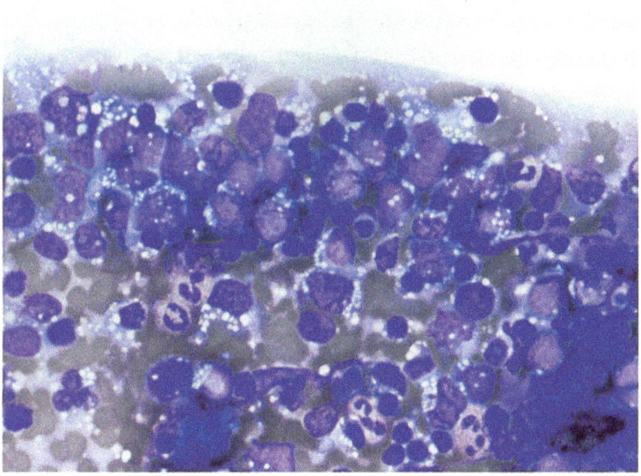

FIGURE 9.6. Burkitt lymphoma. The small clear lipid-containing vacuoles are evident in the cytoplasm (DiffQuik stain, high magnification).

Precursor B- and T-Cell Lymphomas

These neoplasms are composed of precursor B or T cells involving bone marrow (BM) and peripheral blood (PB), and occasionally are accompanied by primary nodal or extranodal site involvement. By consensus, the term lymphoblastic lymphoma (LBL) is used when the process is confined to a mass lesion with minimal or no evidence of PB and BM involvement. Whereas the B-cell lineage predominates in lymphoblastic leukemia, only 10% of LBLs have a B-cell phenotype.

Clinical Findings. Lymphoblastic lymphomas are seen often in children and adolescents. The most frequent sites of involvement in B-LBL are skin, soft tissue, bone, and lymph nodes. Mediastinal masses are infrequent in B-LBL. Mediastinal (thymic) involvement is often present in T-LBL, and patients may have respiratory distress. Any extranodal site may be involved in T-LBL, usually with lymph node and mediastinal involvement. Lymphadenopathy, hepatomegaly, and splenomegaly are frequent in B- and T-LBL. Patients may be asymptomatic in the absence of BM involvement.

Cytology. In smears and imprint preparations, the lymphoblasts in B- and T-LBL are indistinguishable cytologically. Cells may be of small or intermediate size. The small cells are uniform and have scant cytoplasm that may be difficult to recognize, round nuclei with occasional clefting and indentations, homogeneous, fine, and delicate chromatin, and multiple variably prominent nucleoli. When intermediate-sized cells predominate, the pattern shows more anisocytosis, and cells have variable, often moderate cytoplasm, basophilic fine and delicate chromatin, often irregular, clefted, and indented nuclear contours, and two to three small nucleoli. Mitotic figures are often numerous, and azurophilic, coarse cytoplasmic granules and vacuoles can occasionally be seen in both B- and T-LBL. In general, the nuclear clefting is more difficult to observe in cytology than in tissue sections (Fig. 9.7).

Immunophenotype. TdT is positive in most cases of B- and T-LBL. The lymphoblasts in B-LBL are almost always positive for the B-cell markers CD19, CD22, cytoplasmic CD79a, and PAX5. The lymphoblasts in T-LBL are positive for the T-cell markers CD7, CD99, CD34, and CD1a.

Cytogenetics. Almost all cases of B-LBL have cytogenetic abnormalities. Some groups of precursor B-cell leukemia/lymphoma

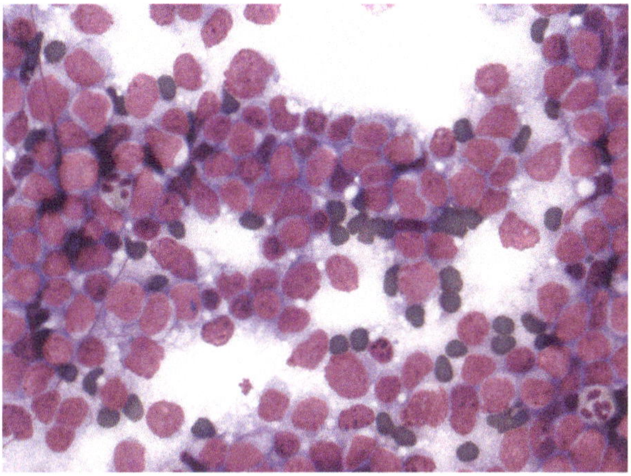

FIGURE 9.7. Precursor T-cell lymphoma. Monotonous population of intermediate-sized lymphocytes is seen, some with slight nuclear irregularities (Giemsa stain, high magnification). Courtesy Roberto Miranda MD, Associate Professor, Department of Pathology, MD Anderson Cancer Center.

have characteristic recurrent genetic abnormalities and distinctive clinical and phenotypic features, which have prognostic implications. T-LBL almost always has T-cell-receptor gene rearrangements, commonly of α and δ loci.

Key Points. The prognosis of B-LBL appears to be better in children than in adults. The prognosis of T-LBL depends on the age of the patient, the stage, and LDH levels.

Adult T-Cell Leukemia/Lymphoma

The distribution of the disease parallels the prevalence of human T-cell leukemia virus type-I (HTLV-I) in the population and is endemic in southwestern Japan, the Caribbean basin, and Central Africa.

Clinical Findings. Adult T-cell leukemia/lymphoma (ATLL) occurs in adults between the ages of 20 and 80 years, with a male to female ratio of 1.5:1. Most patients have generalized disease with lymph node and peripheral blood involvement. The skin is the most commonly involved extranodal site. Generalized lymphadenopathy, skin rash, leukocytosis, eosinophilia, and hypercalcemia are common in acute ATLL. Strongyloidiasis may be seen as the result of T-cell immunodeficiency. Generalized lymphadenopathy without peripheral blood involvement is seen in the lymphomatous variant of ATLL. Patients with the chronic variant of ATLL frequently show skin involvement with mild lymphadenopathy, lymphocytosis, and normal calcium levels. Abnormal circulating lymphocytes with normal count, skin involvement without lymphadenopathy, and normal calcium levels are the only manifestations in the smoldering variant.

Cytology. The predominant neoplastic lymphocytes are of intermediate to large size with marked nuclear irregularities, coarse chromatin, and distinct nucleoli. Giant cells with convoluted nuclei may be present.

Immunophenotype. The tumor cells express T-cell-associated antigens (CD2, CD3, and CD5) and lack CD7. Most cases are CD4+. The large cells may be CD30+, but are negative for ALK. The tumor cells frequently express CCR4 and FOXP3.

Cytogenetics. Neoplastic cells have clonal rearrangement of T-cell-receptor genes and monoclonal integration of HTLV-I.

Key Points. Prognostic factors include age, clinical presentation, serum calcium levels, and LDH. Most patients with the acute variant die of infectious complications within 1 year after the diagnosis.

Peripheral T-Cell Lymphoma

Peripheral T-cell lymphoma (PTCL) is rare, comprises 6% of all non-Hodgkin lymphomas, and is especially common in African-American males in the sixth decade of life or older. The etiology and pathogenesis are unknown.

Clinical Findings. Patients commonly have lymphadenopathy, extranodal (skin, GI tract, liver, spleen, bone marrow) involvement, and systemic symptoms. Pruritus, eosinophilia, and hemophagocytic syndrome may be present, but leukemia is uncommon.

Cytology. The neoplasm is composed of small, intermediate, and large cells in various combinations resulting in a polymorphous pattern or may be monotonous when one cell pattern predominates.

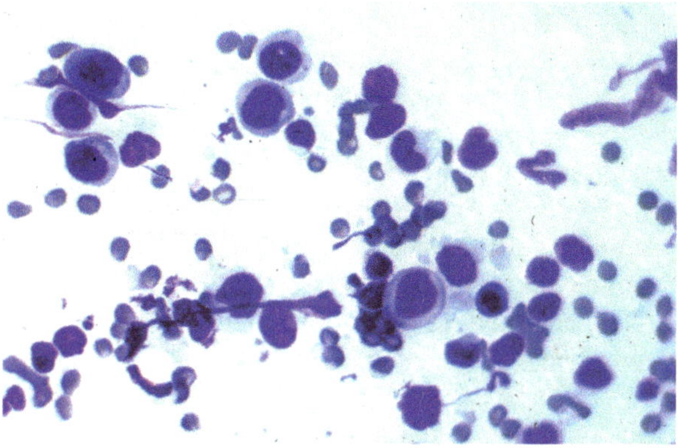

FIGURE 9.8. Peripheral T-cell lymphoma. Prominent nuclear irregularities are seen in this case. The intermediate-sized cell pattern is the least common (DiffQuik stain, high magnification).

The intermediate-cell pattern is the least common (Fig. 9.8). The neoplastic cells range in size from 12 to 28 μm and exhibit clear cytoplasm, irregular nuclei, prominent nucleoli, and numerous mitoses. Clear cells and Reed-Sternberg-like cells may be seen. In addition, small lymphocytes, histiocytes, eosinophils, and plasma cells are present. Tight sarcoid-like granulomas can be seen.

Immunophenotype. The neoplastic cells express pan-T-cell and T-cell-associated antigens including CD2, CD3, CD5, CD7, CD43, and CD45RO and are negative for B-cell antigens. Most are CD4+ and express TCR-αβ. Ki67 is usually high; however, it may be low in a subset of small-cell PTCL.

Cytogenetics. T-cell-receptor genes are clonally rearranged in most cases. Compared to large-cell PTCL, small-cell PTCL has a lesser frequency of abnormal clones and more numerous and complex genetic abnormalities.

Key Points. The diagnosis of PTCL should be made when other entities have been excluded. Small-cell PTCL has a better prognosis than large-cell PTCL, although in general PTCLs are aggressive neoplasms with <50% 5-year survival. Cytologically, PTCL and ATLL can be indistinguishable; however, ATLL occurs with leukemia, hypercalcemia, and HTLV-1-positive serology.

Sezary Syndrome

Sezary syndrome is rare and occurs in adults, usually older than 60 years, and has a male predominance (see Chap. 7). It is an aggressive disease with an overall survival of 20% at 5 years.

Clinical Findings. Patients have erythroderma and generalized lymphadenopathy. Patients may have palmar and plantar hyperkeratosis and onychodystrophy.

Cytology. The neoplastic T cells have cerebriform nuclei (Sezary cells) and are found in the skin, lymph nodes, and peripheral blood. The cells have moderate amounts of basophilic cytoplasm, and the nucleus may have a monocytoid appearance with one to three nucleoli. The smear background may show melanin-laden histiocytes as manifestation of dermatopathic lymphadenopathy (Fig. 9.9).

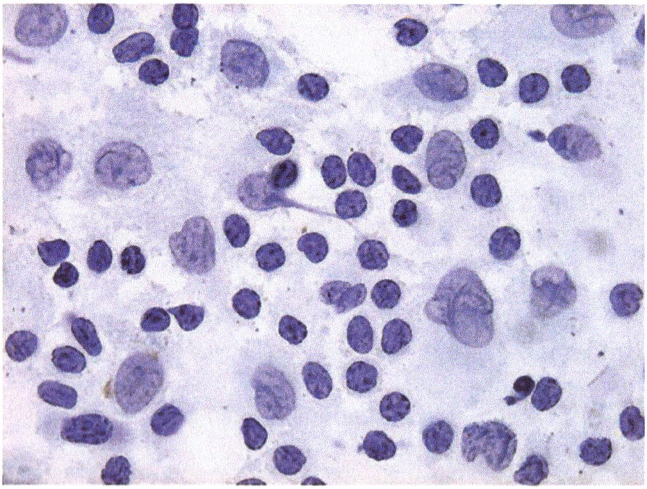

FIGURE 9.9. Sezary syndrome. Intermediate-sized nuclei with cerebriform nuclei are seen. A coexistent dermatopathic lymphadenopathy, as in this case should not be a distractor (Papanicolaou stain, high magnification). Courtesy Dr. Javier Saenz de Santamaria, Pathologist, Department of Pathology, Complejo Universitario de Badajoz, Spain.

Immunophenotype. Tumor cells are CD2+, CD3+, TCRβ+, CD5+, and often CD4+. They express cutaneous lymphocyte antigen (CLA) and the skin-homing receptor CCR4.

Cytogenetics. Tumor cells have T-cell-receptor gene rearrangement. High rates of unbalanced translocations and associated deletions have been detected.

Key Points. In addition to the clinical parameters, the diagnosis of Sezary syndrome is based on the following: an absolute Sezary cell count of 1,000 cells/mm^3 in the peripheral blood, CD4/CD8 ratio >10, and/or loss of one or more T-cell antigens.

Metastatic Small-Cell Malignancies

A lymph node with lymphoma or leukemia does not preclude involvement by a metastasis. The topography of lymph node chains and their territories of lymphatic drainage are helpful clues for determining the primary site of malignancy and are covered in Chap. 3. Regional lymph node metastasis will categorize a malignancy as being stage III.

When possible, the original tumor should be reviewed for comparison of the cytomorphology. In some instances, the cytomorphology may be similar to that of primary lymphoid malignancies, and the final diagnosis is made by use of ancillary tests along with clinical data. Briefly, neurofibrils are seen in neuroblastomas, neurosecretory granules in neuroendocrine tumors, melanin pigment in melanomas, and argyrophil granules in carcinoid tumors.

In the next section, we summarize the metastases that show a monotonous small/intermediate-sized cell pattern.

Neuroendocrine Tumors. These tumors arise from neuroendocrine cells present predominantly in the gastroenteropancreatic system and lung and less commonly in other organs. All neuroendocrine tumors express both epithelial (pankeratin cocktail) and neuroendocrine (neuron-specific enolase, chromogranin, synaptophysin, CD56, and CD57) markers. All carcinoid tumors are negative for vimentin. Lung carcinoid tumor and small-cell carcinoma are positive for TTF-1.

Carcinoid Tumors. Well-differentiated neuroendocrine tumor is a synonym for carcinoid tumor that is capable of invasion and

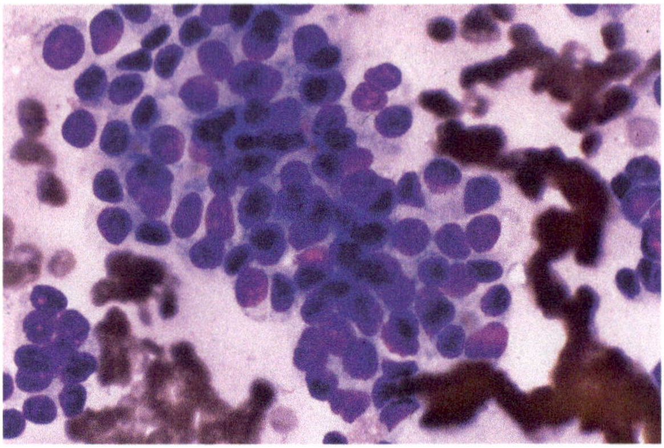

FIGURE 9.10. Carcinoid tumor. Occasionally carcinoid tumors (well-differentiated neuroendocrine carcinomas) may metastasize. Cell aggregates with coarse and uniform chromatin and no nucleoli are characteristic features (DiffQuik stain, high magnification).

metastasis, with a clinical course that depends on the organ location and the tumor size. Carcinoid syndrome (flushing or cyanosis, watery diarrhea, tachycardia, bronchospasm) is present in 10% of patients with carcinoid of all types and is particularly frequent in small-bowel carcinoids. At low-power view, carcinoid tumors have a neuroendocrine architecture with a nesting and/or trabecular pattern showing microacini and aggregates. The neoplastic cells are uniform, cuboidal, with central nuclei, inconspicuous nucleoli and finely granular cytoplasm (Fig. 9.10). Mitoses are rare. Electron microscopy shows numerous pleomorphic dense-core secretory granules along the cytoplasmic membrane.

Atypical Carcinoid Tumors. The atypical carcinoid tumor is less common and lymph node metastases are more frequent than in carcinoid tumor. The smear pattern is similar to that of typical carcinoid tumors. The cells are atypical and slightly spindled, and there are scattered mitoses. However, the distinction from typical carcinoid may not be possible even in excised lymph nodes (Fig. 9.11).

Small-Cell Carcinoma. Small-cell carcinoma of the lung falls in the category of poorly differentiated neuroendocrine carcinoma and is highly malignant with an aggressive clinical course. This tumor occurs in adults in the sixth decade or older who have mediastinal

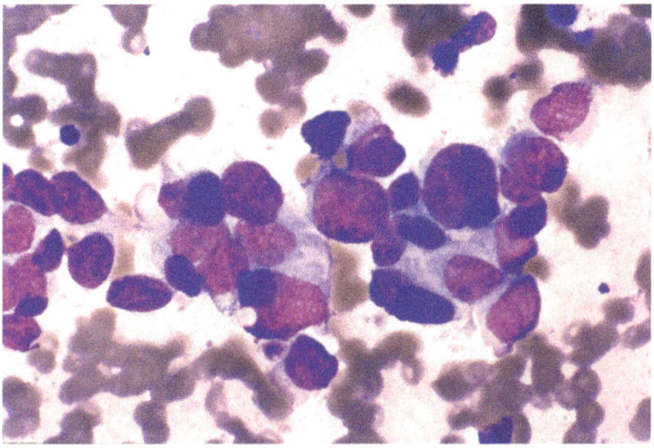

FIGURE 9.11. Atypical carcinoid. Aggregates of intermediate-sized cells, some with elongate nuclei and absence of nucleoli (DiffQuik stain, high magnification).

adenopathy and a history of smoking. The smear is cellular and shows small-cell aggregates, numerous isolated cells, stripped nuclei, and a necrotic background. The neoplastic cells are twice the size of small lymphocytes; they have hyperchromatic nuclei, fragile scant cytoplasm, and inconspicuous nucleoli. Numerous mitoses and apoptotic nuclei are seen. Nuclear molding and "crushing artifact" are characteristic (Figs. 9.12 and 9.13). Some cases show admixed squamous carcinoma or adenocarcinoma. Rare lymphoglandular bodies may be seen in the background. By electron microscopy, the cells show neuroendocrine (cytoplasmic neurosecretory granules) and epithelial (desmosomes and bundles of tonofilaments) characteristics.

Merkel Cell Carcinoma. Merkel cell carcinoma is a rare primary neuroendocrine tumor of the skin and occurs particularly in the head and upper extremities of elderly individuals. This tumor is aggressive and may produce multiple distant metastases including lymph nodes. The aspirates from this tumor are cellular and show scattered small aggregates and predominantly single cells with scant cytoplasm, round to oval nuclei, fine chromatin, and several small nucleoli. A small perinunuclear dot-like cytoplasmic condensation may be found. Cell molding is not a feature. Scattered mitoses and apoptotic nuclei are present, and the background

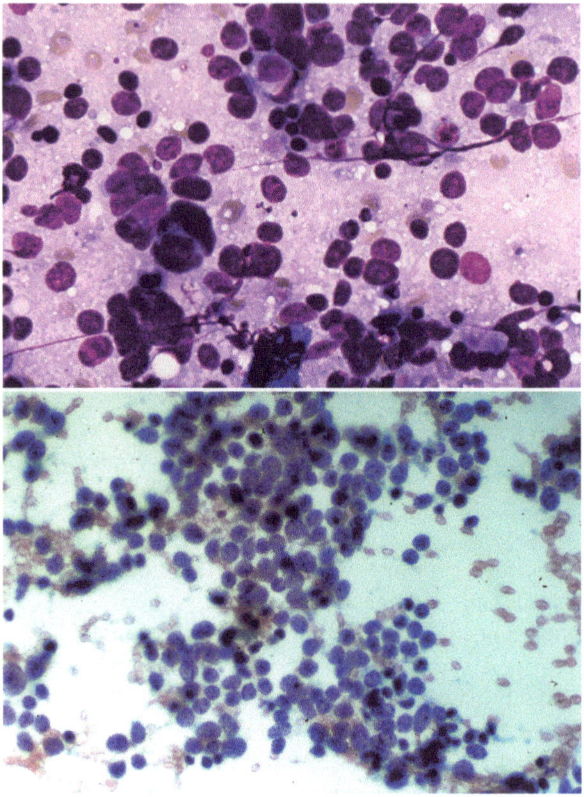

FIGURES 9.12–9.13. Small-cell carcinoma. Inconspicuous cellular aggregation, cell molding, coarse uniform chromatin, and nucleolar absence are characteristic (*Top,* DiffQuik and *bottom* Papanicolaou stains, high magnification).

lacks lymphoglandular bodies. The cells show a positive immunostain for low-molecular-weight keratin, neurofilaments, and NSE. The keratin stain highlights the cytoplasmic condensation (Figs. 9.14–9.16).

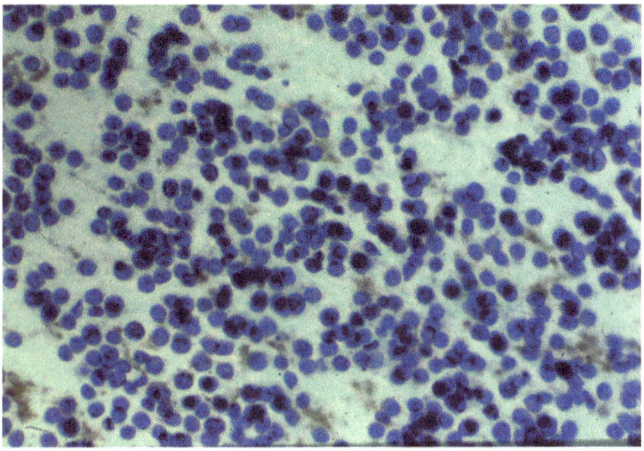

FIGURE 9.14. Merkel cell carcinoma. Cellular smear with prominent cellular dissociation is seen (Papanicolaou stain, high magnification).

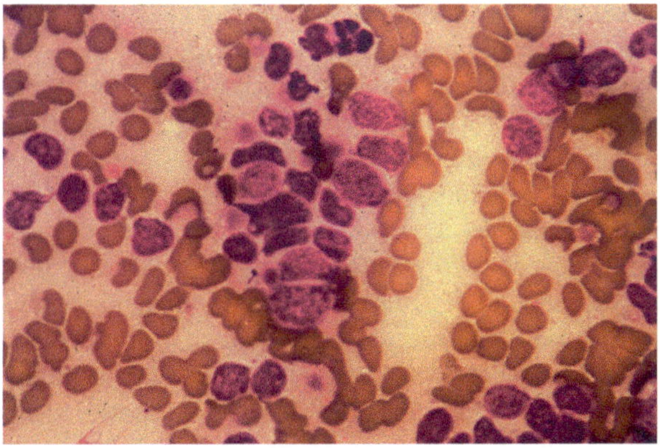

FIGURE 9.15. Merkel cell carcinoma. Perinuclear dot-like cytoplasmic condensations are present in the central cell aggregate. (DiffQuik stain, high magnification).

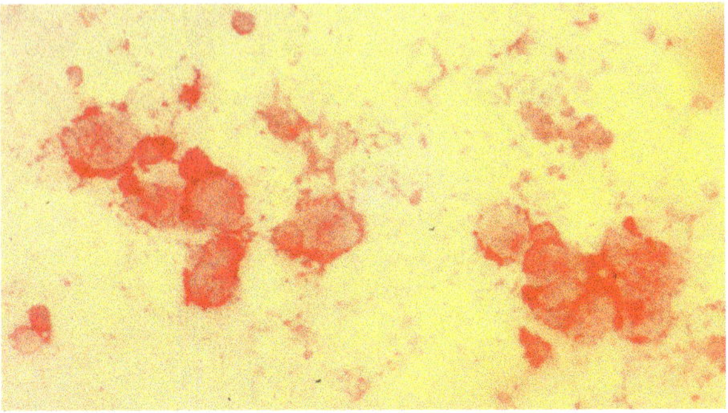

FIGURE 9.16. Merkel cell carcinoma. The perinuclear dot-like cytoplasmic condensations are best evidenced by immunocytochemistry (Keratin immunocytochemical stain, high magnification).

Basal Cell Carcinoma. The smears have moderate cellularity with scattered tightly cohesive cell clusters with sharp irregular borders and smaller numbers of discohesive cells in a clean background without lymphoglandular bodies. Nuclear palisading may be seen in the cellular borders. The cells have "basaloid" or slightly spindled dark nuclei with coarse chromatin and small inconspicuous nucleoli. No nuclear molding is seen.

Melanoma. Melanoma is more frequent in Caucasians than in Blacks, Hispanics, or Asians. If the thickness of cutaneous melanoma exceeds 0.76 mm, the risk of lymph node metastasis increases parallel to the tumor thickness. The regional lymph nodes are involved before the melanoma spreads more distally. However, approximately 4% of melanomas show axillary, cervical, and inguinal lymph node metastasis, in decreasing order of frequency, with occult primary tumor (spontaneous regression). The rare amelanotic melanoma with lymphocyte-like or plasmacytoid-like cytomorphology may resemble lymphoma or plasmacytoma; however, the smear background lacks lymphoglandular bodies (Figs. 9.17 and 9.18). Special stain with S100 protein must be accompanied by Melan A and/or HMB-45 stain, because the S100 protein stain is also positive in the interdigitating reticulum cells of the lymph node.

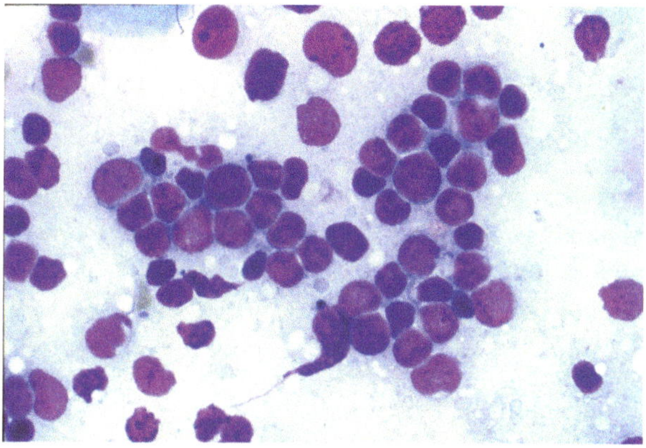

FIGURE 9.17. Melanoma. Amelanotic melanoma with lymphocyte-like cytomorphology resembles lymphoma (DiffQuik stain, high magnification).

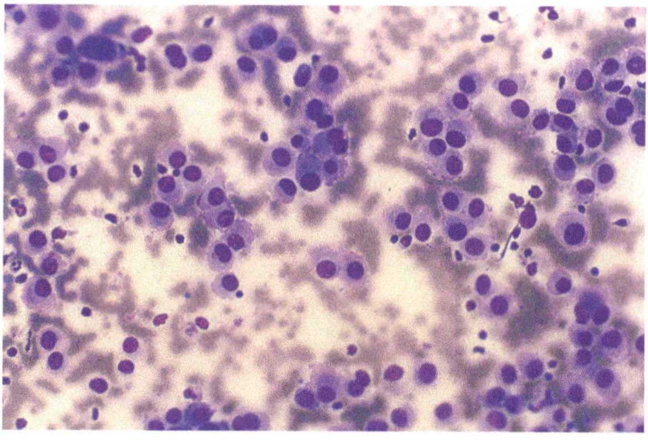

FIGURE 9.18. Melanoma. Amelanotic melanoma with plasmacytoid-like cytomorphology resembles plasmacytoma (DiffQuik stain, high magnification).

Small Blue Cell Tumors. Metastatic neuroblastoma, Ewing sarcoma/peripheral neuroectodermal tumor, and rhabdomyosarcoma occur in children and young adults.

Metastatic Neuroblastoma. Neuroblastoma is derived from primitive sympathetic nervous system cells, is the most common solid tumor in infants, is rare after the age of 5 years and in adults, and arises commonly (75% of cases) in the adrenal medulla and extra-adrenal sympathetic areas. Common sites of metastasis include bone marrow, lymph nodes, liver, skin, orbit, and bone and commonly occur within 2 years after diagnosis. Smears show sheets and aggregates of cells with round nuclei, scant cytoplasm, and minimal nuclear pleomorphism. Apoptotic nuclei and rare mitoses are present in a background that usually lacks lymphoglandular bodies (Fig. 9.19). Neoplastic cells form Homer-Wright rosettes (nuclei are circumferentially arranged and the center is occupied by cytoplasmic processes). Neurosecretory granules and neuritic processes that reflect neural crest derivation can be detected by electron microscopy. Immunohistochemistry-positive markers include synaptophysin, chromogranin, neurofilaments, neuron-specific enolase, and CD57. Neuroblastomas are negative for keratins, LCA, and T- and B-cell markers.

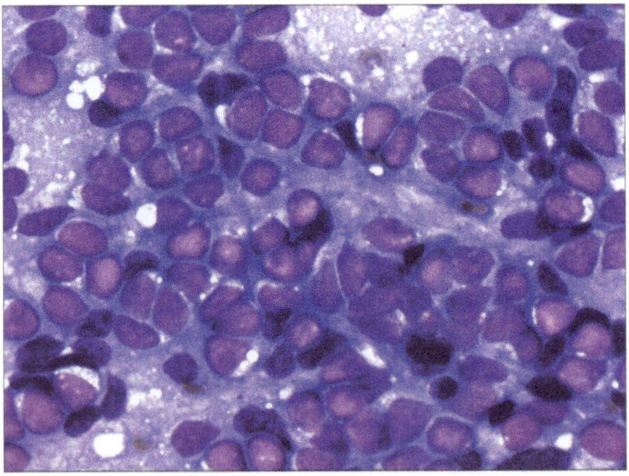

FIGURE 9.19. Neuroblastoma. This common pediatric neoplasm may show cellular dissociation and minimal nuclear pleomorphism. Homer-Wright rosettes are characteristic (not seen in this figure) (Giemsa stain, high magnification).

Ewing Sarcoma/Peripheral Neuroectodermal Tumor. Ewing sarcoma/peripheral neuroectodermal tumor is the second most common bone tumor in children and also affects the soft tissue, with a male predominance. The cell of origin is unknown. Most tumors have *ews* gene translocations, the most common being t(11;22)(q24;q12)/*ews-fli*1. The most common sites of metastasis include the lungs, other bones, lymph nodes, and the central nervous system. Smears show clusters and single uniform cells with round or oval nuclei, scant cytoplasm, and inconspicuous nucleoli (Fig. 9.20). Scattered mitoses and necrosis are present. Classical PNET involving the soft tissue has some neuroepithelial features. The cells are positive for vimentin, CD99 (a protein product of the *MIC2* gene), and FLI-1. Some cases may express neuroendocrine markers and low-molecular-weight keratins.

Rhabdomyosarcoma. This is the most common sarcoma in children and young adults. Rhabdomyosarcomas have a high metastatic potential through hematogenous and lymphatic routes affecting predominantly regional lymph nodes. Cytologically, embryonal rhabdomyosarcoma shows small- to intermediate-sized commonly spindled cells, numerous mitoses, and necrosis. Cells of alveolar rhabdomyosarcoma are often cuboidal, not spindled,

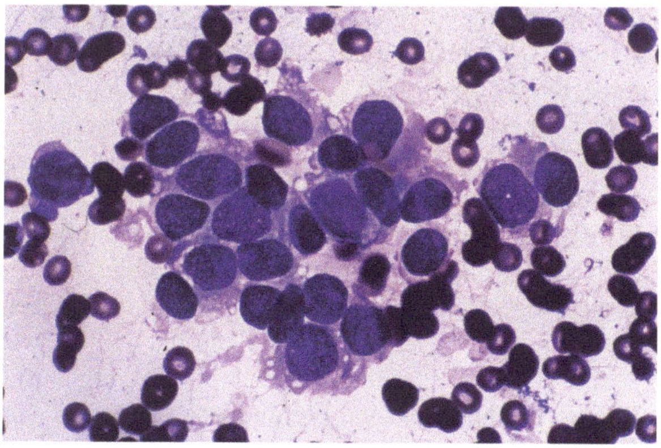

FIGURE 9.20. Ewing sarcoma. High cellularity and uniform oval or round nuclei are present (Giemsa stain, high magnification).

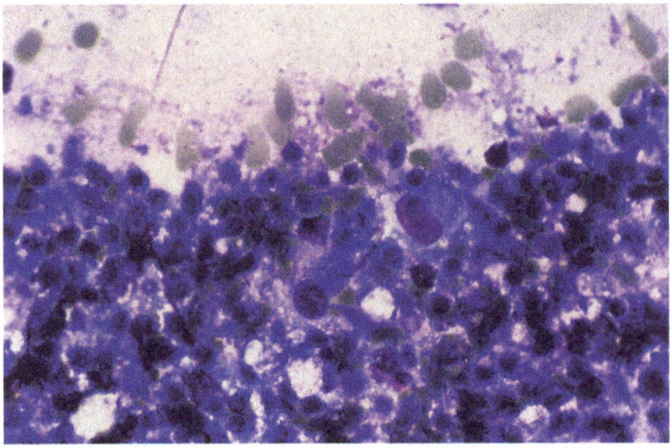

FIGURE 9.21. Rhabdomyosarcoma. Small- and intermediate-sized cells are seen in this cluster. There is mild pleomorphism and no visible nucleoli (Giemsa stain, high magnification).

and of intermediate size with eosinophilic cytoplasm and visible nucleoli. Mitoses and necrosis are also present (Fig. 9.21). Alveolar rhabdomyosarcoma is positive for muscle-specific markers (desmin, myogenin, MyoD1, and muscle-specific actin). CD45 and T- and B-cell markers are negative. There is a characteristic network of cytoplasmic filaments measuring 7 and 10 nm found by electron microscopy. Cytogenetics show t(2;13)(q35;q14) and t(1;13)(p36;q14) involving *PAX3-FKHR* and *PAX7-FKHR* fusion genes, respectively.

Nasopharyngeal Carcinoma. Nasopharyngeal carcinoma has a high incidence in Asia and comprises 15–20% of all malignant neoplasms in southern China. Environmental and genetic factors and EBV infection play a role in the pathogenesis. In non-endemic regions, EBV may be absent. In the United States, the patients with nasopharyngeal carcinoma have a bimodal age presentation with one peak between 15 and 25 years and the other between 60 and 70 years. Common clinical manifestations are unilateral (35% bilateral) superior deep cervical lymphadenopathy, and nasal and ear dysfunction. Tumors with similar histomorphology can arise in the palatine and lingual tonsils, thymus, and larynx. The smears of the undifferentiated type have small reactive lymphocytes in the background and within the neoplastic cell clusters (Fig. 9.22).

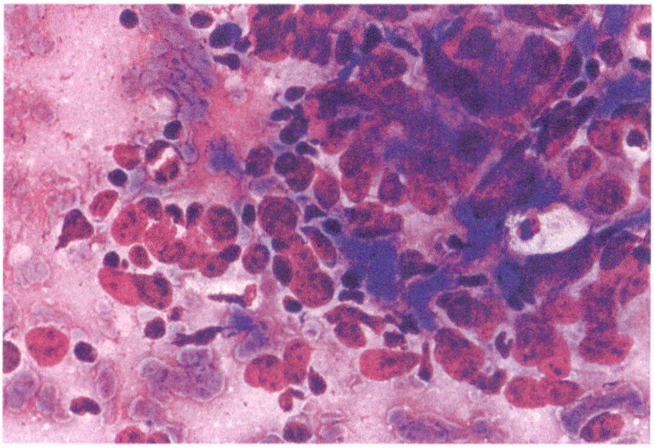

FIGURE 9.22. Nasopharyngeal carcinoma. The neoplastic cells are round, cuboidal and elongated admixed with small lymphocytes (DiffQuik stain, high magnification).

The cells are cuboidal or slightly spindled with scant fragile cytoplasm, indistinct cellular borders, dark coarse chromatin, and small nucleoli. Numerous dissociated malignant cells as well as stripped nuclei are in the background. Mitoses are usually numerous. The immunophenotype is positive for keratin and epithelial membrane antigen, and negative for CD45 and B- and T-cell markers. The neoplastic cells are positive for EBV-associated markers such as EBV-latent membrane protein type 1 and in situ hybridization for EBV small-encoded RNA.

Suggested Reading

Bangerter M, Brudler O et al (2007) Fine needle aspiration cytology and flow cytometry in the diagnosis and subclassification of non-Hodgkin's lymphoma based on the World Health Organization classification. Acta Cytol 51(3):390–398

Dahmoush L, Hijazi Y et al (2002) Adult T-cell leukemia/lymphoma: a cytopathologic, immunocytochemical, and flow cytometric study. Cancer 96(2):110–116

Grenko RT, Shabb NS (1991) Metastatic nasopharyngeal carcinoma: cytologic features of 18 cases. Diagn Cytopathol 7(6):562–566

Jacobs JC, Katz RL et al (1992) Fine needle aspiration of lymphoblastic lymphoma. A multiparameter diagnostic approach. Acta Cytol 36(6):887–894

Koo CH, Rappaport H et al (1989) Imprint cytology of non-Hodgkin's lymphomas based on a study of 212 immunologically characterized cases: correlation of touch imprints with tissue sections. Hum Pathol 20(12 Suppl 1):1–137

Matsushima AY, Hamele-Bena D et al (1999) Fine-needle aspiration biopsy findings in marginal zone B cell lymphoma. Diagn Cytopathol 20(4):190–198

Nizze H, Cogliatti SB et al (1991) Monocytoid B-cell lymphoma: morphological variants and relationship to low-grade B-cell lymphoma of the mucosa-associated lymphoid tissue. Histopathology 18(5):403–414

Pai RK, Mullins FM et al (2008) Cytologic evaluation of lymphadenopathy associated with mycosis fungoides and Sezary syndrome: role of immunophenotypic and molecular ancillary studies. Cancer 114(5):323–332

Richmond J, Bryant R et al (2006) FISH detection of t(14;18) in follicular lymphoma on Papanicolaou-stained archival cytology slides. Cancer 108(3):198–204

Troxell ML, Bangs CD et al (2005) Cytologic diagnosis of Burkitt lymphoma. Cancer 105(5):310–318

10 The Monotonous Large Cell Pattern

Smears showing a monotonous (monomorphic) large cell pattern usually contain more than 50% large cells and frequently show more than 80% large cells. The remaining cells in such smears are usually small lymphocytes. Large lymphocytes measure more than 20 μm (or about 2.5–3 small lymphocyte diameters) in diameter in Romanovsky stained air-dried smears and appear slightly smaller in alcohol-fixed Papanicolaou or H&E-stained smears and cell block sections. The nuclei of large cells are by definition the same size or larger as the nuclei of histiocytes or endothelial cells.

The following is a list of entities that may show a monotonous large cell pattern:

- Diffuse large B-cell lymphoma and its variants
- Follicular lymphoma, grade 3
- Richter transformation of small lymphocytic lymphoma
- Blastoid variant of mantle cell lymphoma
- Peripheral T-cell lymphoma
- NK/T cell lymphoma
- Granulocytic sarcoma
- Nodal Langerhans cell histiocytosis (LCH)
- Dendritic cell neoplasms
- Metastatic carcinoma

S.E. Pambuccian and R.H. Bardales, *Lymph Node Cytopathology*, Essentials in Cytopathology 10, DOI 10.1007/978-1-4419-6964-4_10,

- Metastatic melanoma
- Metastatic sarcoma
- Metastatic seminoma

Diffuse Large B-Cell Lymphoma

Diffuse large B-cell lymphomas (DLBCL) are a rather heterogeneous group of lymphoid tumors with varying clinical presentations, cytomorphology, immunophenotypes, cytogenetics and prognosis that have in common the large size of the lymphocytes, diffuse growth pattern and the B-cell lineage.

Cytologically, the cells of DLBCL may be centroblastic, immunoblastic or anaplastic. However, these cytomorphologic types have little clinical significance since they do not represent distinct entities with the possible exception of the immunoblastic cytomorphology that confers a poor prognosis.

Gene expression profiling has separated two distinct groups among DLBCL, the germinal center B-cell (GCB) – like with a better prognosis and the activated B-cell (ABC) – like with a poor prognosis. These molecularly defined groups roughly correlate with the centroblastic and the immunoblastic cytomorphology. They also roughly correlate with germinal center B-cell like and non-germinal center B-cell like immunophenotypes that may be determined by immunohistochemical stains. A small subgroup of DLBCL that is only characterized by its distinctive immunophenotype is the de novo $CD5^+$ large B-cell lymphoma.

T-cell/histiocyte-rich large B-cell lymphoma is a clinicopathologically distinct type of diffuse large B-cell lymphoma.

Other special types of large B-cell lymphomas that are not included in the category of DLBCL, not otherwise specified and may be encountered in lymph node or mediastinal aspirates, are as follows:

- Primary mediastinal (thymic) large B-cell lymphoma
- Lymphomas with a predominantly plasmablastic cytomorphology:
  - ALK-positive large B-cell lymphoma
  - Plasmablastic lymphoma (PBL)
  - Large B-cell lymphoma arising in HHV8 associated multicentric Castleman disease
  - Primary effusion lymphoma

Some cases defy exact classification among B-cell lymphoma entities and are classified as borderline cases:

- B-cell lymphoma, unclassifiable, with features intermediate between DLBCL and Burkitt lymphoma (Fig. 10.1)
- B-cell lymphoma, unclassifiable, with features between DLBCL and classical Hodgkin lymphoma

Clinical Findings. DLBCL accounts for about 25–40% of lymphomas in adults and about 20% of pediatric lymphomas. In adults, the typical age at diagnosis is during the sixth and seventh decade. Most cases arise de novo, i.e., represent primary large cell lymphomas, whereas in other cases large cell lymphoma represents the progression or transformation of a less aggressive lymphoma such as CLL/SLL (Richter syndrome), follicular lymphoma, marginal zone lymphoma and nodular lymphocyte-predominant Hodgkin

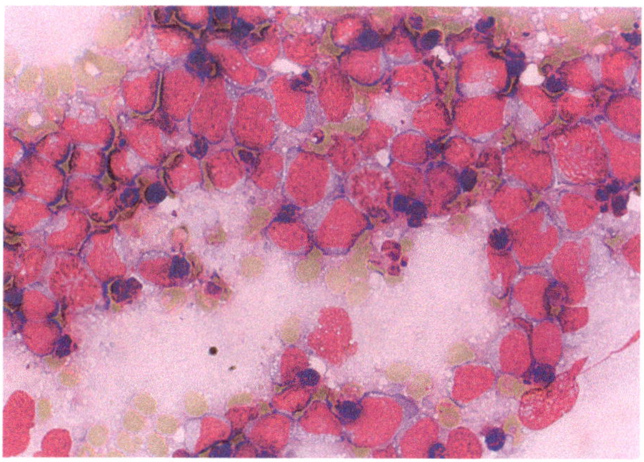

FIGURE 10.1. Fine-needle aspirate of a lymph node involved by neoplastic cells of intermediate to large size with *blue-gray* finely vacuolated cytoplasm, nuclear size and shape variability, numerous mitoses and apoptotic bodies. Immunophenotyping showed a B-cell phenotype and expression of CD10, while cytogenetic studies showed MYC rearrangement as part of a complex karyotype. Because of the size variability, presence of large cells and the presence of MYC rearrangement as part of a complex karyotype, the neoplasm was diagnosed as B-cell lymphoma unclassifiable, with features intermediate between diffuse large B-cell lymphoma and Burkitt lymphoma (Diff-Quik stain, ×1,000).

lymphoma. Some DLBCL arise in patients with immunodeficiencies such as AIDS or as part of the post-transplant lymphoproliferative disorders. Such cases are frequently EBV-positive, whereas only about 10% of DLBCL cases not arising in a background of overt immunodeficiency are EBV-positive.

The presentation is usually with an asymptomatic rapidly enlarging nodal mass but up to 40% of cases have exclusively extranodal involvement at presentation, with symptoms related to the affected organ.

Cytology. Lymph node aspirates show a monotonous population of large lymphoid cells, which typically make up 50–80% of cells present on the smears and a variable admixture of small round lymphocytes and histiocytes (Fig. 10.2). The smears are usually abundantly cellular; however, in some cases where there is sclerosis, they may be paucicellular.

- The *centroblastic variant* of DLBCL is the most common and shows a predominance of centroblasts or an admixture of centroblasts and immunoblastic cells where immunoblastic cells represent less than 90% of neoplastic cells. Neoplastic

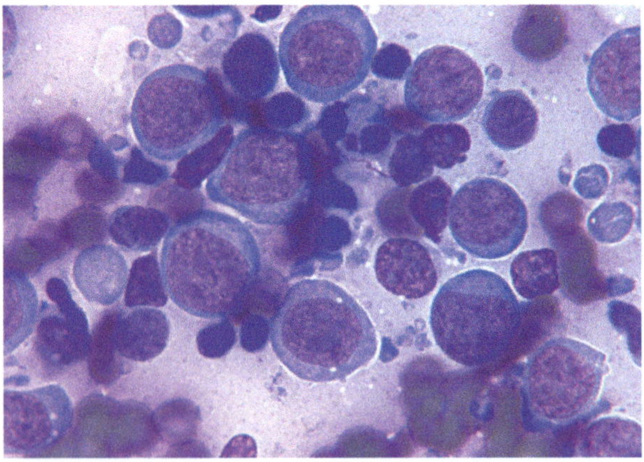

FIGURE 10.2. Fine-needle aspirate of nodal diffuse large B-cell lymphoma. The neoplastic cells represent the majority of cells present and show nuclei that are two to three times larger than those of the small lymphocytes present. Note the nuclear contour abnormalities and plasmacytoid differentiation of the cells with *dark blue* cytoplasm and vague perinuclear halos (Diff-Quik stain, ×1,000).

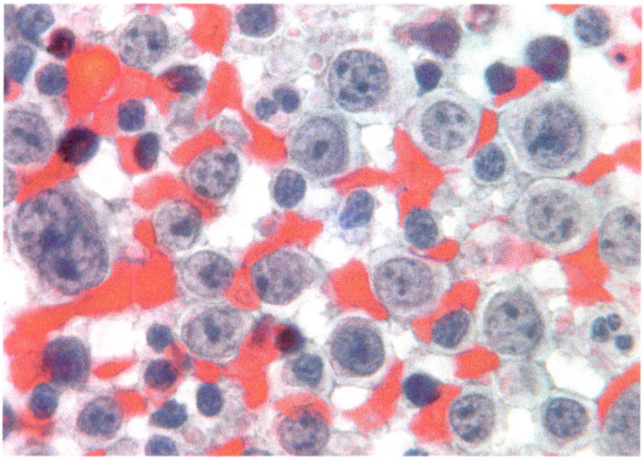

FIGURE 10.3. Fine-needle aspirate of nodal diffuse large B-cell lymphoma with centroblastic cytology. The neoplastic cells represent the majority of cells present and show nuclei that are two to three times larger than those of the small lymphocytes present. They have a scant to moderate amount of ill-defined cytoplasm, smooth nuclear contours, open chromatin and two to four visible to prominent nucleoli (Papanicolaou stain, ×1,000).

centroblastic cells are morphologically similar to normal centroblasts and are medium-to-large cells with scant-to-moderate cytoplasm, central round-to-ovoid nuclei with smooth nuclear contours and possible nuclear infoldings, a vesicular chromatin and two to four nucleoli, frequently located close to the nuclear border (Fig. 10.3). Centroblastic cells may show irregular nuclear contours and nuclear multilobation; in some cases they may resemble spindle cells (Fig. 10.4). Cytoplasmic vacuolation can be prominent and include the lymphoglandular bodies present (Fig. 10.5).

- The *immunoblastic variant* of DLBCL is by definition composed almost exclusively (over 90%) of immunoblastic cells that are larger than centroblasts, have round nuclei with a prominent central nucleolus and a moderate amount of basophilic cytoplasm, well seen in Romanowsky-stained air-dried smears. The cytoplasm is frequently vacuolated. Plasmacytoid differentiation may be present (Fig. 10.6).
- The *anaplastic variant* of DLBCL is composed of large to very large pleomorphic cells (Fig. 10.7) that bear at least a

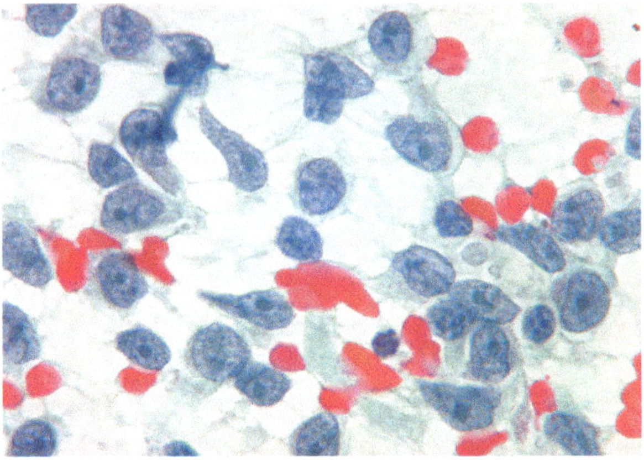

FIGURE 10.4. Fine-needle aspirate of nodal diffuse large B-cell lymphoma with centroblastic cytology. The neoplastic cells represent the majority of cells present and show nuclei that are two to three times larger than those of the small lymphocytes present. They have a scant to ill-defined cytoplasm, irregularly shaped elongated nuclei with irregular contours with deep cleaves, open chromatin and prominent nucleoli (Papanicolaou stain, ×1,000).

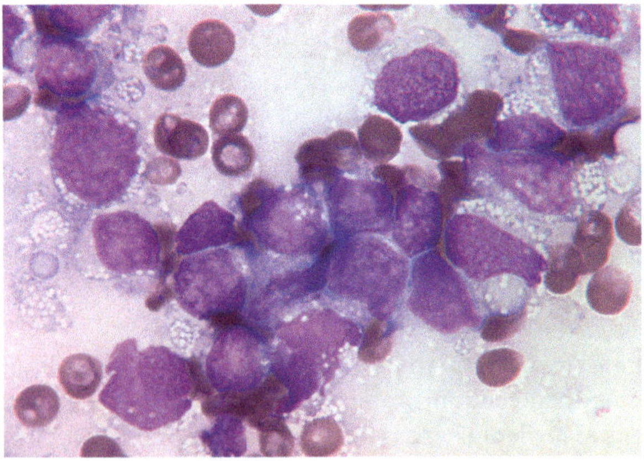

FIGURE 10.5. Fine-needle aspirate of nodal diffuse large B-cell lymphoma with prominent cytoplasmic vacuolation and vacuolated lymphoglandular bodies (Diff-Quik stain, ×1,000).

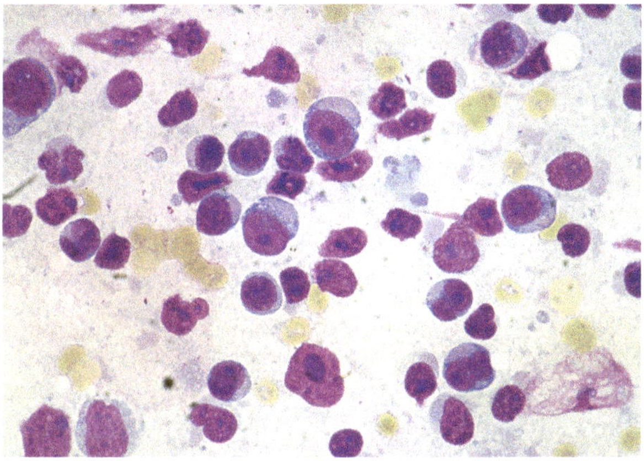

FIGURE 10.6. Fine-needle aspirate of nodal diffuse large B-cell lymphoma with immunoblastic cytology and plasmacytoid differentiation. Note the prominent central nucleoli and the eccentric location of the nuclei (Diff-Quik stain, ×400).

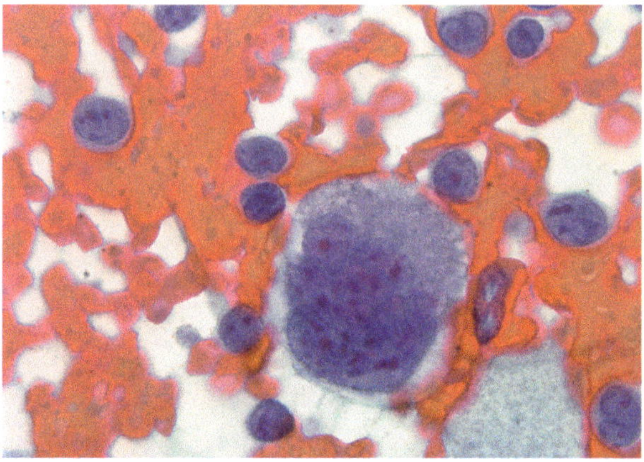

FIGURE 10.7. Fine-needle aspirate of nodal diffuse large B-cell lymphoma, anaplastic variant showing very large pleomorphic cells (Papanicolaou stain, × 1,000).

superficial resemblance to Hodgkin and Reed-Sternberg cells (HRS) or to the cells of anaplastic large cell lymphoma (ALCL), a neoplasm of T-cell lineage.

- A rare *spindle cell variant* belonging to the germinal center B-cell-like immunophenotype has also been described

All cytologic variants of DLBCL can have a variable admixture of epithelioid histiocytes; unless the neoplastic cells constitute a minority of the cells present in the aspirate, such cases should not be designated as T-cell/histiocytes-rich B-cell lymphoma. Mast cells may also be present, appear to be a reflection of the host inflammatory response and are associated with a better outcome. The presence of mast cells is also associated with fibrosis. Since the cytoplasm of large lymphocytes is very fragile, large cell lymphomas usually show abundant lymphoglandular bodies and numerous naked atypical nuclei and cells damaged during smearing. Crush artifact may be prominent. Clumping together of naked nuclei may occur artifactually (Fig. 10.8), mimicking the nuclear molding seen in small cell carcinomas. Apparent clustering of intact neoplastic cells may also occur (Fig. 10.9). Necrosis, in the form of background necrotic debris and shadow cells (Fig. 10.10), can be present and can be extensive. Mitoses and apoptotic bodies

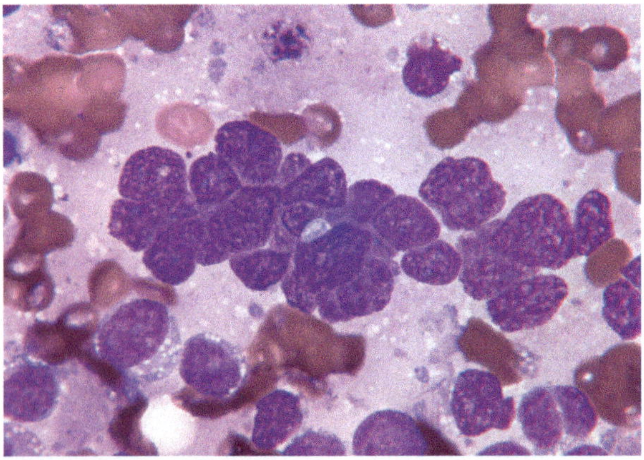

FIGURE 10.8. Fine-needle aspirate of nodal diffuse large B-cell lymphoma showing a clump of naked nuclei, which should not be confused with the molding seen in small cell carcinoma (Diff-Quik stain, ×1,000).

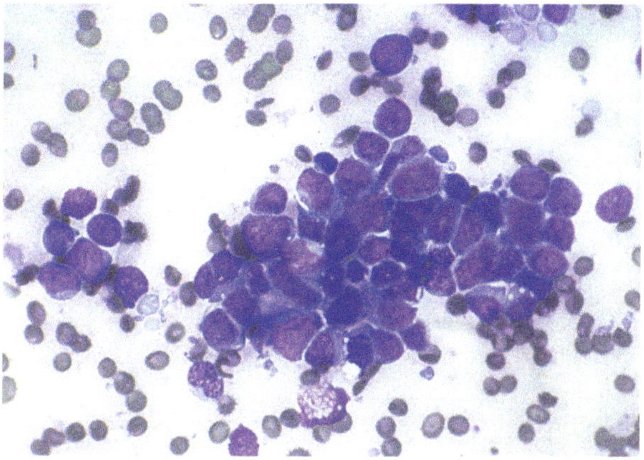

FIGURE 10.9. Fine-needle aspirate of nodal diffuse large B-cell lymphoma showing apparent clustering of intact neoplastic cells; such clusters may mimic metastatic malignancies (Diff-Quik stain, ×400).

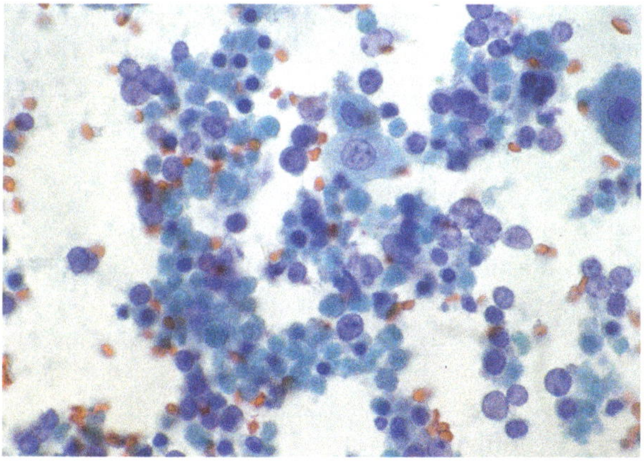

Figure 10.10. Fine-needle aspirate of nodal diffuse large B-cell lymphoma showing necrosis. Necrotic debris is present in the background, the nuclei are pyknotic and shadow (ghost) cells and naked nuclei are present. Cell size may be underestimated in such aspirates (Papanicolaou stain, ×400).

are frequent in all cytomorphologic variants of large B-cell lymphoma (Fig. 10.11) and tingible body macrophages may occur or even be frequent.

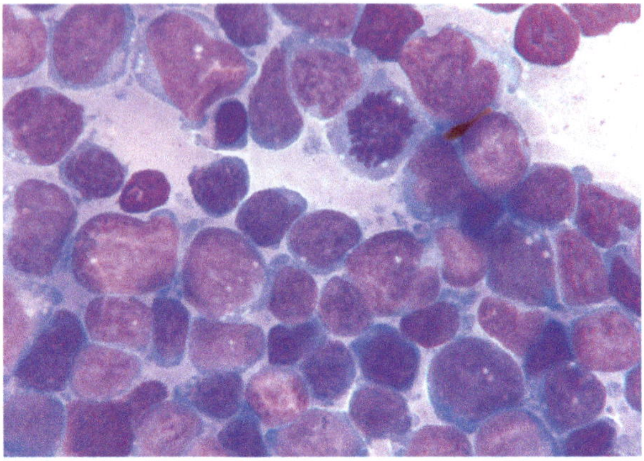

FIGURE 10.11. Fine-needle aspirate of nodal diffuse large B-cell lymphoma showing a mitosis and several apoptotic bodies. Note the nuclear contour irregularities with nose-like protrusions (Diff-Quik stain, ×1,000).

Immunophenotype. All cases of DLBCL express at least one of the pan B-cell markers (CD19, CD20, CD22 and CD79a). PAX5 and CD45 but may lack one or more of these markers. CD20 expression is frequently lost after rituximab treatment. CD5 is expressed in about 10% of the case, most of which are de novo DLBCL rather than cases of transformed small lymphocytic lymphoma. The anaplastic variant frequently expresses CD30. DLBCL with a centroblastic cytomorphology frequently show a germinal center phenotype, i.e. are CD10+, or, if CD10– are positive for bcl6 and negative for MUM1. DLBCL with immunoblastic cytomorphology usually show a non-germinal center, activated B-cell phenotype, i.e. are CD10–/ bcl6– or CD10-/bcl6+/MUM1+ according to the Hans algorithm.

Immunophenotyping by flow cytometry may be false negative, i.e. may not demonstrate the presence of clonal population by light chain restriction in 15–25% of cases of DLBCL. This most likely occurs due to selective loss of the neoplastic large cells through disruption of their fragile cytoplasm during fine-needle aspiration, storage in RPMI or processing for flow cytometry. In such cases, the flow cytometry forward-scatter versus side-scatter plot shows an almost complete absence of large cells (increased forward scatter and side scatter) despite the presence of numerous such cells in the aspirate smears. In such cases, the diagnosis can be confirmed by immunostains performed on cell block sections, if available or a diagnosis of suspicious for large cell lymphoma may be made with a recommendation for excisional biopsy. Another potential source of difficulty to establish light chain restriction by flow cytometry is the rather common absence of surface immunoglobulin on the neoplastic cells of DLBCL (especially in primary mediastinal B-cell lymphomas). In such cases, a large cell population that shows B-cell lineage markers is highly suggestive of DLBCL.

Cytogenetics. The most common cytogenetic abnormalities occurring in DLBCL are involving the BCL6 gene (*3q27*) which are found in about 30% of cases, especially in activated B-cell (ABC) DLBCL, followed by the BCL2 translocation, t(14;18)(q32;q21), which is found in 20–30% of cases, particularly in germinal center B-cell (GCB) DLBCL. About 10% of cases of DLBCL have MYC abnormalities, and in some of these cases, an accurate differentiation from Burkitt lymphoma may not be possible (B-cell lymphoma, unclassifiable, with features between DLBCL and Burkitt lymphoma).

Key Points. The cytomorphologic diagnosis of large cell lymphoma is usually straightforward in the presence of a dispersed monotonous large cell lymphoid population. The potential pitfall created by a false-negative immunophenotyping result can be avoided by always correlating flow cytometry results with morphology.

T-Cell/Histiocyte-Rich Variant of DLBCL

This variant of DLBCL represents less than 10% of all DLBCL cases. Because the large B-cells are vastly outnumbered by reactive T-cells and histiocytes, the smear pattern is usually a monotonous small cell pattern or a polymorphous pattern. This variant is discussed in Chap. 8.

Primary Mediastinal (Thymic) Large B-Cell Lymphoma

Primary mediastinal B-cell lymphoma (PMBCL) is a distinctive large B-cell lymphoma most likely arising from the asteroid B cells of the thymic medulla. It accounts for about 2–4% of all non-Hodgkin lymphomas and shares morphologic, immunophenotypic and molecular genetic features with both DLBCL and classic Hodgkin lymphoma (cHL), nodular sclerosis subtype.

Clinical Findings. Primary mediastinal lymphoma is a rapidly progressive neoplasm that usually presents with a bulky, anterosuperior mediastinal mass and symptoms related to local invasion or pressure effects (superior vena cava syndrome). Invasion of adjacent structures is common and involvement of regional (supraclavicular and cervical) lymph nodes may occur. The disease tends to occur in younger adults than DLBCL, with an age (fourth and fifth decade) and sex (female) predilection similar to cHL. The prognosis is also more favorable than that of DLBCL.

Cytology. Because PMBCL may show extensive sclerosis, the aspirates may be hypocellular or show numerous damaged large cells lacking cytoplasm. Aggregates of such large cells may be present and mimic a carcinoma or melanoma. When adequately cellular and devoid of artifacts, the smears consist of dispersed large lymphocytes with round to oval nuclei that may have smooth or irregular borders, displaying one or more prominent nucleoli. Nuclei are usually 5–6 times larger than those of small lymphocytes, but may be much larger, up to 20 times the size of a small lymphocyte and may be multilobated, mimicking Hodgkin lymphoma or ALCL. The amount of cytoplasm varies from scant to abundant and is typically intensely basophilic in air-dried stained with a Romanowsky-type stain and may be vacuolated. Lymphoglandular bodies and mitotic figures are present. Fragments of connective tissue may be present. Benign entrapped thymic epithelial cells may be present in about a third of cases as loose clusters and dispersed cells, and represent a potential pitfall both in the cytomorphologic assessment of the aspirate and in immunohistochemistry.

Immunophenotype. The neoplastic cells of PMBCL express CD45 and pan-B-cell markers (CD 19, 20, 22 and 79a), usually express CD23, bcl6 and MUM1 and are generally negative for CD10 and CD21. CD30 is usually present, but the expression is weak and is not present in all neoplastic cells. Differentiation from classic Hodgkin lymphoma is possible by the absence of CD15 and cyclin E and the presence of CD79a and p63.

Cytogenetics. PMBCL is lacking the chromosomal translocations seen in DLBCL but may show amplification of chromosome regions 2p (c-REL) and 9p (JAK2).

Key Points. The cytologic diagnosis of PMBCL is difficult when sclerosis is present and the smears are hypocellular. The possibility that entrapped thymic epithelium may be present should be taken into account to avoid misdiagnosis as thymoma or metastatic carcinoma.

Neoplasms with Predominantly Plasmablastic Cells

- Plasmablastic lymphoma
- Primary effusion lymphoma (PEL)
- PBL arsing in HHV8-related multicentric Castleman disease (PBL-MCD)
- ALK+ diffuse large B-cell lymphoma (ALK+ DLBCL)

New large B-cell lymphoma types that were recently proposed by the 2008 WHO classification include lymphomas composed predominantly of immunoblastic or plasmablastic cells that share a similar morphology but differ in clinical features, association with HIV, EBV and HHV8 (human herpesvirus 8) and immunophenotype.

Clinical Findings. PBL, PEL and PBL-MCD occur predominantly in HIV+ individuals, immunosuppressed patients and elderly patients and have a poor prognosis. Both PBL and PEL are also associated with EBV infection; PEL is additionally associated with HHV8 infection. PBL-MCD is associated with HHV8 but not with EBV. EBV can be demonstrated in tumor cells by EBER in situ hybridization, while HHV8 can be demonstrated in tumor cells using *LANA-1* immunohistochemistry. ALK+ DLBCL is not associated with HIV, EBV or HHV8.

PBL and PEL occur predominantly in extranodal location: PBL most commonly in the oral mucosa and PEL in pleural effusions. However, both can also occur in lymph nodes.

PBL-MCD and ALK+ DLBCL are primarily nodal diseases, but can also occur extranodally.

Cytology. All these lymphomas share a plasmablastic or immunoblastic cytomorphology. Plasmablastic cytomorphology may be

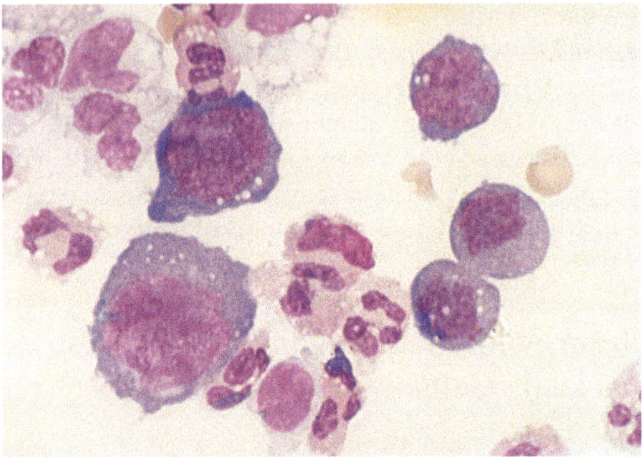

FIGURE 10.12. Plasmablastic cells in primary effusion lymphoma (Wright stain, ×1,000, courtesy of Robert W. McKenna, M.D., Division of Hematopathology, Department of Laboratory Medicine and Pathology, University of Minnesota).

difficult to differentiate from immunoblastic cytomorphology, both sharing the prominent central nucleoli. It is characterized by cells that resemble large plasma cells but have no or minimal nuclear clumping, less abundant cytoplasm with no or minimal hof region (Fig. 10.12). The smears from these lymphomas show a monomorphic proliferation of large, round-to-oval cells, with moderate amounts of cytoplasm and eccentrically placed vesicular nuclei, usually with a single prominent central nucleolus. The plasmacytoid appearance is more prominent in air-dried Romanowsky-stained smears. Numerous mitoses, apoptotic bodies and tingible body macrophages are usually present. The differential diagnosis of such plasmacytoid neoplastic cells in fine-needle aspirates is with plasma cell neoplasms (Fig. 10.13), plasmacytoid cells of metastatic carcinomas from the breast and urothelium, neuroendocrine carcinomas, tumors with a rhabdoid phenotype and melanomas.

Immunophenotype. Plasmablastic differentiation usually results in the loss of the lymphocytic and B-cell markers CD45, CD20 and PAX5, preservation of CD79a and acquisition of plasma cell markers (CD138 and CD38). The neoplastic cells usually express cytoplasmic immunoglobulins; interestingly different classes of

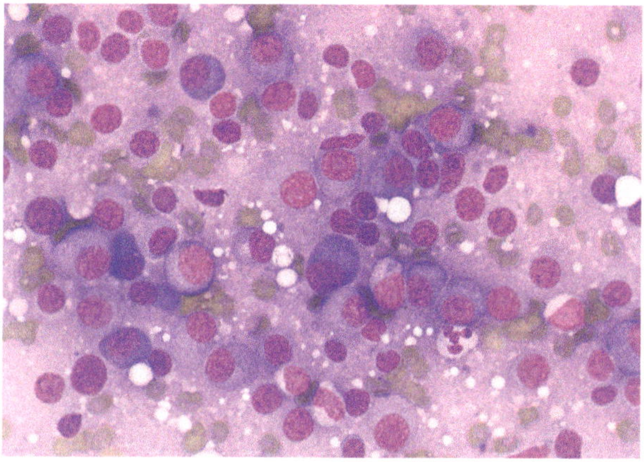

FIGURE 10.13. Fine-needle aspirate of a lymph node involved by a plasma cell neoplasm (myeloma). Note the more abundant eccentric cytoplasm and better defined hof (Diff-Quik stain, ×600).

immunoglobulins are expressed in different lymphomas: IgG in PBL, IgM in PBL-MCD and IgA in ALK+ DLBCL. The neoplastic cells of PEL express CD30 and EMA; the neoplastic cells of ALK+ DLBCL are defined by strong granular cytoplasmic ALK staining.

Expression of CD56 indicates a plasma cell neoplasm rather than a plasmacytoid lymphoma.

Key Points. PBLs usually occur in the setting of HIV infection and immunosuppression and may be caused by EBV, HHV8 or both.

Follicular Lymphoma, Grade 3

Follicular lymphoma, grade 3 (FL-3) accounts to about a third of follicular lymphomas and is clinically distinct from grades 1 and 2 follicular lymphomas because of its marked differences in therapeutic response and prognosis. FL-3 is defined histologically as a lymphoma of follicular center cells with at least focal follicular (nodular) growth pattern and a mean of more than 15 centroblasts per high power field. The neoplastic cells of grade 3A follicular lymphomas are an admixture of centroblasts and centrocytes, whereas grade 3B follicular lymphomas are composed almost entirely of sheets of centroblasts. Grade 3B follicular lymphoma shows cytomorphologic, immunophenotypic and genetic similarities to diffuse large B cell lymphoma. Since the distinction relies exclusively on finding at least focal nodular growth pattern histologically, it may not be possible to distinguish grade 3B follicular lymphomas from diffuse large B cell lymphomas on fine-needle aspirates. Although DLBCL and grade 3 follicular lymphomas are treated similarly, the risk of recurrence of grade 3 follicular lymphomas is higher.

Smears of grade 3 follicular lymphomas usually show about 40–60% centroblasts, also referred to as "transformed cells" and an admixture of variable proportions of centrocytes and small lymphocytes. Cells are predominantly dispersed but rare lymphocytic (follicular) aggregates may be present. It is not always possible to classify a cell as centroblasts or centrocytes by size, since both show a spectrum of sizes that overlap; however, in Papanicolaou-stained slides, we classify all cells with rounded (rather than angular) nuclei, open chromatin, no prominent cleaves or groves and visible multiple nucleoli as centroblasts. These features are more difficult to appreciate in Romanowsky-stained air-dried smears. Mitoses can be frequent, in contrast to grade 1 and 2 follicular lymphomas in which they are uncommon.

Cell block sections may show follicles and allow the demonstration of follicular dendritic cells ($CD21^+$) within the neoplastic follicles in which centroblasts predominate.

Immunophenotyping and cytogenetic features are similar to those of lower grade follicular lymphomas, but FL-3 are less commonly positive for CD10 (50–75%) and bcl2 (50–75%) and the t(14;18) translocation. On the contrary, there is more frequent MUM1 expression (75%) and a higher proliferation rate (Ki67 of about 20%).

Large Cell (Richter) Transformation of Small Lymphocytic Lymphoma

Transformation to DLBCL occurs in up to 10% of patients with small lymphocytic lymphoma (SLL/CLL). Clinically, there is an abrupt change in the patient's clinical condition after a long

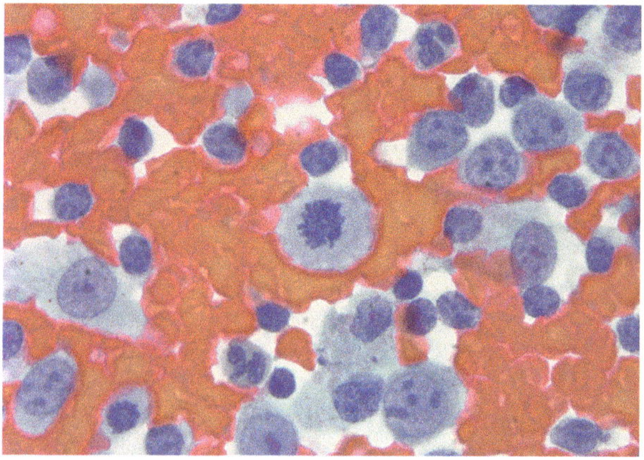

FIGURE 10.14. Fine-needle aspirate of large cell transformation of small lymphocytic lymphoma (Richter syndrome). About 50% of cells have centroblastic features while the smaller cells have cytologic features of CLL/SLL (Papanicolaou stain, ×1,000).

course of stable disease, marked by increasing lymphadenopathy and fever and elevation of serum lactate dehydrogenase or alpha-2 microglobulin. The cytomorphology is either centroblastic (Fig. 10.14) or immunoblastic. Similar large cell transformation can occur in other indolent lymphomas (follicular lymphoma, mantle cell lymphoma, lymphoma of mucosa-associated lymphoid tissue and nodular lymphocyte predominant Hodgkin lymphoma). The resulting large cell lymphoma usually preserves the immunophenotypic and cytogenetic characteristics of the indolent lymphoma. The prognosis is poor.

Blastoid (Large Cell) Variant of Mantle Cell Lymphoma

Cases of mantle cell lymphoma where the neoplastic cells are larger and show higher proliferative rates are designated as blastoid, large cell or pleomorphic variants. Such variants may be associated with a more aggressive clinical course. The smears show cells

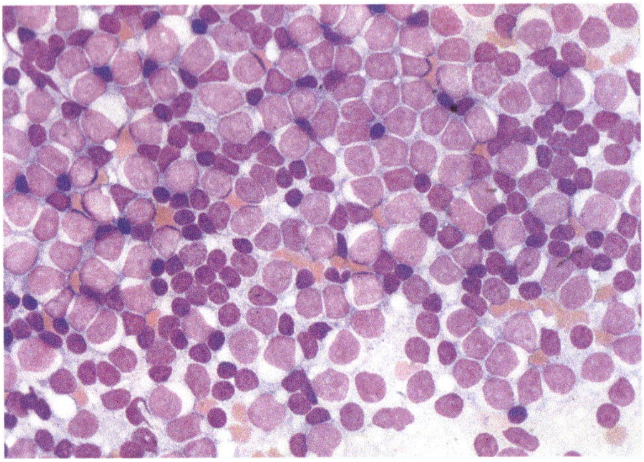

FIGURE 10.15. Fine-needle aspirate of mantle cell lymphoma, blastoid type. The neoplastic cells are more than twice the size of small lymphocytes and have an open finely granular chromatin (Diff-Quik stain, ×400).

that resemble either lymphoblasts (scant cytoplasm and vesicular chromatin) (Fig. 10.15) or centroblasts (scant cytoplasm, folded, cleaved or oval nuclei and prominent nucleoli). Immunophenotypic and cytogenetic features are similar to the usual variant of mantle cell lymphoma.

Peripheral T-Cell Lymphoma, NOS

Peripheral T-cell lymphomas, not otherwise specified, are a group of neoplasms with variable morphology. The typical features of these neoplasms are discussed in Chap. 9. In about a third of such cases, the aspirate smears show a predominance of large atypical cells (Fig. 10.16). Pleomorphic cells may also be present suggesting Hodgkin lymphoma. The neoplastic cells are dispersed, sometimes binucleated, with irregularly shaped, convoluted nuclei and coarse chromatin, small to prominent nucleoli and scant pale cytoplasm. Mitotic figures are usually present. An admixture of lymphocytes, plasma cells, histiocytes, neutrophils and eosinophils in various proportions may be present and may give the aspirate a pleomorphic appearance.

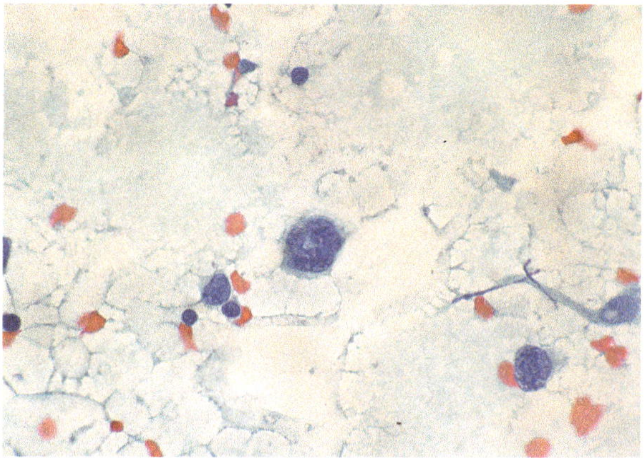

FIGURE 10.16. Fine-needle aspirate of peripheral T-cell lymphoma extending into perinodal fat. Note the multilobated and convoluted nuclei, and the coarse chromatin (Papanicolaou stain, ×400).

NK/T Cell Lymphoma

Natural killer/T-cell (NK/T-cell) lymphomas are rare neoplasms affecting preferentially Asian and Central and South American populations. This neoplasm characteristically arises in the nasal cavity, nasopharynx or surrounding structures, but nodal involvement may occur in the absence of overt nasal involvement. The clinical course of NKTCL is typically aggressive.

The cytological spectrum on NKTCL is very broad, from a predominance of small cells to a predominance of large cells (Fig. 10.17). Neoplastic cells show irregularly shaped nuclei, sometimes assuming a cucumber-like shape, with granular chromatin, multiple small, inconspicuous nucleoli and pale cytoplasm. Azurophilic granules may be seen in the cytoplasm (Fig. 10.18) in high-quality air-dried smears stained with the Wright stain or similar Romanowsky-type stains. A polymophous background of small lymphocytes, plasma cells, histiocytes, neutrophils, and eosinophils may also be present.

The immunophenotype of the neoplastic cells is similar to that of normal natural killer cells: CD2+, CD56+, surface CD3−, cytoplasmic CD3e+, CD7−/+, CD8−/+, CD4−. They frequently express

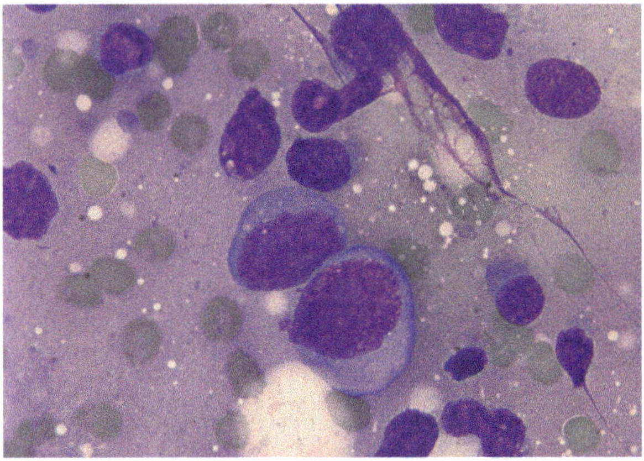

FIGURE 10.17. Fine-needle aspirate of NK/T-cell lymphoma showing large neoplastic cells with coarse chromatin and sparsely vacuolated cytoplasm (Diff-Quik stain, ×1,000).

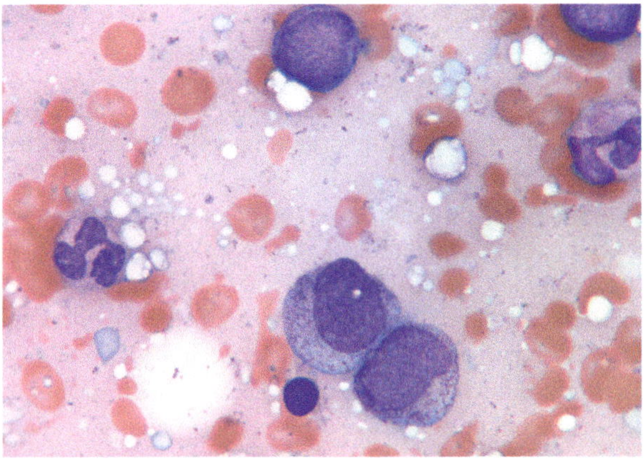

FIGURE 10.18. Fine-needle aspirate of NK/T-cell lymphoma showing numerous cytoplasmic granules (Diff-Quik stain, ×1,000).

granule proteins such as granzyme B, TIA-1 and perforin. Positivity for EBV (EBER in situ hybridization) and cytotoxic granule protein expression are required for the diagnosis.

Myeloid (Granulocytic) Sarcoma

Myeloid (granulocytic) sarcoma or extramedullary myeloid tumor is an extramedullary proliferation of myeloid blasts with or without maturation that occurs at an extramedullary location, including the lymph nodes. Aspirates from such lymph nodes may show a monotonous large cell pattern (Fig. 10.19). The diagnostic features of myeloid sarcoma are discussed in Chap. 13.

Nodal Langerhans Cell Histiocytosis (LCH)

LCH is a rare idiopathic proliferative disorder of Langerhans cells that occurs predominantly in childhood. Histologically, there is a proliferation of Langerhans cells accompanied by a variable number of normal inflammatory cells such as eosinophils, lymphocytes (T cells) and macrophages, along with osteoclast-type multinucleated giant cells.

Although the Langerhans cells are clonal, overexpress p53 and show loss of heterozygosity in multiple loci (chromosomes 1, 4, 6, 7, 9, 16, 17 and 22), all features strongly suggestive of a

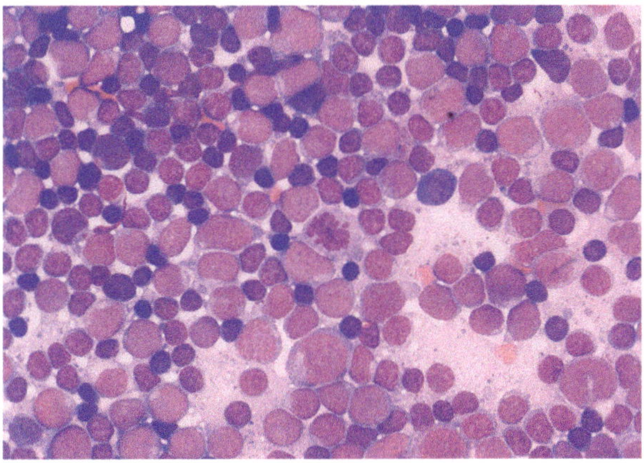

FIGURE 10.19. Fine-needle aspirate of nodal myeloid sarcoma showing large cells with blastic features (Diff-Quik stain, ×600).

neoplastic process, some authors consider that LCH may be a reactive, possibly immunologically mediated condition with similarities to sarcoidosis, in which Langerhans cells are victims of a "cytokine storm."

Clinical Findings. LCH characteristically involves bones, but may also involve skin, lung, liver, spleen, the hypothalamic–pituitary region, bone marrow and lymph nodes either as a single system or as multisystem involvement. Multiple lymph nodes may be involved (multifocal involvement). The most characteristic presentation is with a painless lump in a single bone, frequently of the skull, in a 3- to 6-year-old child. When extraosseous involvement occurs, lymph nodes are involved in about 25% of cases. Lymph nodes draining the affected bone are frequently involved. The lymph node groups most frequently involved are cervical, followed by inguinal, axillary and mediastinal.

Cytology. Fine-needle aspirates from LCH involving lymph nodes usually show a predominance of large atypical cells (Langerhans cells) (Fig. 10.20), admixed with various numbers of small lymphocytes, eosinophils (Fig. 10.21), neutrophils, osteoclast-like giant cells (Fig. 10.22) and plasma cells. The background shows lymphoglandular bodies and may also show eosinophilic granules.

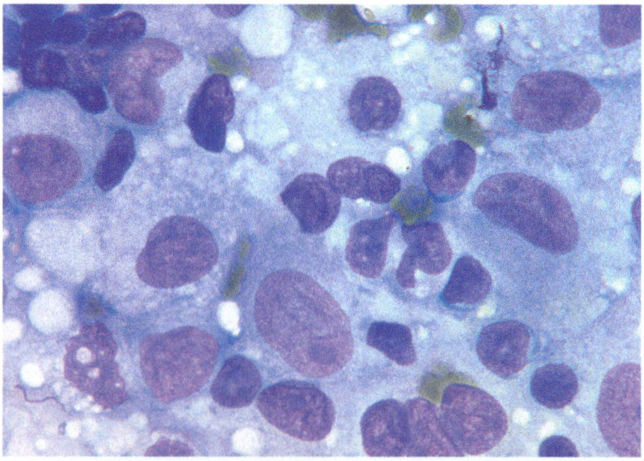

FIGURE 10.20. Fine-needle aspirate of nodal LCH showing large cells with abundant *light blue* faintly wrinkled cytoplasm, elongated, grooved nuclei with fine chromatin and visible nucleoli (Diff-Quik stain, ×1,000).

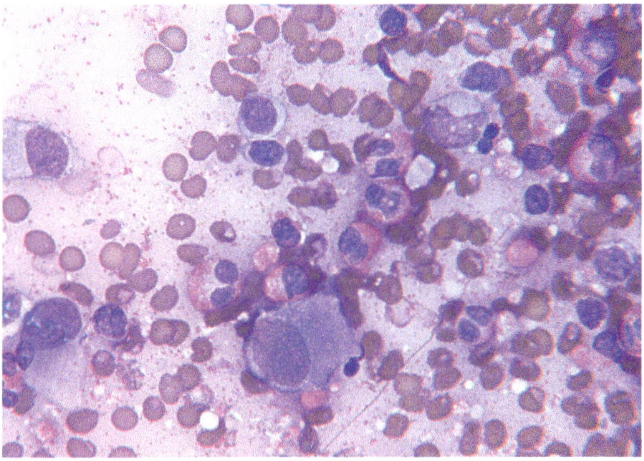

FIGURE 10.21. Fine-needle aspirate of nodal LCH showing numerous eosinophils. Eosinophilic granules are seen in the background most likely due to the disruption of the eosinophils' cytoplasm during smearing (Diff-Quik stain, ×600).

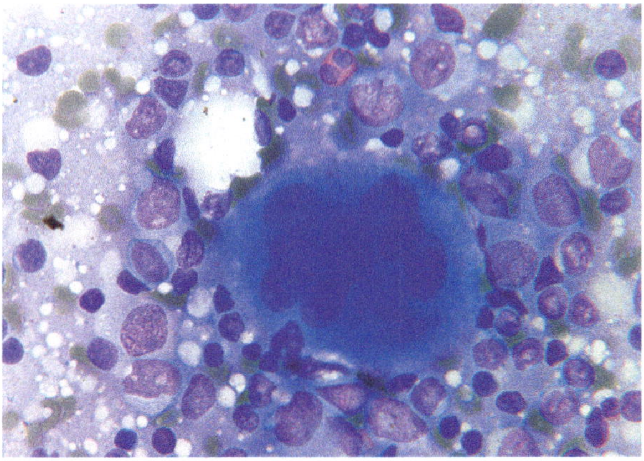

FIGURE 10.22. Fine-needle aspirate of nodal LCH showing an osteoclastic giant cell surrounded by Langerhans cells, small lymphocytes and a single eosinophil. Numerous lymphoglandular bodies are seen in the background (Diff-Quik stain, ×600).

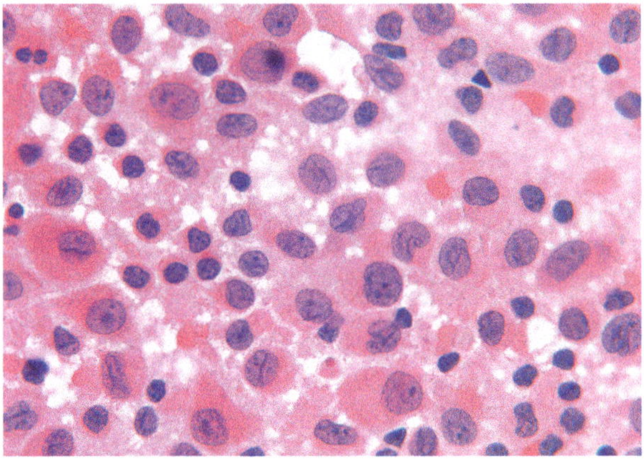

FIGURE 10.23. Touch imprint of calvarial LCH showing the characteristic extensively grooved nuclei (Hematoxylin and eosin stain, ×1,000).

Capillary fragments may also be present. Langerhans cells are large cells, measuring about three to five times the size of a small lymphocyte with round-to-oval nuclei and a moderate-to-large amount of eccentric cytoplasm. Occasional cytoplasmic vacuoles may be present. The most characteristic cytologic feature of Langerhans cells is their irregularly contoured, deeply grooved nucleus (Fig. 10.23). Multiple grooves may occur at angles to each other in a nucleus, resulting in intersecting grooves. Grooves are better seen in Papanicolaou or H&E-stained smears. The nuclear chromatin is finely granular and nucleoli are usually small but may be prominent. Langerhans cells may be distinguished from typical histiocytes by the lack of nuclear grooves in histiocytes and their more vacuolated cytoplasm, frequently containing phagocytic debris. The number of lymphocytes, plasma cells, eosinophils and neutrophils is variable and eosinophils, a hallmark of the condition ("eosinophilic granuloma"), may be entirely absent. When present, osteoclast-type giant cells are very distinctive. The large and atypical appearance of Langerhans cells and the presence of eosinophils and other reactive cells may suggest Hodgkin lymphoma. (see also Chap. 13).

Immunophenotype. Langerhans cells are positive for CD1a, S100 and langerin (CD207). The latter is a component of the Birbeck granules, zipper-like or racquet-shaped structures that are the ultrastructural hallmark of Langerhans cells and is more sensitive and specific for Langerhans cells than CD1a.

Key Points. Identification of the characteristic deep grooves in the nuclei of large cells in lymph node aspirates of children should prompt for the evaluation of LCH by performing immunohistochemical stains for S100, CD1a and langerin on cell block sections.

Dendritic Cell Neoplasms

Dendritic cell neoplasms involving lymph nodes may show variable cytomorphologic patterns, including a monotonous large cell pattern. They are discussed in Chap. 13.

Metastatic Malignancies

- Metastatic carcinoma
- Metastatic melanoma
- Metastatic sarcoma
- Metastatic seminoma

Metastatic carcinomas may in rare cases show few malignant cells admixed with numerous lymphocytes in lymph node aspirates, but when the lymph node sampled by fine-needle aspiration is enlarged because of the presence of metastatic disease the aspirate is usually composed of numerous malignant cells and few lymphoid cells. In such cases, a dispersed monotonous large cell aspirate pattern may be present, especially when the metastatic cells are from a poorly differentiated malignancy and are dyshesive. Such metastatic malignancies may be encountered in lymph node fine-needle aspirates from patients without a known history of malignancy. In addition to metastatic neuroendocrine carcinomas, already discussed in Chap. 9, metastatic carcinomas that may mimic the aspirate cytomorphology of lymphomas include prostate carcinomas and breast carcinomas. Metastatic sinonasal undifferentiated carcinomas (SNUC) and lymphoepithelioma-type nasopharyngeal carcinomas may closely mimic large cell lymphomas.

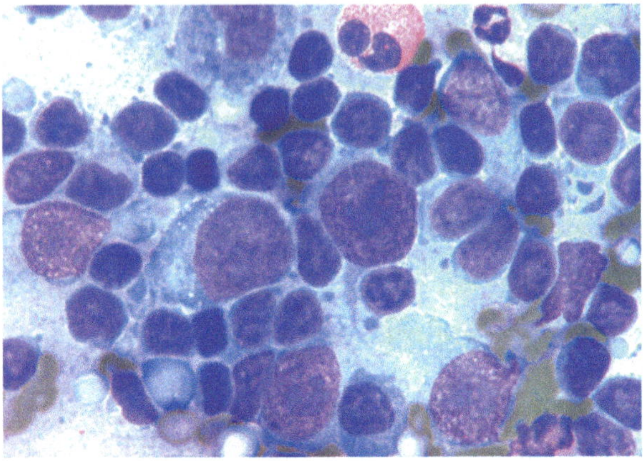

FIGURE 10.24. Fine-needle aspirate of nodal metastasis from undifferentiated nasopharyngeal carcinoma (lymphoepithelioma, Schmincke-type) showing large cells intermingled with lymphoid cells. The neoplastic cells have eccentric vacuolated cytoplasm, large nuclei with smooth outlines and single central, prominent, angular nucleoli (Diff-Quik stain, ×1,000).

The neoplastic cells may appear similar to large cell lymphoma cells (particularly immunoblastic or PBL cells) (Fig. 10.24) and lymphoglandular bodies may be present in the background. The differential diagnosis between metastatic carcinomas and lymphoid neoplasms is even more complicated when smears show widespread loss of the fragile cytoplasm of the neoplastic cells, resulting in predominantly naked nuclei. Metastatic carcinoma cells tend to be in general much larger and have more cytoplasm than lymphoma cells (Fig. 10.25). When cytoplasmic vacuoles occur they are usually larger (Fig. 10.26) than those seen in lymphoma cells and are seen in both Papanicolaou-stained and Romanowsky-stained smears as they contain mucin rather than lipid. At least focal cellular adhesion is frequently present and small clusters of tumor cells may be seen in a smear with predominantly dispersed cells, suggesting an epithelial neoplasm. Nuclear molding may also be present. However, since both clusters of tumor cells and molding may occasionally be present in lymphomas, the diagnosis of metastatic carcinomas showing a dispersed monotonous large cell pattern should be confirmed by correlation with clinical history, comparison with

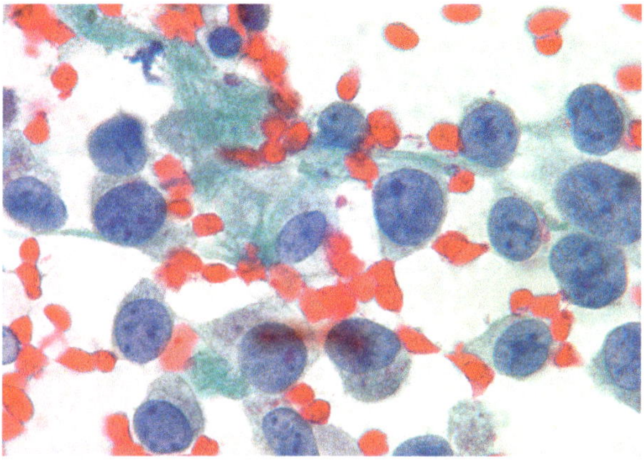

FIGURE 10.25. Fine-needle aspirate of metastatic adenocarcinoma to a mediastinal lymph node showing loosely cohesive large cells with moderate amounts of cytoplasm, open chromatin and multiple visible nucleoli (Papanicolaou stain, ×1,000).

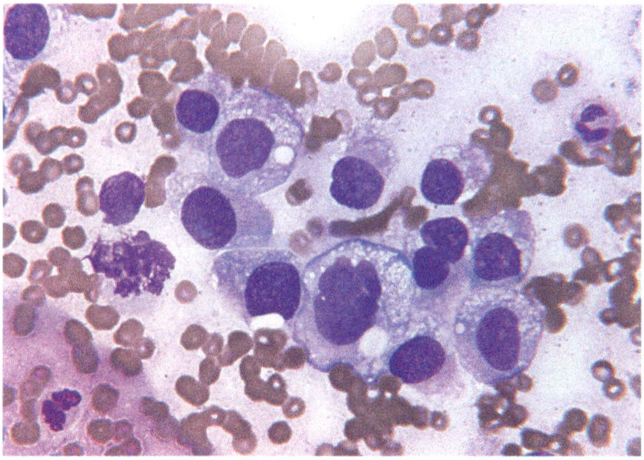

FIGURE 10.26. Fine-needle aspirate of a nodal metastasis of a pulmonary adenocarcinoma showing dispersed pleomorphic large cells with ample amounts of vacuolated cytoplasm (Diff-Quik stain, ×1,000).

any available previous pathology material, and immunoperoxidase stains. Metastatic carcinomas usually express cytokeratins and may express EMA and markers characteristic for their origin.

For example, TTF1 is expressed in the nuclei of metastatic thyroid and pulmonary carcinomas, PSA in prostatic carcinomas and BRST2 and estrogen receptors in metastatic breast carcinomas. Markers of viral infection of neoplastic cells may be found in lymphoepithelioma-type nasopharyngeal carcinomas (EBV), where they may further contribute to differential diagnostic difficulties with lymphomas and in metastatic Merkel cell carcinomas, where the demonstration of the Merkel cell polyomavirus is diagnostic.

Metastatic melanoma may also show a monotonous large cell pattern in smears of fine-needle aspirates of lymph nodes (Fig. 10.27). It may mimic the cytomorphology of any neoplasm, including lymphoma although metastatic melanoma cells are usually larger and more pleomorphic. The diagnosis is facilitated by the clinical history and the demonstration of melanin pigment in tumor cells or associated histiocytes (melanophages) (Fig. 10.28), but melanin may be entirely absent and the history of melanoma may not be available. Metastatic melanoma is further discussed in Chap. 9.

Metastatic sarcomas. Sarcomas rarely metastasize to lymph nodes, and when they do, usually show a spindle cell pattern or a

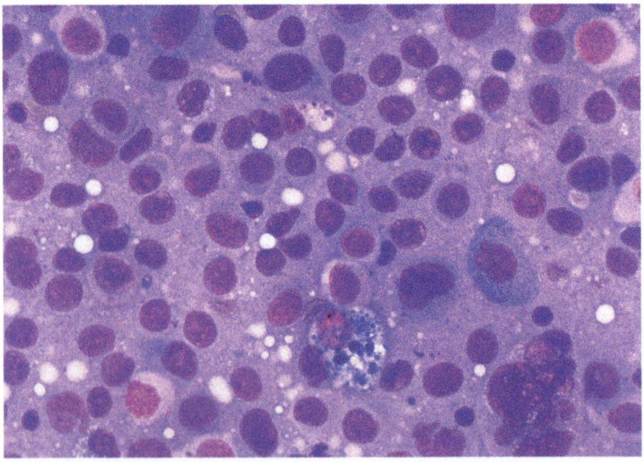

FIGURE 10.27. Fine-needle aspirate of a nodal metastasis of malignant melanoma showing dispersed large plasmacytoid cells and a melanophage (Diff-Quik stain, ×600).

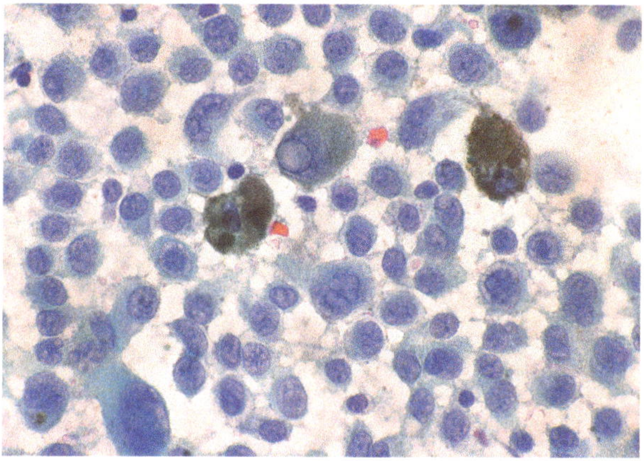

FIGURE 10.28. Fine-needle aspirate of a nodal metastasis of malignant melanoma showing dispersed pleomorphic large cells and melanophages. Note the characteristic binucleated cells, intranuclear pseudoinclusion and fine pigmentation of the cytoplasm of some of the neoplastic cells (Papanicolaou stain, ×600).

pleomorphic pattern. However, sarcomas with a "small blue cell" or epithelioid morphology can occasionally show a monotonous large round cell pattern in fine-needle aspiration smears of lymph nodes and can closely mimic lymphomas. The most common mesenchymal tumors to mimic large cell lymphomas are metastatic rhabdomyosarcoma (Fig. 10.29), neuroblastoma (including esthesioneuroblastoma) (Fig. 10.30) and Ewing sarcoma/peripheral neuroectodermal tumor (Fig. 10.31), all discussed in Chap. 9.

Metastatic seminoma/dysgerminoma. Seminomas and dysgerminomas are germ cell tumors of the testis and respectively of the ovary that usually occur in young adults. They have a high metastatic rate at presentation and may present with lymph node metastases from occult primary tumors, especially in retroperitoneal lymph nodes. Extragonadal seminomas may also occur in the midline, frequently in the mediastinum of young adults and may be sampled by fine-needle aspiration of the mediastinum, posing differential diagnostic considerations with lymphomas.

Metastatic seminomas usually have a distinctive fine-needle aspiration cytomorphology. Smears are usually moderately to highly

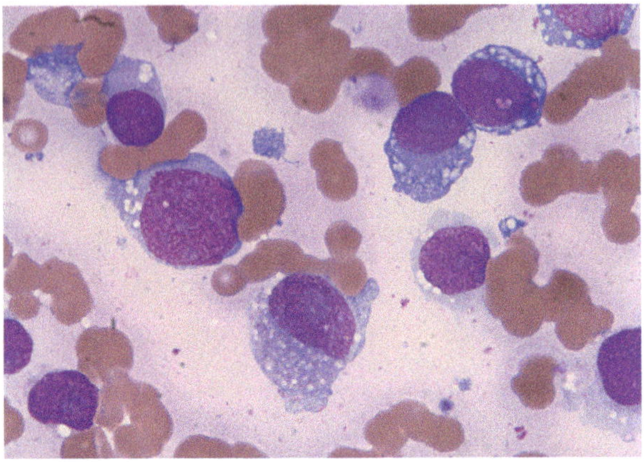

FIGURE 10.29. Fine-needle aspirate of a nodal metastasis of alveolar rhabdomyosarcoma showing dispersed large cells with vacuolated cytoplasm, showing a striking resemblance to lymphoid neoplastic cells (Diff-Quik stain, ×1,000).

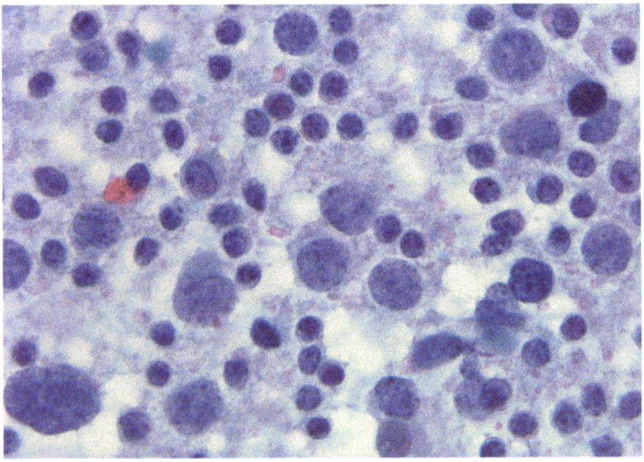

FIGURE 10.30. Fine-needle aspirate of a nodal metastasis of neuroblastoma showing dispersed large cells admixed with lymphocytes. Note the characteristic salt-and-pepper chromatin (Papanicolaou stain, ×1,000).

cellular and show a predominance of large cells with prominent nucleoli, against a background of small lymphocytes (Fig. 10.32). Collections of histiocytes and well-formed epithelioid granulomas

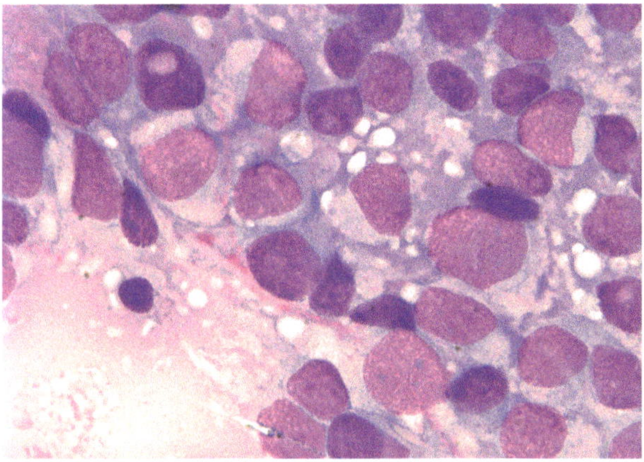

FIGURE 10.31. Fine-needle aspirate of a nodal metastasis of Ewing sarcoma showing dispersed large cells with blastic appearance admixed with lymphocytes (Diff-Quik stain, ×1,000).

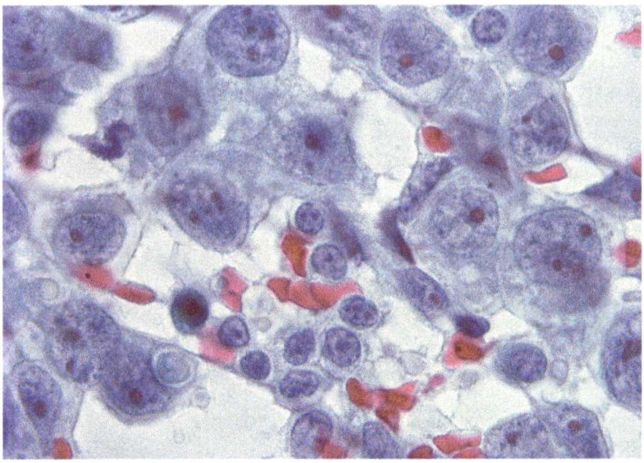

FIGURE 10.32. Fine-needle aspirate of a nodal metastasis of seminoma showing very large cells admixed with lymphocytes. Note the abundant vacuolated or clear cytoplasm, smooth nuclear contours, open chromatin and prominent central nucleoli (Papanicolaou stain, ×1,000).

may be present. The large tumor cells have scant to moderately abundant, but very fragile vacuolated eccentric cytoplasm, which is frequently disrupted in most or all of the tumor cells, which appear as naked nuclei. The smearing of this vacuolated (glycogenated) cytoplasm results in the characteristic "tigroid" or finely lace-like background (see Fig. 5.11). This background is only seen in air-dried Romanowsky-stained smears and not in Papanicolaou-stained smears. The smear pattern is often dispersed, but small two to three cell clusters of neoplastic cells may occur in cells with intact cytoplasm. The nuclei are usually round but show irregular contours and mild-to-marked anisonucleosis, open chromatin and a single prominent macronucleolus. Nuclei are also fragile and smears may show crush artifact with nuclear threads. Mitotic figures and apoptotic bodies are usually present.

The characteristic but not pathognomonic tigroid background is only present in about half of lymph node fine-needle aspirates from metastatic seminomas and its presence appears to be directly proportional to the cellularity of the sample and inversely proportional to the amount of blood present. The differential diagnosis with large cell lymphoma and metastatic melanoma or poorly differentiated carcinomas may be difficult when the tigroid background is not seen or when only fixed aspirate smears are available for the diagnosis. The immunohistochemical staining pattern of seminomas is characteristic, including positivity for PLAP, D2–40 and OCT3/4 and CD117 and can help the differential diagnosis.

Suggested Reading

Yao JL, Cangiarella JF, Cohen JM, Chhieng DC (2001) Fine-needle aspiration biopsy of peripheral T-cell lymphomas. A cytologic and immunophenotypic study of 33 cases. Cancer 93(2):151–159

Saqi A, McGrath CM, Skovronsky D, Yu GH (2002) Cytomorphologic features of fine-needle aspiration of metastatic and recurrent melanoma. Diagn Cytopathol 27(5):286–290

Wakely PE Jr (2002) Cytopathology-histopathology of the mediastinum: epithelial, lymphoproliferative, and germ cell neoplasms. Ann Diagn Pathol 6(1):30–43

Lin O, Gerhard R, Zerbini MC, Teruya-Feldstein J (2005) Cytologic features of plasmablastic lymphoma. Cancer 105(3):139–144

Das DK (2006) Serous effusions in malignant lymphomas: a review. Diagn Cytopathol 34(5):335–347

Young NA (2006) Grading follicular lymphoma on fine-needle aspiration specimens – a practical approach. Cancer 108(1):1–9

Reid-Nicholson M, Kavuri S, Ustun C, Crawford J, Nayak-Kapoor A, Ramalingam P (2008) Plasmablastic lymphoma: cytologic findings in 5 cases with unusual presentation. Cancer 114(5):333–341

Swerdlow SH, Campo E, Harris NL, Jaffe ES, Pileri SA, Stein H, Thiele J, Vardiman JW (2008) WHO classification of tumours of haematopoietic and lymphoid tissues. In: Bosman FT, Jaffe ES, Lakhani SR, Ohgaki H (ed) Lyon, IARC

de Leval L, Hasserjian RP (2009) Diffuse large B-cell lymphomas and Burkitt lymphoma. Hematol Oncol Clin North Am 23(4):791–827

Gurbaxani S, Anastasi J, Hyjek E (2009) Diffuse large B-cell lymphoma – more than a diffuse collection of large B cells: an entity in search of a meaningful classification. Arch Pathol Lab Med 133(7):1121–1134

Ioachim HL, Medeiros LJ (2009) Ioachim's lymph node pathology, 4th edn. Wolters Kluwer Health/Lippincott Williams & Wilkins, Philadelphia

Skoog L, Tani E (2009) Lymphoma look-alike. Monogr Clin Cytol 18:64–75

Skoog L, Tani E (2009) T cell neoplasms. Monogr Clin Cytol 18:38–48

Skoog L, Tani E (2009) B cell neoplasms. Monogr Clin Cytol 18:19–37

Sun T (2009) Atlas of hematologic neoplasms, Springer, Boston, MA

11
The Pleomorphic Cell Pattern

The pleomorphic cell pattern is characterized by the presence of pleomorphic or anaplastic cells in a background of lymphoid cells. Pleomorphic cells present in lymph node aspirates measure 40–60 μm or more and show marked nuclear abnormalities, characterized by irregular nuclear shape, multinucleation and prominent nucleoli.

The following is a list of entities showing a pleomorphic pattern. Hodgkin lymphoma (HL) and anaplastic large-cell lymphoma (ALCL) are discussed in detail, while the other entities are discussed here only inasmuch as they enter the differential diagnosis and were not discussed elsewhere.

- Hodgkin lymphoma
- Anaplastic large-cell lymphoma
- Hodgkin-type Richter transformation of SLL/CLL
- Diffuse large B-cell lymphoma variants
- Thymoma
- Metastatic carcinoma
- Metastatic melanoma
- Metastatic mesenchymal malignancies

S.E. Pambuccian and R.H. Bardales, *Lymph Node Cytopathology*, Essentials in Cytopathology 10, DOI 10.1007/978-1-4419-6964-4_11,

Hodgkin Lymphoma

Hodgkin lymphoma has been historically separated from all other lymphomas (non-HLs) because of its distinctive clinical presentation and progression, its characteristic histology and the long debate about the neoplastic or nonneoplastic nature of the condition, which also accounts for the less committing designation as "Hodgkin disease." The cell of origin of HLs has eluded recognition until relatively recently when it became apparent that the neoplastic cells in HLs are B cells that have lost most of their B-cell markers in classic HL (cHL) while preserving them in nodular lymphocyte predominant HL.

Hodgkin lymphomas account for 10–30% of all lymphomas. Two main types of HL are currently recognized, which may represent different disease entities. The first type, cHL, accounts for about 95% of all HL cases, includes the nodular sclerosing, mixed cellularity, lymphocyte-rich and lymphocyte-depleted subtypes, whereas the second type, nodular lymphocyte predominant Hodgkin lymphoma (NLPHL), accounts only for about 5% of cases.

Histologically, all types of HL are characterized by the presence of a few large atypical cells in a background of numerous reactive cells, including variable proportions of lymphocytes, plasma cells, eosinophils, mast cells, neutrophils and histiocytes, which may form granulomas. In cHL the mononuclear neoplastic cells are named Hodgkin cells and the multinucleated ones Reed–Sternberg cells (collectively termed HRS cells), whereas in NLPHL they are termed popcorn cells or lymphocyte predominant (LP) cells (formerly called L&H cells).

Although the neoplastic cells of cHL are positive for EBV in about 40% of cases in developed countries and in up to 100% in tropical countries, no EBV positivity is found in the neoplastic cells of NLPHL.

Classic Hodgkin Lymphoma

The nodular sclerosis (60–70% of cases) and mixed cellularity (20% of cases) account for the majority of cases, while the lymphocyte-rich (5% of cases) and the lymphocyte-depleted (1% of cases) subtypes are rare.

Many cases diagnosed as the lymphocyte-depleted subtype in the older literature were later recognized to be other neoplasms, including ALCL and anaplastic variants of diffuse large B-cell lymphoma (DLBCL).

Clinical Findings. CHL has a bimodal age distribution, with the first peak occurring in the second and third decades and the second peak occurring in the sixth decade. The nodular sclerosis subtype, which occurs mostly in young adults, is largely responsible for the first peak in incidence.

Apart from the presence of enlarged, nontender lymph nodes, patients are frequently asymptomatic at presentation. The enlarged lymph nodes are most commonly found in the neck region (75% of cases), followed by the mediastinum, axilla or inguinal areas. HL tends to spread contiguously from one lymph node group to a neighboring one. Constitutional symptoms (type B symptoms) usually occur in patients with widespread disease and consist of fever, night sweats and weight loss. Other less common symptoms include anorexia, pruritus and alcohol-induced pain in the involved areas.

The stage of disease is usually determined by the Cotswold modification of the Ann Arbor classification, where stage I represents involvement of a single lymph node region, stage II the involvement of two or more lymph node regions on the same side of the diaphragm, stage III involvement of lymph node regions on both sides of the diaphragm and stage III, IV disseminated (multifocal) disease. The disease is also classified as limited, intermediate and advanced based on both stage and the presence of B symptoms. Treatment of cHL with multiagent chemotherapy, radiation therapy or both is very effective, resulting in a cure rate of over 85%.

Cytology. In the typical case, the cytologic findings of cHL are very characteristic; very large (40–60 μm and larger) Reed–Sternberg cells or their mononuclear variants, the Hodgkin cells (HRS cells), stand out against a reactive background.

Not much can be added to the classical description of HRS cells given by Dorothy Reed in 1902: very large cells with usually round, bean-shaped or indented nucleus or nuclei that are very large in proportion to the cell. The nucleus usually shows one or more very large nucleoli (macronucleoli) which may reach diameters up to 7 μm

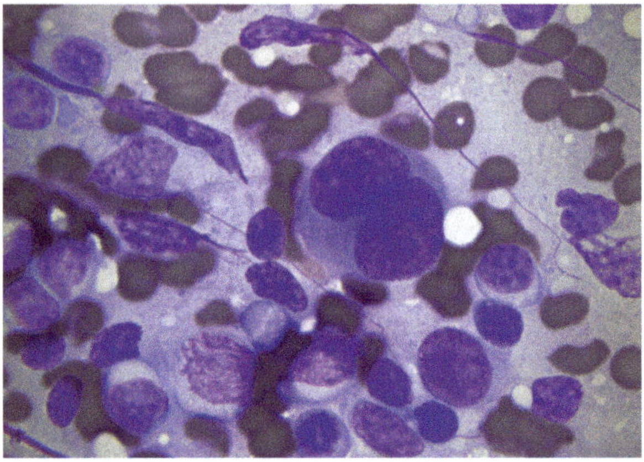

FIGURE 11.1. Classic binucleated Reed–Sternberg cell in a lymph node aspirate (Diff-Quik stain, ×1,000).

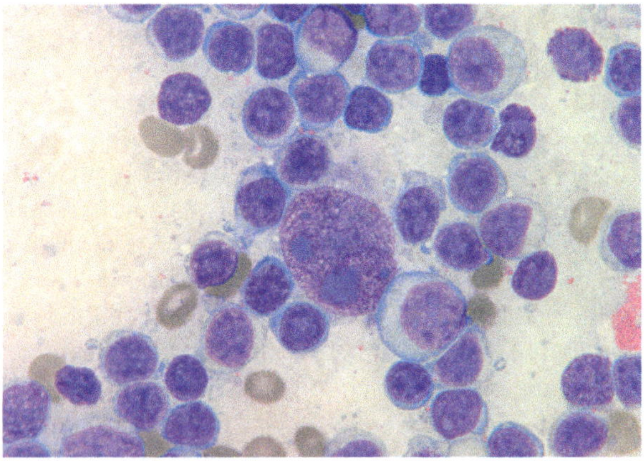

FIGURE 11.2. Reed–Sternberg cell showing prominent inclusion-like nucleoli and reticulated chromatin pattern (Diff-Quik stain, ×1,000).

and stand out because they usually stain differently than does the nucleus and are surrounded by a narrow paler halo (Fig. 11.1). The nuclear chromatin is arranged in small irregularly distributed angular heterochromatin fragments alternating with lighter euchromatin, in a pattern described as reticular (Fig. 11.2).

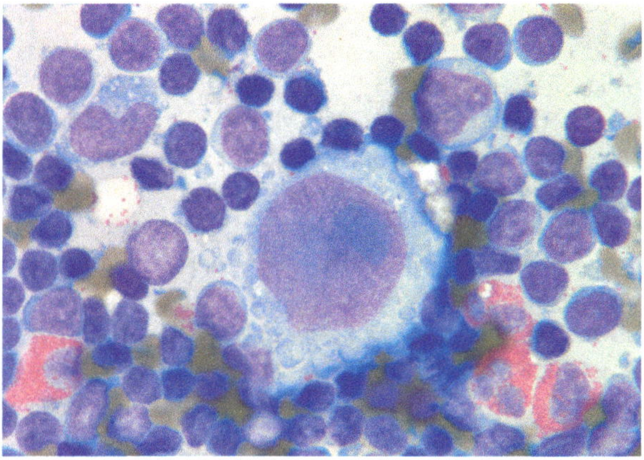

FIGURE 11.3. Mononuclear variant of Reed–Sternberg cell (Hodgkin cell) showing peripheral cytoplasmic blebs. Note the surrounding eosinophils (Diff-Quik stain, ×1,000).

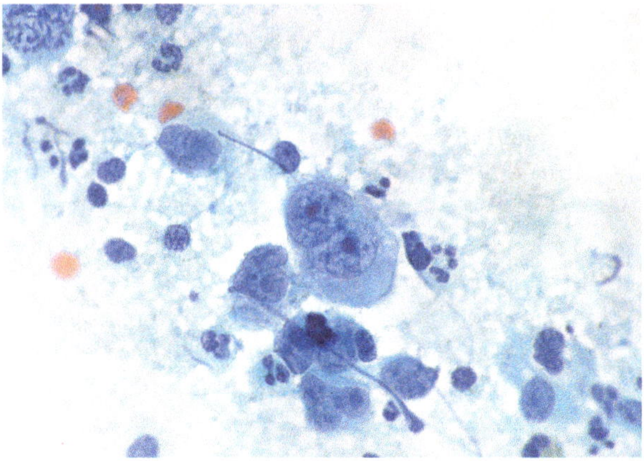

FIGURE 11.4. Classic binucleated Reed–Sternberg cell in a lymph node aspirate. Note the mitotic figure in the left upper corner (Papanicolaou stain, ×1,000).

The cytoplasm of HRS cells is abundant, usually homogeneous, but may show granules, vacuoles or contain pigment. The membrane may show cytoplasmic blebs (Fig. 11.3). The cytologic features of HRS cells are well seen in both air-dried Romanowsky-type stains and alcohol-fixed Papanicolaou-stained (or H&E) smears (Fig. 11.4).

Classic Reed–Sternberg cells are bilobed, binucleated or multinucleated cells with abundant cytoplasm and prominent macronucleoli. Frequently the two nuclei or lobes appear as mirror images of each other. In Romanowsky-type stains, RS cells have ample pale blue–gray cytoplasm, large multiple or single polylobed nuclei and prominent inclusion-like macronucleoli in each nucleus or nuclear lobe. In Papanicolaou-stained smears HRS cells have clear, ill-defined cytoplasm, even more prominent nucleoli and prominent nuclear chromatin and contour abnormalities. HRS cells are frequently found at the edges of the smears. Since the cytoplasm of HRS cells is very fragile it may be lost during smearing or the preparation of cytospins with resultant large naked nuclei with prominent nucleoli.

The number of HRS cells is variable from case to case. They may be so few as to be overlooked on the smears or may be so many as to mimic other conditions, especially in the so-called syncytial variant of nodular-sclerosis HL and in the lymphocyte-depleted variant of HL. Usually they represent 1–5% of cells in the smear, with mononuclear variants predominating over classic RS cells. Occasional HRS in mitosis and apoptotic HRS cells with smudged chromatin and indistinct nucleoli (mummified or zombie cells) can be found in smears from all types of cHL, although the latter are more common in NSHL.

The background most frequently is composed of small lymphocytes with occasional eosinophils, plasma cells and mast cells (Fig. 11.5). Neutrophils are usually sparse, but rarely may be the dominant background cell type which the designation "suppurative" HL reflects (Fig. 11.6). Single epithelioid histiocytes or well-formed epithelioid granulomas and lymphocytic tangles may be present. The presence of numerous eosinophils and of discrete epithelioid cells may serve as cytomorphologic clues for the diagnosis of HL. Mast cells are more common in the nodular sclerosis variant, and their number correlates with the degree of fibrosis. Bundles of fibroblasts and fragments of collagen may rarely be present in smears and cell block sections and orient the diagnosis toward the nodular sclerosis variant.

Differential diagnostic considerations include suppurative and granulomatous lymphadenitides and all conditions that may show RS-like cells, including reactive lymphadenopathies (infectious

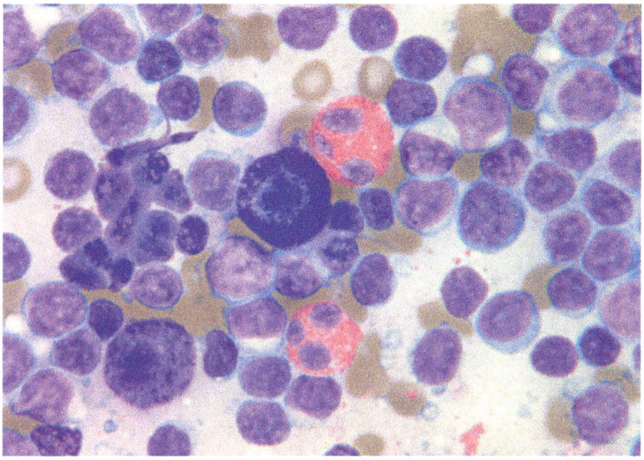

FIGURE 11.5. Fine-needle aspirate of Hodgkin lymphoma showing the characteristic background eosinophils and mast cells (Diff-Quik stain, ×1,000).

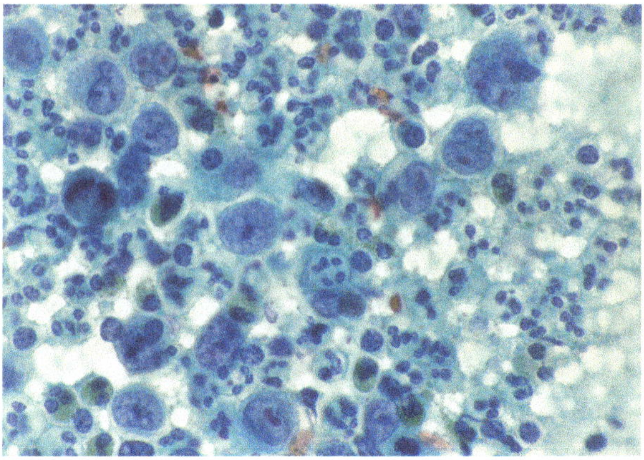

FIGURE 11.6. Fine-needle aspirate of Hodgkin lymphoma, suppurative-type showing numerous Hodgkin–Reed–Sternberg cells in a background of neutrophils (Papanicolaou stain, ×1,000).

mononucleosis), B- and T-cell lymphomas, and metastatic malignancies, especially carcinomas and melanomas. Cells that may, on occasion, be confused with HRS cells include immunoblasts found in reactive conditions, cytomegalovirus (CMV) and herpes simplex virus-infected cells, the multinucleated Warthin–Finkeldey cells (polykaryocytes), occasionally seen in measles, HIV and other viral lymphadenitides, binucleated follicular dendritic cells and the "dysplastic" follicular dendritic cells sometimes found in aspirates of the hyaline vascular variant of Castleman disease.

Subtyping Classic HL

Although separating cHL from NPLHL is important due to their different treatment and prognosis, subtyping cHL on fine-needle aspirates is difficult, potentially inaccurate and may lack clinical significance as staging almost entirely determines prognosis and therapy. The distinction between cHL and NLPHL is possible through determining their different immunoperoxidase staining profile on cell block sections. Although we are not subtyping cHL on FNA samples, we present the cytologic features of the four subtypes of cHL separately to highlight the subtle differences in their cytologic features.

a. *Nodular sclerosis HL.* NSHL is usually diagnosed in aspirates from cervical and mediastinal lymph nodes from young patients. Histologically this subtype is characterized by nodules separated by collagen bands, and by the HRS cell variant, the lacunar cell. Smears are frequently hypocellular and diagnostic HRS cells may be hard to find due to the difficulty in obtaining an aspirate from such fibrotic lymph nodes. Since the lacunae around lacunar cells are the result of a formalin fixation shrinkage artifact, they are not seen in cytologic preparations but may be seen in cell block sections. However, HRS cells of NSHL tend to have smaller nuclei, smaller nucleoli and more abundant cytoplasm than have the HRS cells of other HL subtypes.
   The syncytial variant is an unusual variant of NSHL, and is characterized by cohesive aggregates or sheets of RS cells; due to the abundance of HRS cells and their cohesiveness this variant could be mistaken for metastatic malignancies and anaplastic large-cell lymphoma.

b. *Mixed cellularity HL.* Most frequently encountered in peripheral (rather than mediastinal) lymph nodes of middle-aged men, this subtype is most commonly showing EBV positivity of the HRS cells (75%). It is also more frequent in HIV-infected patients and in developing countries. Since there is less fibrosis in this variant, the smears are more cellular and may show more frequent eosinophils, neutrophils and histiocytes than other variants and numerous classic RS cells. Epithelioid histiocytes and granulomas are also more common in this subtype.

c. *Lymphocyte-rich cHL.* This subtype typically occurs in peripheral lymph nodes of older men. HRS cells are seen in a background typical of a reactive lymph node with polymorphous lymphocytes, without eosinophils or histiocytes. Morphologically, the distinction from NLPHL is difficult or impossible and immunostains are needed to make that distinction.
d. *Lymphocyte-depleted cHL.* This rare subtype of HL is usually seen in middle-aged male patients; as MCHL, it is more common in HIV-infected individuals and in developing countries. About 50% of cases are EBV-related. This subtype commonly presents with advanced disease and has the worst prognosis.

HRS cells with pleomorphic or anaplastic nuclei tend to dominate the smears due to the relative paucity of lymphocytes. Fibroblasts and collagen fragments may also be present.

Nodular Lymphocyte Predominant HL

NLPHL usually involves one or two lymph node groups in the cervical axillary or inguinal region of adults aged 30–50. A very high cure rate is achieved with therapy, but about 10% of patients eventually relapse, usually progressing to DLBCL at relapse.

The cytologic features of NLPHL have been only rarely described. The diagnosis is difficult due to the rarity of LP (popcorn) cells, which typically represent less than 1% of cells. LP cells are also less conspicuous than HRS cells of cHL and show a highly twisted or multilobed nucleus with prominent but smaller nucleoli. Large lymphocytic aggregates may also be present, most likely representing the nodules that define this variant histologically (Fig. 11.7).

Immunophenotype. When the immediate on-site evaluation of the aspirate suggests HL, obtaining a cell block is preferable to

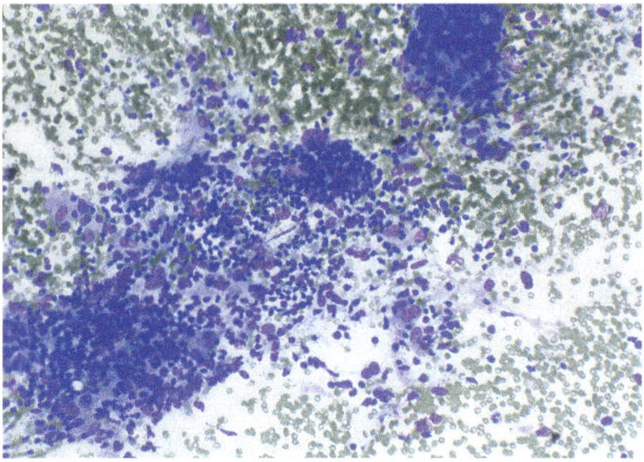

FIGURE 11.7. Fine-needle aspirate of nodular lymphocyte predominance Hodgkin lymphoma showing clusters of small lymphocytes with admixed large atypical cells (Diff-Quik stain, ×100).

sending an aliquot for flow cytometry since flow cytometry has traditionally not been helpful in the diagnosis of HL. Conventional flow cytometry usually shows an elevated CD4/CD8 ratio of the background lymphocytes, but this is a nonspecific finding. Advances in multiparameter flow cytometry may allow the diagnosis of cHL by demonstrating coexpression of CD30 and CD40, mostly with the expression of surface and/or cytoplasmic CD15 in HRS cells. However, this flow cytometry approach is not widely available currently, and performing immunoperoxidase stains on cell block sections is currently the preferred method to confirm the diagnosis of HL and rule out its mimics.

Although the HRS cells of cHL are B-cells, they usually lack most B-cell markers, including CD19, CD20, CD22 and CD79a. However, about 20–25% of cHL cases may show some expression of these markers. The only B-cell marker that is almost invariably, even if weakly expressed by HRS cells of cHL, is PAX5, the main B-cell lineage commitment and maintenance factor. As opposed to other B-cell markers which show membranous expression, PAX5 shows nuclear expression and is therefore very reliable, even in cases where the fragile cytoplasm of HRS cells has been damaged.

In addition to the loss of B-cell markers, HRS cells consistently express lineage-inappropriate markers, such as CD15 and fascin, and show strong positivity for MUM1/IRF4. The typical immunophenotype of cHL HRS cells is CD30+ (>90%), CD15+ (>80%), CD45−, as well as EMA−, and usually allows differentiation of cHL from NLPHL, B-cell lymphomas and T-cell lymphomas, including ALCL (Table 11.1). The neoplastic cells of NLPHL show an almost opposite staining pattern: CD45+, CD15−, CD30− (occasionally positive), EMA+ (about 50% cases) and CD20+. T-cell lymphomas are not PAX5 positive, while most cases of B-cell lymphomas are negative for CD15 and CD30. Positivity for EBV that occurs in about 40% of cHL cases and can be demonstrated by in-situ hybridization (EBER) or by immunohistochemistry (EBNA1, LMP1 and LMP2A) can be used to differentiate cHL (especially the lymphocyte-depleted subtype) from ALCL and other entities entering the differential diagnosis (Table 11.1).

Cytogenetics. Sensitive PCR-based methods for clonality detection can identify clonal B-cell rearrangements in the majority of cases of cHL. Although HRS cells have been shown to have complex cytogenetic abnormalities, including hyperploid karyotypes, no diagnostically useful specific abnormalities have been demonstrated.

Key Points. Aspirates with rare pleomorphic cells clearly standing out against a background of normal lymphoid elements, eosinophils, neutrophils and histiocytes are characteristic of cHL. The presence of numerous neutrophils or granulomas is rather common and may cause diagnostic difficulties.

Anaplastic Large-Cell Lymphoma

Anaplastic large-cell lymphoma is a mature T cell lymphoma that accounts for approximately 20% of all T-cell lymphomas and 2% of adult and 20–30% of childhood non-HLs in North America. According to the presence or absence of ALK protein expression it can be divided into the morphologically indistinguishable but clinically distinct ALK+ ALCL (50–80% of cases) and ALK− ALCL.

TABLE 11.1. Immunohistochemical markers useful in the differential diagnosis of Hodgkin lymphoma.

	CD3, CD5, CD7	CD20	PAX5	CD15	CD30	CD45	EMA	EBV
cHL	–	– (80%)	+	+	+	–	–	+/–
NLPHL	–	+	+	–	–	+	+/–	–
TC/HRLBCL	–	+	+	–	–	+/–	–/+	–
ALCL	+/–	–	–	–	+	+	+	–
pTCL	+/–	–	–	–	–	+	–	–
PMBL	–	+	+	–	+ (weak)	+	–	–

cHL classic Hodgkin lymphoma, *NLPHL* nodular lymphocyte predominant Hodgkin lymphoma, *TC/HRLBCL* T-cell/histiocyte-rich large B-cell lymphoma, *ALCL* anaplastic large-cell lymphoma, *pTCL* peripheral T-cell lymphoma, *PMBL* primary mediastinal B-cell lymphoma

Clinical Findings. ALK+ ALCL involves both lymph nodes and extranodal sites (skin, musculoskeletal system, lungs, liver) of young, predominantly male patients, whereas ALK− ALCL tends to affect elderly patients. In children the vast majority of ALCL cases are ALK+. ALCL patients typically present with advanced-stage disease and type B-symptoms.

ALK− ALCL involves extranodal tissues less frequently than ALK+ ALCL, but has been recently increasingly reported in the breast, in association with silicone implants. Response to treatment and prognosis of patients with ALK+ ALCL is good, much better than that of other peripheral T-cell lymphomas; the prognosis of ALK− ALCL is much worse, but still slightly better than that of other peripheral T-cell lymphomas.

Cytology. ALCL has a number of morphologic variants or patterns, the most frequent (75%) being the *common* (or *classic*) pattern, the *lymphohistiocytic* (10%) and the *small cell* variant (5–10%). The small cell variant is composed of neoplastic cells that are neither large, nor anaplastic, and may enter the differential diagnosis of small blue cell tumors and of lymphomas composed of intermediate-sized neoplastic cells.

Common to all morphologic variants is the presence of "hallmark" cells, large or very large cells, with diameters of 40 to over 70 μm, with horseshoe-shaped or kidney-shaped nuclei, abundant clear or basophilic cytoplasm and prominent perinuclear clear hofs, corresponding to the Golgi regions (Fig. 11.8). Nucleoli are round or angular, eosinophilic in the Papanicolaou stain and prominent but are usually smaller than those of HRS cells and do not have their inclusion-like appearance. The cytoplasm may show peripheral blebs, small vacuoles (Fig. 11.9) and occasionally also small azurophilic granules. A continuum of cell sizes of the abnormal cells can usually be seen (Fig. 11.10). Other characteristic neoplastic cells include "half-doughnut cells," "doughnut cells," multinucleated giant cells with nuclei arranged in a ring abutting the cytoplasmic border ("wreath cells"), "embryo cells" "tennis racket" or "hand mirror" cells, cells with polylobed nuclei and Reed–Sternberg-like cells. A large number of smaller neoplastic cells without such characteristic nuclear shapes, with nondescript or plasmacytoid appearance, are also present. Frequent mitoses and apoptotic cells are present in aspirate smears. Erythrophagocytosis

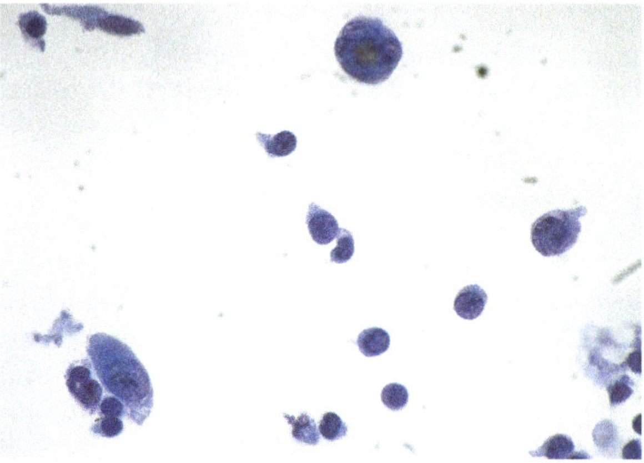

FIGURE 11.8. Fine-needle aspirate of anaplastic large-cell lymphoma showing a hallmark cell with distinct hof (Papanicolaou stain, ×400).

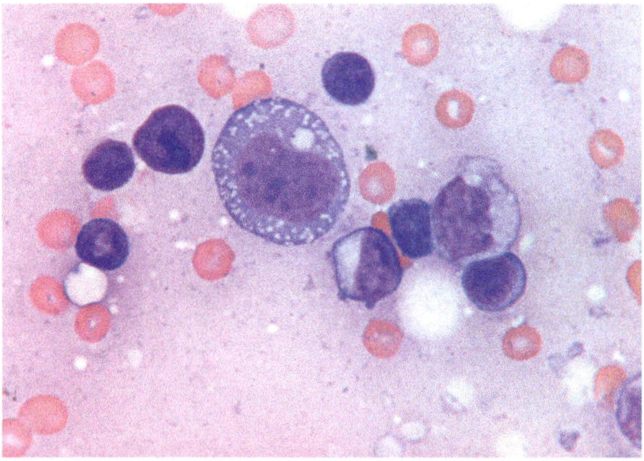

FIGURE 11.9. Fine-needle aspirate of anaplastic large-cell lymphoma showing a very large atypical cell with prominent cytoplasmic vacuolation (Diff-Quik stain, ×1,000).

or cell cannibalism by the large cells can occasionally be seen. The background usually shows reactive lymphocytes, but may be dominated by neutrophils, histiocytes or eosinophils.

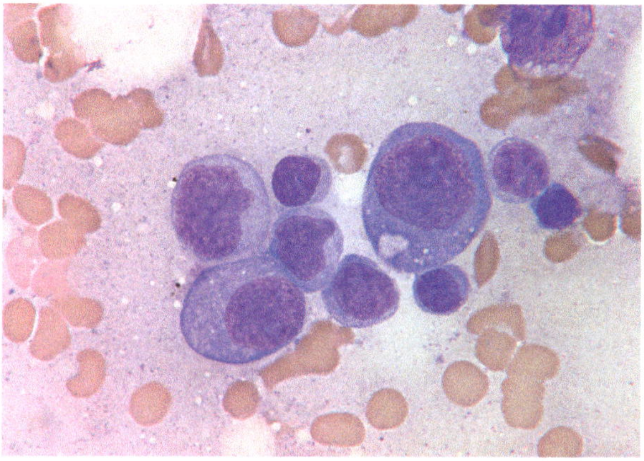

FIGURE 11.10. Fine-needle aspirate of anaplastic large-cell lymphoma showing atypical cells with a spectrum of sizes from medium-sized to large and very large (anaplastic) (Diff-Quik stain, ×1,000).

Due to its pleomorphic neoplastic cells, ALCL may pose difficult differential diagnostic considerations with both lymphomas (especially HL) and metastatic malignancies. In contrast to cHL where neoplastic cells are usually rare and stand out against a clearly benign background, neoplastic ALCL cells are more numerous and show a gradation of sizes and atypicality. Immunohistochemistry is useful in the differentiation from other lymphomas (Table 11.1) and from metastatic malignancies.

Immunophenotype. Immunoperoxidase stains on cell block sections are the most practical way to determine the immunophenotype of ALCL neoplastic cells since flow cytometry, which may be useful in some cases, is hampered by technical difficulties.

ALK usually shows both nuclear and cytoplasmic staining in cases that are positive. The large, pleomorphic neoplastic cells of ALCL are by definition positive for CD30 in a membranous and Golgi pattern. The vast majority of cases express one or more T-cell markers (CD2, CD4, CD5) although CD3 is frequently lost. The neoplastic cells are consistently CD45 and EMA positive (Table 11.1).

Cytogenetics. The t(2;5) (p23;q35) translocation fusing the receptor tyrosine kinase anaplastic lymphoma kinase (*ALK*) gene to the nucleophosmin (*NPM1*) gene is the most frequently encountered (>80%) cytogenetic abnormality in ALK+ ALCL. At least six additional translocations involving the *ALK* gene with different partners have been described and result in different ALK immunostaining patterns: nuclear, cytoplasmic, membranous or combination of these patterns.

The t(2;5) translocation can be detected by FISH and the translocation product by molecular studies. ALK– ALCL shows no recurrent chromosomal abnormalities.

Key Points. ALCL should be suspected when smears show a gradation of neoplastic cells from intermediate to large bizarre cells with marked nuclear shape abnormalities and multinucleation. The diagnosis should be confirmed by immunostains, cytogenetic studies (FISH) or molecular studies.

Hodgkin-Type Richter Transformation of SLL/CLL

The transformation of small lymphocytic lymphoma/chronic lymphocytic leukemia to an aggressive lymphoma is called Richter syndrome in honor of Maurice N. Richter, who first described it in 1928.

While the transformation most commonly occurs to DLBCL, it may occur to cHL in less than 1% of SLL/CLL cases. In such cases large pleomorphic cells morphologically and immunophenotypically consistent with Reed–Sternberg cells are found in a background of cells consistent with SLL/CLL. The Reed–Sternberg cells are usually clonally related to the SLL/CLL cells. As opposed to de novo cHL, the prognosis of these patients is poor with a median survival of less than 1 year. Therefore these patients should not be diagnosed with HL, but with Hodgkin-type Richter syndrome.

Patients usually have a longstanding history of SLL/CLL and develop large lymph nodes (>5 cm), or rapidly enlarging lymph nodes, extranodal lesions or the appearance of B symptoms or sudden LDH elevation.

De novo cHL may also occur in patients with SLL/CLL in which the HRS cells are not clonally related to the SLL/CLL clone; this form has a better prognosis. Morphologically, such de novo cHLs show HRS cells against a reactive cellular background rather than the monotonous SLL/CLL background.

Diffuse Large B-Cell Lymphoma Variants

Of the DLBCL types, the most likely to enter the differential diagnosis of the pleomorphic cell pattern are primary mediastinal B-cell lymphoma and T-cell/histiocyte-rich B-cell lymphoma. While they have many similarities to cHL, they do not usually show HRS cells in the aspirate. When such Reed–Sternberg-like cells are present, the differential diagnosis requires immunophenotyping by flow cytometry or immunoperoxidase stains (Table 11.1).

Another differential diagnostic consideration is a rare type of DLBCL with plasmablastic or immunoblastic features that expresses ALK protein. However, these lymphomas do not usually show pleomorphic cells and do not express CD30. The anaplastic cytologic variant of DLBCL may pose differential diagnostic difficulties with ALCL; however, the neoplastic cells express B-cell markers rather than T-cell markers. Anaplastic plasma cell tumors may also enter the differential diagnosis; clinical correlation and demonstration of cytoplasmic light chain restriction are diagnostic.

Peripheral T-Cell Lymphoma, Not Otherwise Specified

Peripheral T-cell lymphoma, not otherwise specified (PTCL, NOS), may occasionally show bizarre pleomorphic cells; the diagnosis is based on the immunophenotype (Table 11.1).

NK/T-Cell Lymphoma

While the majority of NK/T-cell lymphomas are extranodal, primarily nasal neoplasms, nodal involvement may occur. The smears are most often dominated by intermediate to large cells, but may also show pleomorphic cells. The diagnosis is made by demonstrating cytoplasmic CD3 positivity in addition to CD56 positivity; the neoplastic cells are usually negative for CD30 and CD15.

Extramedullary Hematopoiesis

The megakaryocytes found in extramedullary hematopoiesis and the adrenal myelolipoma may mimic Reed–Sternberg cells or ALCL cells. Correct identification of the background of erythroid and myeloid precursors is essential for the diagnosis.

Thymoma

Thymoma, an epithelial tumor of the thymus, may pose differential diagnostic difficulties in mediastinal fine-needle aspirates since large epithelial cells, which may have prominent nucleoli, are seen in the background of a reactive lymphoid population, and may therefore mimic HL or ALCL (Fig. 11.11). The correct diagnosis depends on the demonstration of cytokeratin staining of the neoplastic cells.

Metastatic Malignancies with Pleomorphic Cells

In lymph node enlargement caused by metastatic malignancies, the lymphoid structures are usually largely replaced by metastatic

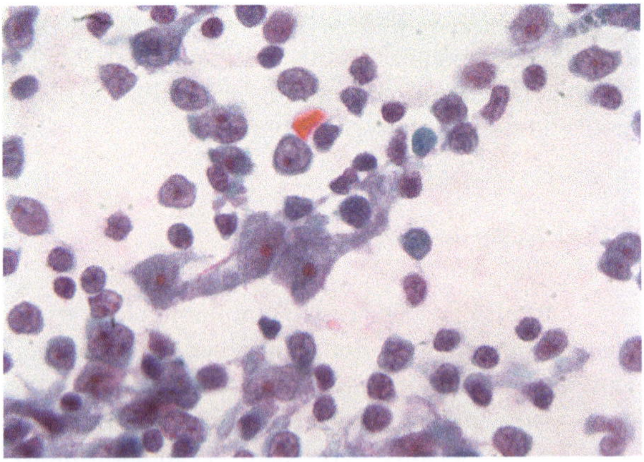

Figure 11.11. Fine-needle aspirate of thymoma showing the large neoplastic epithelial cells with prominent nucleoli in a background of small lymphocytes (Papanicolaou stain, ×1,000).

tumor; the needle aspirate will therefore show a predominance of large pleomorphic tumor cells with few background lymphocytes. Such aspirates may enter the differential diagnosis of ALCL. Occasionally, however, rare pleomorphic cells are seen in the background of a reactive lymphoid population, mimicking HL.

Metastatic Carcinomas

Metastatic carcinomas usually show at least loosely cohesive clusters of tumor cells; these may enter the differential diagnosis of HL and ALCL since both the syncytial variant of cHL and ALCL may show apparently cohesive groups of neoplastic cells.

Less differentiated metastatic carcinomas may show a single cell pattern, with pleomorphic cells which may mimic HL and ALCL (Figs. 11.12 and 11.13).

Metastatic carcinomas that are close mimics of HL and ALCL are metastatic lymphoepithelioma-type nasopharyngeal carcinomas and anaplastic carcinomas of the thyroid and lung. However, other metastatic carcinomas may at times show Reed–Sternberg-like cells or anaplastic multinucleated cells. The diagnosis is aided

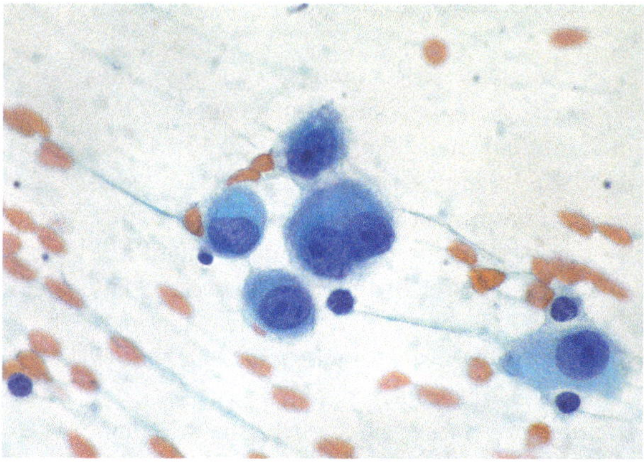

FIGURE 11.12. Fine-needle aspirate of a retroperitoneal lymph node showing metastatic urothelial carcinoma with Reed–Sternberg-like cells (Papanicolaou stain, ×1,000).

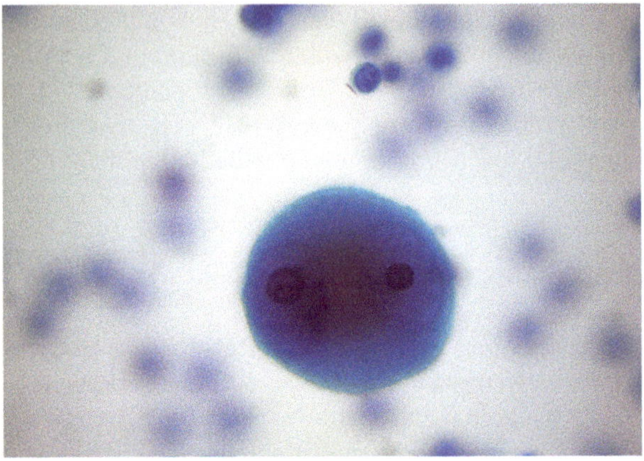

FIGURE 11.13. Fine-needle aspirate of a nodal metastasis of endometrial carcinoma with Reed–Sternberg-like cells (Papanicolaou stain, ×1,000).

by the clinical context, in particular, by a history of previous malignancy. The neoplastic cells are positive for cytokeratin in addition to EMA and lack lymphoid markers.

Metastatic Melanoma

Metastatic malignant melanomas frequently show very large binucleated cells with dual mirror image nuclei (DMIN or "demon cells") or multinucleated giant cells (Fig. 11.14). Such cells may mimic Reed–Sternberg cells or ALCL cells, especially since they also show very prominent macronucleoli. The correct diagnosis is helped by the identification of melanin pigment in the cytoplasm of the neoplastic cells or of the accompanying histiocytes. However melanin may be absent in metastatic melanomas. The demonstration of intranuclear pseudoinclusions which are not a feature of HL or ALCL is also helpful.

In difficult cases, immunohistochemistry will demonstrate S100 positivity, with or without additional HMB45 and Melan A staining, while lymphoid markers are negative.

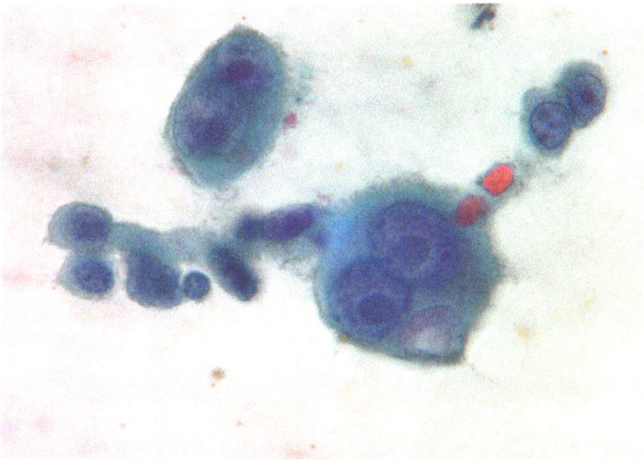

FIGURE 11.14. Fine-needle aspirate of malignant melanoma metastatic to lymph node; the large binucleated cells with prominent macronucleoli surrounded by halos can closely mimic Reed–Sternberg cells (Papanicolaou stain, ×1,000).

Metastatic Mesenchymal Malignancies

Lymph node metastases from sarcomas are unusual; however, when they occur they may mimic HL or ALCL due to the presence of pleomorphic single cells or loose clusters in a lymphoid background. Of the metastatic mesenchymal neoplasms, the most likely to be confused with HL or ALCL are metastatic high-grade undifferentiated sarcomas (malignant fibrous histiocytomas) (Fig. 11.15), metastatic rhabdomyosarcomas and metastatic neuroblastomas. Metastatic neuroblastoma may show a spectrum of neuroblastic to ganglion cell differentiation, with large, frequently multinucleated ganglion-like cells which may mimic HRS cells or ALCL cells. The identification of neuropil-like material in the background is diagnostically useful. The correct diagnosis is made by clinical correlation and the appropriate immunostains (desmin and myogenin in rhabdomyosarcoma and NSE in neuroblastoma).

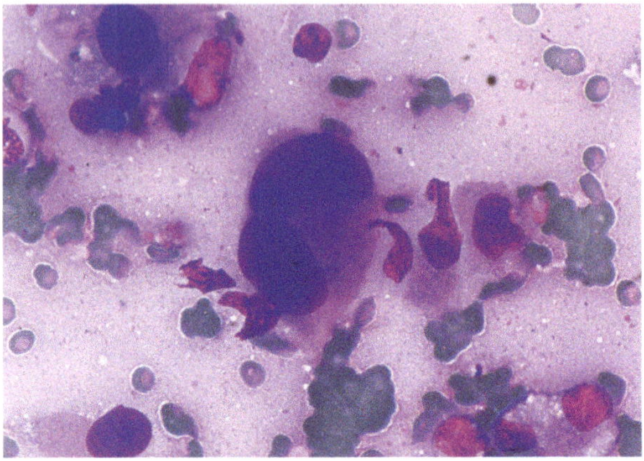

FIGURE 11.15. Fine-needle aspirate of high-grade undifferentiated sarcoma (malignant fibrous histiocytoma) metastatic to lymph node; bizzarre large binucleated cells may mimic Reed–Sternberg cells (Papanicolaou stain, ×1,000).

Suggested Reading

Das DK, Francis IM, Sharma PN, Sathar SA, John B, George SS, Mallik MK, Sheikh ZA, Haji BE, Pathan SK, Madda JP, Mirza K, Ahmed MS, Junaid TA (2009) Hodgkin's lymphoma: diagnostic difficulties in fine-needle aspiration cytology. Diagn Cytopathol 37(8):564–573

Fromm JR, Thomas A, Wood BL (2009) Flow cytometry can diagnose classical Hodgkin lymphoma in lymph nodes with high sensitivity and specificity. Am J Clin Pathol 131(3):322–332

Iacobuzio-Donahue CA, Clark DP, Ali SZ (2002) Reed-Sternberg-like cells in lymph node aspirates in the absence of Hodgkin's disease: pathologic significance and differential diagnosis. Diagn Cytopathol 27(6):335–339

Ioachim HL, Medeiros LJ (2009) Ioachim's lymph node pathology, 4th edn. Wolters Kluwer Health/Lippincott Williams & Wilkins, Philadelphia

Mourad WA, al Nazer M, Tulbah A (2003) Cytomorphologic differentiation of Hodgkin's lymphoma and Ki-1+ anaplastic large cell lymphoma in fine needle aspirates. Acta Cytol 47(5):744–748

Ng WK, Ip P, Choy C, Collins RJ (2003) Cytologic and immunocytochemical findings of anaplastic large cell lymphoma: analysis of ten fine-needle aspiration specimens over a 9-year period. Cancer 99(1):33–43

Rapkiewicz A, Wen H, Sen F, Das K (2007) Cytomorphologic examination of anaplastic large cell lymphoma by fine-needle aspiration cytology. Cancer 111(6):499–507

Skoog L, Tani E (2009) Hodgkin lymphoma. Monogr Clin Cytol 18:49–52

Strum SB, Park JK, Rappaport H (1970) Observation of cells resembling Sternberg-Reed cells in conditions other than Hodgkin's disease. Cancer 26(1):176–190

Zhang JR, Raza AS, Greaves TS, Cobb CJ (2006) Fine-needle aspiration diagnosis of Hodgkin lymphoma using current WHO classification–re-evaluation of cases from 1999–2004 with new proposals. Diagn Cytopathol 34(6):397–402

12 Infectious and Noninfectious Lymphadenitis

Infectious lymphadenitis can be caused by viral, bacterial, mycobacterial, fungal, and protozoal agents. Non-neoplastic noninfectious lymphadenitis can be associated with systemic processes such as collagen vascular diseases, Rosai–Dorfman disease, sarcoidosis, Castleman disease (CD), drugs, and foreign bodies.

We will mainly focus on entities that have not been covered in previous chapters as part of the differential diagnosis of the hematolymphoid malignancies. When appropriate, the reader will be referred to other sections of this book. The main cytologic clues for diagnosis are listed in Table 12.1. The FNA smear patterns are listed in Table 12.2.

Viral Lymphadenitis

Eight members of the human herpes virus (HHV) family infect humans; they are herpes simplex types 1 and 2 (HHV-1 and 2), herpes-varicella zoster (HHV-3), Epstein–Barr (HHV-4), cytomegalovirus (HHV-5), HHV-6, HHV-7, and Kaposi sarcoma herpes (HHV-8). All are double-stranded DNA viruses. A prominent paracortical hyperplasia with immunoblastic proliferation is seen in viral lymphadenitis.

S.E. Pambuccian and R.H. Bardales, *Lymph Node Cytopathology*, Essentials in Cytopathology 10, DOI 10.1007/978-1-4419-6964-4_12,

TABLE 12.1. Lymphadenitis/lymphadenopathy: cytologic clues for the diagnosis.

Entity	Cytologic feature(s)
Viral	
Infectious mononucleosis	Immunoblasts with marked atypia
Herpes simplex	Cowdry A inclusions, ground-glass nuclei, multinucleation
Cytomegalovirus	Large cells with large eosinophilic nuclear inclusion
Varicella-Herpes Zoster	Rare small intranuclear inclusions
Measles	Polykaryocytes (not specific)
Human immunodeficiency virus	Polymorphous lymphoid cell pattern. Plasma cells in late stages
Bacterial	
Cat scratch	Granulomas, necrosis, acute inflammation
Lymphogranuloma venereum	Granulomas, necrosis, acute inflammation
Syphilis	Small granulomas and plasma cells
Tuberculosis	Granulomas and caseation necrosis
Mycobacterium avium-intracellulare complex	Numerous bacilli within histiocytes and in the background smear (pseudo-Gaucher cells and "negative images")
Leprosy, tuberculoid	Small noncaseating granulomas
Fungal	
Cryptococcus	Yeast with mucoid thick capsule. Mucous background. Narrow-based buds
Pneumocystis	Foamy exudates
Histoplasma	Intracytoplasmic yeasts. Granular calcific background
Coccidioides	Large spherules with yeast forms
Protozoal	
Toxoplasma	Crescent-shaped organisms (2–6 μm)
Leishmania	Amastigotes 1–3 μm with histiocytes (Donovan bodies) and multinucleated giant cells
Filaria	Fragments of dead calcified organisms
Noninfectious	
Kimura lymphadenopathy	Polymorphous lymphoid cell pattern with polykaryocytes (not specific)
Kikuchi disease	Necrosis
Rosai–Dorfman disease	Histiocytes with cytophagocytosis (emperipolesis, erythrocytes, plasma cells)

(continued)

TABLE 12.1. (continued)

Entity	Cytologic feature(s)
Sarcoidosis	Cell damage, non-necrotizing granulomas. Schaumann and cytoplasmic asteroid bodies
Systemic lupus erythematosus	Necrosis. Hematoxylin bodies
Rheumatoid arthritis	Polymorphous lymphoid cell pattern and plasma cells
Castleman disease, plasma cell variant	Plasma cells
Dermatopathic	Lipid or pigment (melanin)-laden histiocytes
Lymphoepithelial lesion	Keratin and lymphocytes
Drug-induced lymphadenopathy	Follicular and/or immunoblastic hyperplasia
Amyloid	Amorphous "waxy" material, lymphocytes, multinucleated giant cells
Silicone	Histiocytes with clear cytoplasmic vacuoles, multinucleated giant cells
Lipid	Histiocytes with small cytoplasmic vacuoles, multinucleated giant cells (lipogranulomas)

TABLE 12.2. The various FNA smear patterns as clues for the diagnosis.

Necrosis	*Granulomas with necrosis*
Infectious mononucleosis (focal)	Cat scratch disease
Herpes simplex (focal)	Mycobacterial infection
Kikuchi disease (marked)	Fungal infection
Systemic lupus erythematosus (marked)	Kikuchi disease
Pneumocystis (marked)	Lymphogranuloma venereum
Infarcted lymph node (marked)	Leishmania
Neutrophils	*Granulomas without necrosis*
Bacterial infection (marked)	Toxoplasma
Anaplastic large cell lymphoma (scattered)	Sarcoidosis (rare with necrosis)
Anaplastic carcinoma (scattered)	Syphilis
	Whipple disease
	Tuberculoid leprosy
	Filaria
	Tumor-associated lymphadenitis

Infectious Mononucleosis

Infectious mononucleosis is an acute self-limited disease caused by the Epstein–Barr virus (EBV) that infects B-cells via the CD3d complement receptor (CD21). Both epithelial cells and B-cells in the oropharynx can be infected by EBV. The viral spread is via direct contact with oral secretions. The EBV produces an antibody response with cell proliferation during the first week of the disease. Infectious mononucleosis affects predominantly adolescents and young adults who have fever, pharyngitis, and cervical or generalized lymphadenopathy. The lymph nodes are enlarged and soft, but not matted. Lymphocytosis with atypical lymphocytes is commonly seen in the peripheral blood. The disease resolves in 3–4 weeks in most patients. Life-threatening disease is seen in immunosuppressed individuals.

The cytology preparations show numerous large reactive immunoblasts, large and small lymphocytes, histiocytes, tingible-body macrophages, and rare plasma cells. Numerous mitoses and apoptotic nuclei are also present. The immunoblasts are large and show a basophilic cytoplasm, a large nucleus, and a single central round or polyhedral nucleolus. Necrosis may be present. The pattern invites one to make the erroneous diagnosis of large cell lymphoma. (Fig. 12.1).

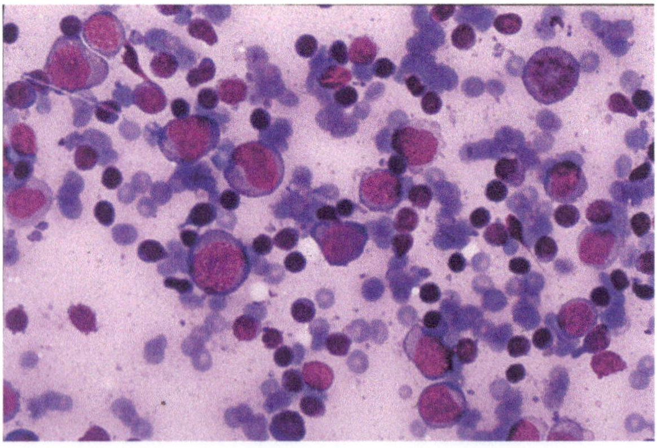

FIGURE 12.1. Infectious mononucleosis. A reactive immunoblastic proliferation with scattered mitoses is characteristic of this Epstein–Barr virus infection (DiffQuik stain, high magnification).

No light chain restriction is identified, and the immunostains for B- and T-cells demonstrate a reactive pattern. EBV can be demonstrated by immunohistochemistry, in situ hybridization, and other molecular analysis in tissue sections. The differential diagnosis includes large cell lymphoma, anaplastic large cell lymphoma, lymphocyte predominance Hodgkin lymphoma, and classical Hodgkin lymphoma.

Herpes Simplex Virus

Herpes simplex virus (HSV) infects human beings and animals, but only humans are symptomatic. HSV-1 is transmitted by oral secretions and causes keratoconjunctivitis, as well as oropharyngeal and esophageal lesions. HSV-2 is sexually transmitted and causes genital lesions. Once primary infection occurs, the virus migrates along sensory nerves and becomes latent in the dorsal root ganglia. When HSV reactivates, it causes recurrent infection. A more chronic and severe course occurs in immunosuppressed patients. HSV lymphadenitis may be associated with hematologic malignancies and may show a regional or generalized lymphadenitis or multiorgan involvement.

Numerous immunoblasts, some with large folded nuclei, are present. Small and medium-sized lymphocytes, macrophages, and eosinophils may be present. Microabscesses or granulomas are not seen; however, areas of necrosis may be seen harboring cells with HSV cytopathic effect (multinucleation, ground glass appearance, and Cowdry type A inclusions).

The HSV can be identified by immunohistochemistry, in situ hybridization, and molecular techniques such as PCR.

When necrosis predominates, the smear pattern has to be differentiated from cat scratch lymphadenitis, Kikuchi lymphadenitis, and SLE lymphadenitis.

Cytomegalovirus

Cytomegalovirus (CMV) is the largest of the human viruses and is transmitted from person to person by blood transfusion, transplacentally, and by saliva and respiratory secretions. The virus infects endothelial cells, T-lymphoid cells, and reticulum cells from lymphoid organs. The CMV remains indefinitely as a latent infection in immunocompetent individuals and reactivates when there is immunosuppression. These patients commonly show multiorgan involvement including lymph nodes.

The cytology preparations show immunoblastic proliferation with monocytoid cells, centrocytes, and centroblasts. The infected cells are large with a single intranuclear eosinophilic inclusion surrounded by a clear space (owl's eye). Small cytoplasmic basophilic inclusions are also present. Infected cells can be detected by immunohistochemistry with use of anti-CMV antibodies and by in situ hybridization.

Varicella-Herpes Zoster

The viruses from patients with chickenpox (varicella) and shingles (herpes zoster) are identical. The varicella-zoster virus (VZV) remains latent in the sensory ganglia of the cranial nerves and the spinal dorsal-root ganglia and spreads centrifugally through the nerves to reactivate years after the primary infection in the setting of immunodeficiency and manifests as maculopapular eruption, vesicles, and generalized lymphadenopathy. The vesicle fluid is highly infectious.

The affected lymph nodes are tender and usually are cervical, supraclavicular, and axillary. The smears show immunoblastic proliferation with lymphocytes, histiocytes, and plasma cells. Some cells are enlarged and show an intranuclear inclusion surrounded by a clear halo. Such cells may be also seen in the scrapings from the base of the vesicles.

Vaccinia

Vaccinia, a poxvirus, is less virulent than smallpox virus and is antigenically similar. Vaccinia lymphadenitis is generally induced by vaccination against smallpox infection and occurs in the draining lymph nodes at the vaccination site. The lymph node shows marked immunoblastic proliferation with scattered mitoses. Occasionally, the immunoblasts resemble the popcorn cells of Hodgkin lymphoma. Lymphocytes, plasma cells, mast cells, and eosinophils are also present.

Measles

Measles is a paramyxovirus that involves the skin, mucous membranes, and reticuloendothelial system, producing an acute syndrome with fever and general symptoms in nonimmunized patients, commonly children. Viral proliferation occurs in lymphocytes and macrophages, which facilitates the systemic dissemination. Lymphadenitis occurs in the presence of infection or recent vaccination for measles. The axillary, cervical, and inguinal lymph nodes are commonly involved.

The lymph node shows immunoblastic proliferation. Multinucleated giant cells or polykaryocytes (Warthin–Finkeldey) with grape-like arranged nuclei usually appear in the prodromal phase of measles and disappear when the cutaneous eruption is established. These cells may be seen in other lymphadenopathies, particularly reactive lymphoid hyperplasia, acute HIV infection, Hodgkin lymphoma lymphocyte-predominant, and low-grade non-Hodgkin lymphomas.

Human Immunodeficiency Virus

See Chap. 7. The human immunodeficiency virus 1 (HIV-1) is the agent of HIV infection and is a lentivirus, a subfamily of retroviruses. HIV-1 infects CD4+ lymphocytes, macrophages, and dendritic cells; the first disseminates the virus and the last two are the reservoirs. In the late stage, the CD4 lymphocytes and the dendritic cells are destroyed, the viremia resurges, and opportunistic infections and tumors develop in the immunosuppressed host.

The acute and chronic phase of HIV infection has generalized lymphadenopathy that harbors processes which may be reactive, infectious (mycobacterial and fungal), or neoplastic (lymphoma, Kaposi sarcoma). In the acute phase, the smear shows a florid reactive lymphoid hyperplasia, as well as scattered large monocytoid cells with clear cytoplasm and round nuclei, neutrophils, multinucleated cells (polykaryocytes of Warthin–Finkeldey), and tingible body macrophages. Less cellular smears and the presence of plasma cells are characteristic in the subacute phase of HIV lymphadenitis. Hypocellular smears with a paucity of lymphocytes and predominance of plasma cells are characteristic of the chronic burned-out phase of HIV infection. The main role of FNA cytology in HIV patients is to rule out opportunistic infections and neoplasms such as lymphoma or Kaposi sarcoma.

Bacterial Lymphadenitis

Bacterial lymphadenitis is most common in the pediatric population and affects regional lymph nodes draining areas of bacterial infections (dental abscess, infected wound, appendicitis, etc.). The lymph nodes are enlarged, soft, and tender. The overlying skin is red and edematous and may result in abscess formation with drainage. The most common pyogenic agent is staphylococcus and rarely tularemia, yersinia, typhoid fever, or melioidosis. In early stages, the smears show a purulent pattern with free or phagocytosed bacteria. Later, the smears show lymphocytes, plasma cells, and tingible-body macrophages. The Gram stain is useful for identifying the bacterial elements. Cultures are definitive for etiologic identification. Occasionally, anaplastic large cell lymphoma may have numerous neutrophils in the background.

Cat Scratch

See Chap. 7. Cat scratch disease is a common cause of chronic lymphadenitis in children and adolescents. In the United States, 55% of cases occur in patients aged 18 years or younger, commonly in the months of September–January. The pathogenic organism is *Bartonella henselae*; a Gram-negative bacillus is transmitted by fleas to kittens and is transmitted to humans by a cat bite or lick. In cats, the organism resides in the erythrocytes and does not cause significant illness. The patients have enlarged, nodular, and matted regional lymphadenopathy that is fixed to surrounding tissues and commonly occurs in the upper extremities and face. The lymphadenopathy develops 1–3 weeks after the primary skin lesion and is usually accompanied by systemic symptoms. In immunocompetent individuals, the disease is self-limited and resolves in 6–12 weeks in the absence of treatment. Suppuration occurs in 10% of cases. A systemic life-threatening disease may occur in AIDS patients.

The smears show a reactive lymphoid hyperplasia pattern with monocytoid cells and scattered tingible-body macrophages in the early stages of the disease. A suppurative granulomatous pattern with necrosis, neutrophils, epithelioid histiocytes, granulomas, and rare multinucleated Langhans-type giant cells is seen in more established processes (Fig. 12.2). Microbiologic detection is difficult, and the diagnosis is supported by the clinical history, serology, and histopathology. The organisms can be visualized by the Warthin–Starry silver stain, immunoperoxidase stain with anti-*B. henselae* antibodies, indirect immunofluorescence, PCR, and enzyme immunoassay. The diagnostic sensitivity of all tests is low. The silver stain is the most sensitive, but is the least specific. Lymphogranuloma venereum is identical cytologically, and immunofluorescence and serology are necessary for the diagnosis. The differential cytologic diagnosis also includes bacterial suppurative lymphadenitis, tularemia, and other granulomatous

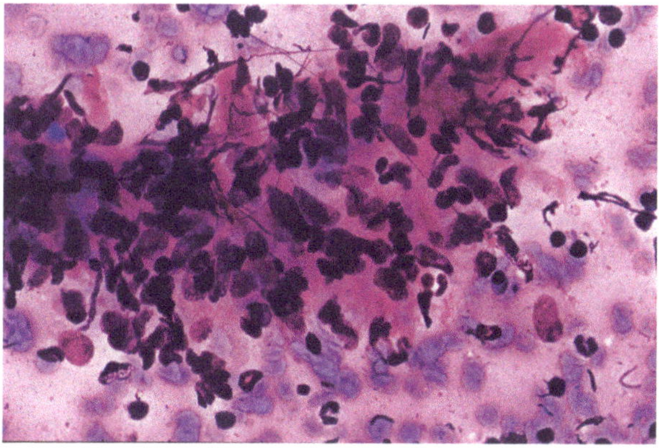

FIGURE 12.2. Cat scratch disease. A suppurative granulomatous pattern is characteristic of cat scratch disease in the appropriate clinical setting (DiffQuik stain, high magnification).

processes including tuberculosis; special stains and cultures are needed for ruling out these processes.

Bacillary Angiomatosis

The pathogenetic organism is *Bartonella henselae* and involves the skin and reticuloendothelial system in immunosuppressed individuals, particularly those with HIV. The skin lesions grossly resemble pyogenic granulomas, and the lymph nodes draining the skin lesions show a proliferation of small blood vessels and scattered neutrophils that replaces the lymphoid tissue. The Gram-negative bacilli are identified by the Warthin–Starry silver stain or by immunohistochemistry with anti-bartonella antibodies (Figs. 12.3 and 12.4). This lesion must be differentiated histologically from Kaposi sarcoma, which affects a similar patient population. The precise diagnosis is important because treatment is curative with antimicrobial agents.

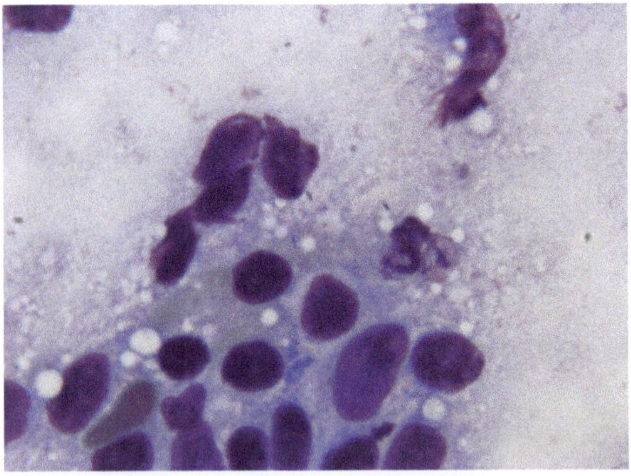

FIGURE 12.3. Bacillary angiomatosis. Small aggregates of oval, round, and spindled cells and rare bacilli are seen in the smears. (Giemsa stain, high magnification). Courtesy of Roberto Miranda MD, Associate Professor, Department of Pathology. MD Anderson Cancer Center.

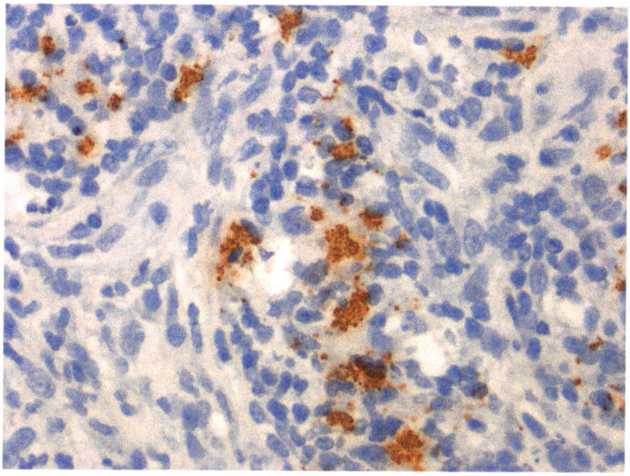

FIGURE 12.4. Bacillary angiomatosis. Small aggregates of spindled cells and bacilli are seen in tissue section. Immunohistochemistry confirms the diagnosis. (Immunohistochemistry with anti-bartonella antibody stain high magnification). Courtesy of Roberto Miranda MD, Associate Professor, Department of Pathology. MD Anderson Cancer Center.

Lymphogranuloma Venereum

This sexually transmitted disease is caused by the intracellular bacterium *Chlamydia trachomatis*, which causes a painless herpetiform lesion at the site of mucosal entry (cervix, anus, and penis) 7–12 days after sexual contact, followed by regional lymphadenitis 1–8 weeks later. The affected lymph nodes are usually pelvic in men, but may be perianal or pelvic when the site of entrance is located in the anus or uterine cervix. The lymph nodes are initially tender, movable, and firm, and then they become matted and fixed to surrounding tissues. Later, the lymph nodes may rupture, forming sinus tracts that often involve the skin. Lymphatic obstruction with edema and anorectal strictures is a late complication.

The lymph nodes have foci of necrosis with neutrophils surrounded by lymphocytes, plasma cells, histiocytes, and multinucleated giant cells, similar to the pattern seen in cat scratch and tularemia lymphadenitis. Macrophages with single or multiple cytoplasmic vacuoles containing the organisms are present. Follicular hyperplasia is seen in the areas without necrosis. Complement fixation is the laboratory test most commonly used for diagnosing active infection. PCR can amplify the chlamydial DNA from the affected organs and, along with serology, help in the differential diagnosis.

Syphilis

See Chap. 7. Syphilitic lymphadenitis is caused by the bacterial spirochete *Treponema pallidum*, acquired by sexual contact or maternal–fetal transmission. Regional and generalized lymphadenitis is present in the primary and secondary stages of infection, respectively. In the primary stage, the inguinal or cervical lymphadenitis is accompanied by the chancre present at the anogenital or oral port of entry and lasts 2–4 weeks. The secondary stage shows skin rash, mucosal macules and papules, and condyloma lata, which occur 6–8 weeks after the onset of the disease. Lymphadenitis may be present in early tertiary syphilis.

The smear pattern in the primary infection shows prominent lymphoid hyperplasia, scattered immunoblasts, and small lymphocytes. Numerous plasma cells are present. Small, noncaseating granulomas may be present. The spirochetes are identified by dark-field examination of exudates and the silver Warthin–Starry stain. Immunofluorescence and immunoperoxidase stains with specific antibodies against *T. pallidum* as well as PCR to amplify *T. pallidum* DNA are also used. The diagnosis is supported by serologic tests for syphilis.

Whipple Disease

Lymphadenitis of Whipple disease is caused by *Tropheryma whipplei*, a rod-shaped bacillus classified as an actinomycete. Whipple disease affects the GI tract and other organs, including peripheral (predominantly axillary and cervical) and mesenteric lymph nodes. Peripheral lymphadenitis may be the first evidence of the disease. The organism is phagocytosed and degraded by macrophages, which infiltrate the lamina propria of the GI tract, producing a malabsorption syndrome, fever, and weight loss. Antibiotic therapy for at least 1 year is recommended.

The lymph nodes show numerous single and loose aggregates of foamy macrophages that contain a PAS positive, diastase resistant material. Small granulomas and multinucleated cells may be seen. The organisms appear granular within the macrophages when stained with anti-*T. whipplei* antibody. The macrophages are CD68+. PCR may be used for amplifying the ribosomal genes.

Mycobacteria

Mycobacteria are aerobic acid-fast bacilli. Organisms that are highly pathogenic to humans include *Mycobacterium tuberculosis*, *Mycobacterium leprae*, and atypical or nontuberculous mycobacteria.

The *M. tuberculosis* is prevalent in HIV-infected individuals and in foreign-born young immigrants to the United States. The most common form of extrapulmonary tuberculosis is lymphadenitis that commonly affects cervical (frequently posterior triangle) and supraclavicular, mediastinal, and axillary chains in decreasing order of frequency. The lymph nodes may be matted and markedly necrotic and fluctuant. Postimmunization with bacillus Calmette–Guerin (BCG) may result in axillary lymphadenitis, which is seen after an interval of 10 weeks up to 3 years after vaccination and which resolves spontaneously or may require surgical excision. The *M. tuberculosis* is engulfed by macrophages and is transported to the lymph nodes or other locations where they can remain quiescent for years. The bacilli activate CD4+ T-cells and produce tissue necrosis, and the macrophages transform into uni- or multinucleated epithelioid macrophages. Thus, the smears of tuberculous lymphadenitis show epithelioid granulomas, caseation necrosis, lymphocytes, and occasional Langhans-type giant cells. The bacilli can be detected by special acid-fast staining and are detected predominantly in the background smear. The presence of acid-fast bacilli in smears is directly proportional to the necrosis and inversely to the granulomas. The bacilli are bright red, slender, and beaded by the Ziehl–Neelsen acid-fast stain (Figs. 12.5 and 12.6); however, only 20% of culture-positive cases have a positive stain. Culture in Lowenstein–Jensen medium can take up to 6 weeks for a definitive diagnosis, thus delaying treatment. Polymerase chain

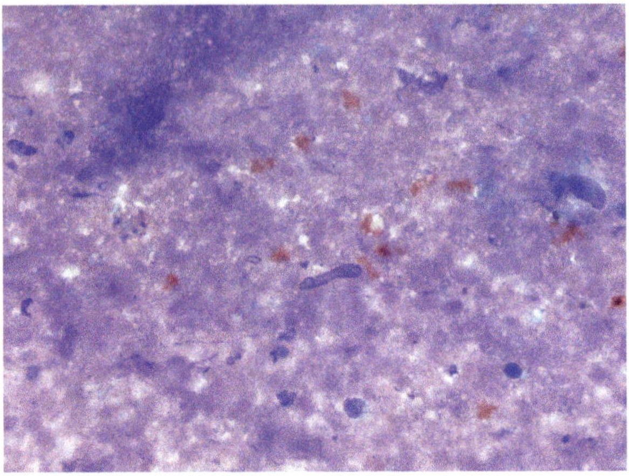

FIGURE 12.5. Mycobacterium tuberculosis. A background of necrosis is present with scattered stripped nuclei of epithelioid cells. (DiffQuik, high magnification).

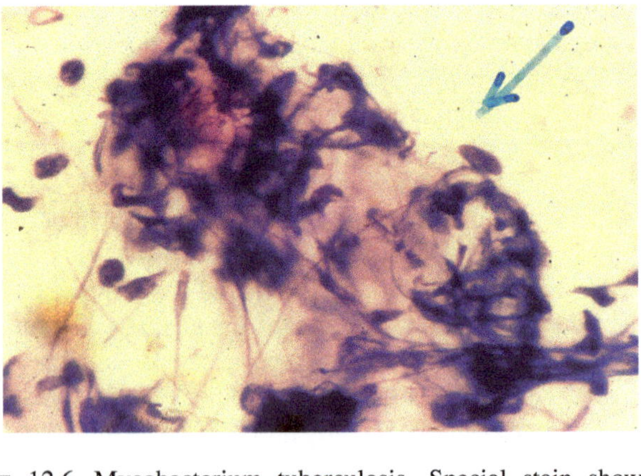

FIGURE 12.6. Mycobacterium tuberculosis. Special stain shows rare bright red, slender, and beaded bacilli (Ziehl–Neelsen acid-fast stain, high magnification).

reaction in fluids, smears, and tissue samples, including paraffin-embedded tissue, can detect the organism in less than 6 h. Indirect evidence of infection is obtained by skin test positivity in infants or recent conversion in adults. The differential diagnosis includes *M. avium*-intracellulare complex (MAI) infection, histoplasma, Kikuchi, and cat-scratch lymphadenitis and sarcoidosis.

Atypical mycobacteria are a cause of chronic granulomatous lymphadenitis in children. In adults, the infection occurs in the presence of immunosuppression. The organisms are widely spread in nature and include *M. marinum*, *M. fortuitum*, *M. scrofulaceum*, and *M. kansasii*. Commonly affected sites include cervical lymph nodes and may be associated with erythema of the overlying skin and abscess formation. MAI, found in the soil and tap water, is highly pathogenic in patients with AIDS and may produce regional or generalized lymphadenitis and systemic disease. The smears show necrosis, poorly formed granulomas, and numerous large histiocytes with foamy cytoplasm (pseudo-Gaucher cells) filled with bacilli (Figs. 12.7 and 12.8). Occasionally, the histiocytes develop a spindle-cell phenotype (MAI spindle-cell pseudotumor). The characteristic negative images within the

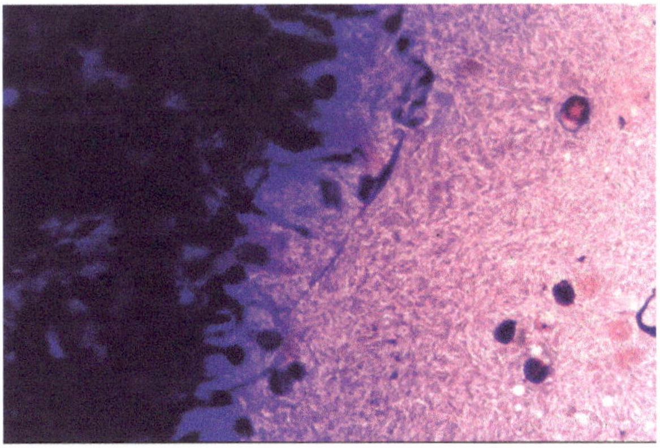

FIGURE 12.7. Atypical mycobacteria. Numerous bacilli seen as negative images are identified in the background along with a poorly formed granuloma (DiffQuik stain, high magnification).

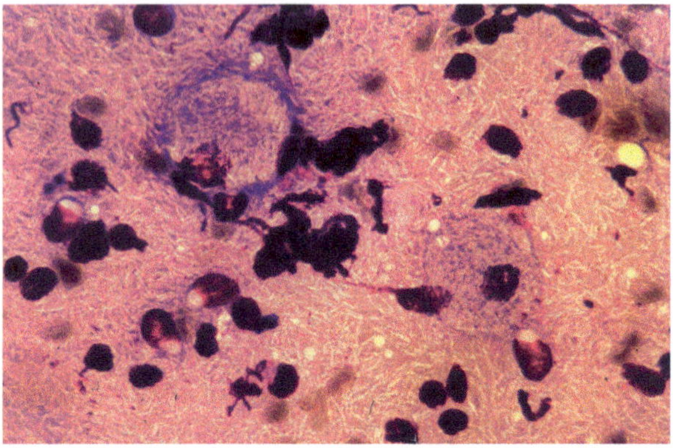

FIGURE 12.8. Atypical mycobacteria. Numerous bacilli seen as negative images are identified in the background and within ballooned histiocytes (DiffQuik stain, high magnification).

cytoplasm of macrophages and in the background are best seen in Romanovsky-stained smears. The definite diagnosis is made by cultures and polymerase chain reaction in smears and formalin-fixed, paraffin embedded tissue.

The *M. leprae* lymphadenitis is usually associated with skin lesions and peripheral nerve involvement, although it may be the initial manifestation of the disease with nonapparent skin or nerve involvement, and occurs in any stage of the disease process from lepromatous to tuberculoid leprosy. Inguinal, cervical, axillary, epitrochlear, and preauricular lymph nodes are commonly affected. In lepromatous leprosy, the lymph nodes are large and show variable numbers of foamy histiocytes laden with bacilli, reactive germinal center lymphocytes, and plasma cells (Figs. 12.9 and 12.10). In tuberculoid leprosy, the lymph nodes are smaller and show non-necrotizing granulomas, Langhans-type giant cells, predominantly small lymphocytes, and rare bacilli. Because the organisms do not grow in vitro, demonstration by acid-fast stain, clinical findings, and skin test (lepromin test) is necessary for diagnosis.

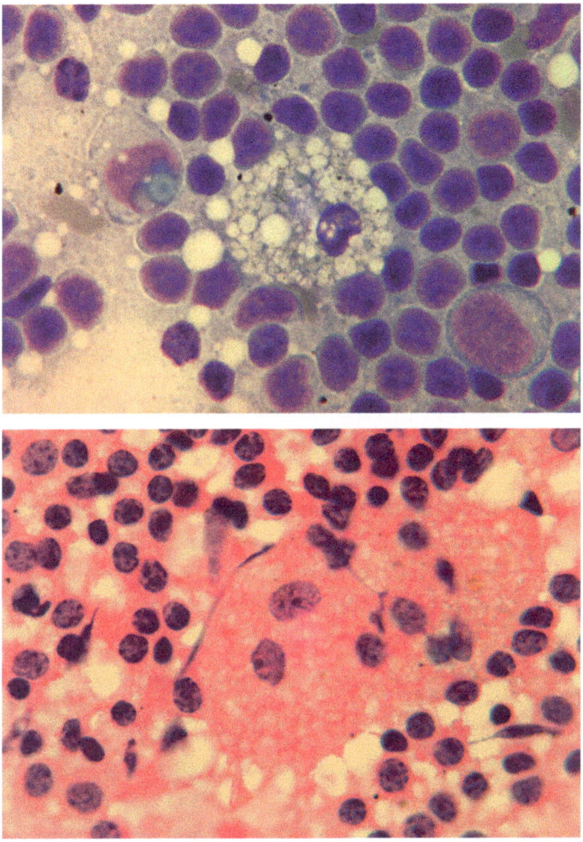

FIGURES 12.9–12.10. Leprosy. Variable numbers of foamy histiocytes in a background of reactive germinal center lymphocytes are present in these cases. The cytoplasmic bacilli may not be readily visible (*Top*, DiffQuik and *bottom*, hematoxylin and eosin stains, high magnification).

Fungal Lymphadenitis

Fungal infections may involve the lymph nodes, particularly when immunocompetency is affected. The prevalence of these infections is influenced by the incidence of mycoses, i.e., histoplasmosis and coccidioidomycosis in certain geographic areas. The identification of the organism in cytologic material permits the application of early antifungal therapy before culture and serologic results are available.

Cryptococcus

Cryptococcus neoformans, a monomorphic fungus that forms only spores, is found in bird nests and pigeon feces. The infection is transmitted by inhaling of the organism and involves the lung and mediastinal lymph nodes, particularly in patients who have AIDS, hematolymphoid malignancies, systemic diseases, or are on corticosteroid therapy. The lymph node smears show scattered yeast forms, both extracellular and within the histiocytes, in a background of abundant mucoid material (Fig. 12.11). Multinucleated cells and granulomas may be seen. The yeasts show frequent narrow-based buds and are surrounded by a thick mucoid capsule that stains with mucicarmine and PAS stains. India ink can also detect the yeasts. Sarcoidosis, regardless of the corticosteroid

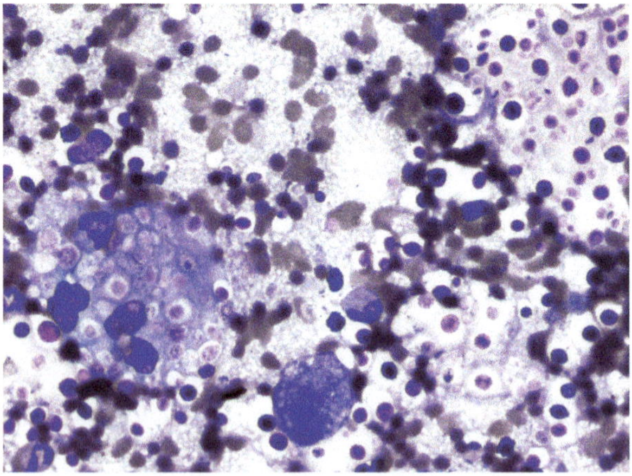

FIGURE 12.11. Cryptococcosis. Features characteristic include abundant intracellular and extracellular mucin. The narrow-based budding organisms are surrounded by a clear hallo (DiffQuik stain, high magnification).

therapy, seems to be a risk factor for cryptococcosis. Culture and serologic tests in peripheral blood and cerebrospinal fluid confirm the diagnosis.

Pneumocystis

This infection is common in AIDS patients and is caused by *Pneumocystis jiroveci*, formerly called *Pneumocystis carinii*, and predominantly causes bilateral pneumonia. Occasionally, the infection is systemic, affecting other organs including lymph nodes, predominantly mediastinal and retroperitoneal. The lymph nodes show necrosis, lymphocytes, rare giant cells, and eosinophilic foamy exudates containing the characteristic cup-shaped organisms that are best seen with Grocott's methenamine-silver stain. Immunofluorescence and polymerase chain reaction methods can be used for diagnosis.

Histoplasma

Histoplasmosis is endemic in the Mississippi and Ohio River valleys in the Midwest and in Central South areas of the United States and in Central America. Histoplasma capsulatum is dimorphic and is transmitted by bats, birds, and chicken feces that contaminate the soil. The airborne yeasts are inhaled. The primary infection is controlled in immunocompetent individuals, or the infection disseminates and involves several organs including mediastinal and cervical lymph nodes in immunosuppressed individuals. The lymph-node cytology preparations show granulomas, multinucleated giant cells, and epithelioid histiocytes containing cytoplasmic yeasts that appear as round, small intracytoplasmic vacuoles measuring 2–4 μm in diameter. Necrosis and calcific deposits are present in the background. A positive silver stain showing yeast forms in a background of necrosis may be sufficient to initiate antifungal therapy in the appropriate clinical setting (Figs. 12.12–12.15). Serologic tests must be supported by culture results for a definitive diagnosis.

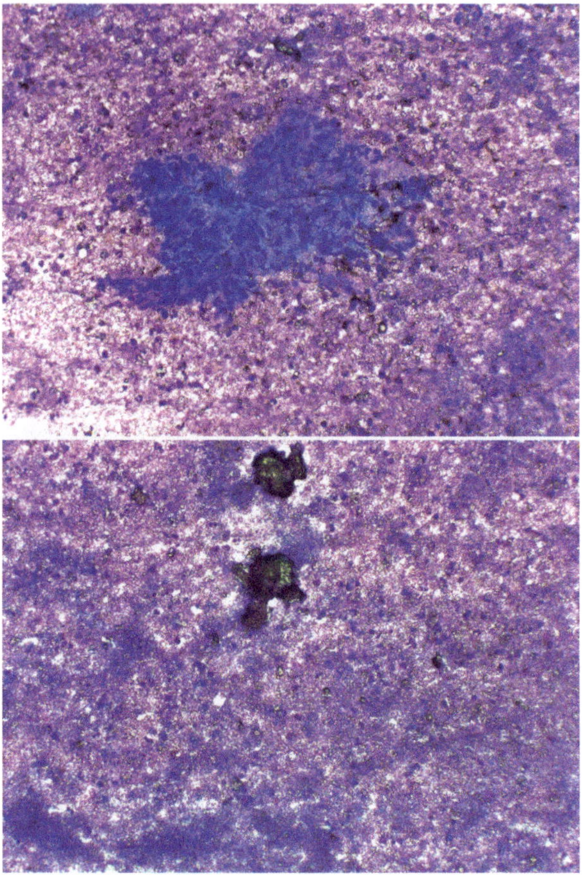

FIGURES 12.12–12.13. Histoplasmosis. Granulomas with extensive necrosis and calcium deposits can be seen in mediastinal lymphadenitis due to *H. capsulatum* (DiffQuik stain, high magnification).

Coccidioides

Coccidioidomycosis is endemic in the southwestern region of the United States, particularly in the San Joaquin Valley of Southern California, New Mexico, and Arizona, Mexico, and South America. *Coccidioidis immitis* is dimorphic and remains in the soil as mycelial infective forms, which are acquired by

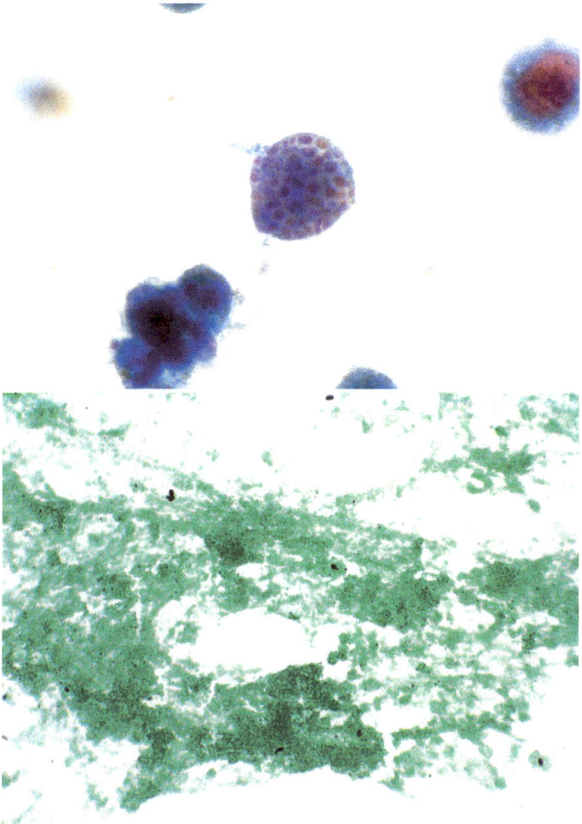

FIGURES 12.14–12.15. Histoplasmosis. The spores are intracellular and can be detected in the necrotic background using a silver stain (*Top*, Papanicolaou stain, and *bottom* Grocott's methenamine-silver stain, high magnification).

inhalation under windy and dry-weather conditions. Like tuberculosis and histoplasmosis, the primary infection is pulmonary. Systemic disease involving various organs including lymph nodes is seen in immunosuppressed individuals, particularly in those with AIDS. Cytology preparations show granulomas, epithelioid histiocytes, Langhans-type giant cells containing the organisms, lymphocytes, plasma cells, and a background of necrosis. The yeast forms or sporangia are present in the form of large spherules which have a thick capsule containing small yeasts (Figs. 12.16 and 12.17). The organisms are best seen with PAS and silver stains. Serologic tests, immunofluorescence, and culture confirm the diagnosis.

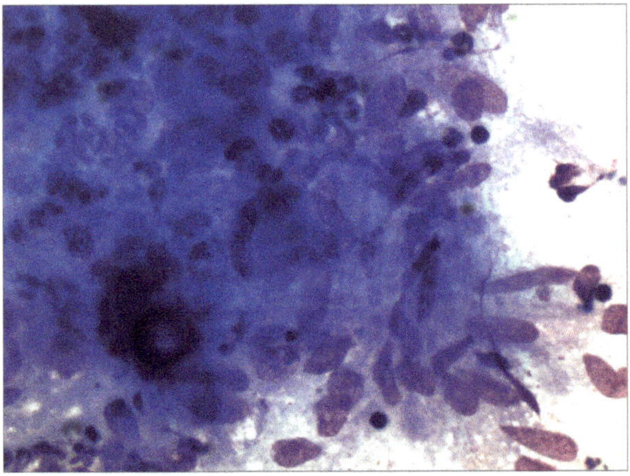

FIGURE 12.16. Coccidioidomycosis. A granuloma with an empty spherule in the left lower quadrant is seen in the Giemsa stained figure. (high magnification).

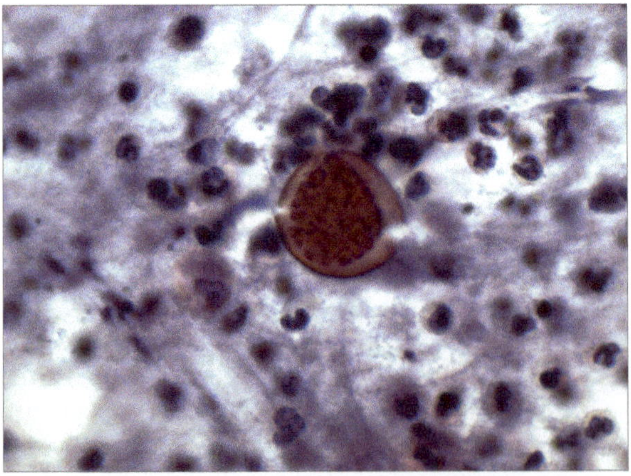

FIGURE 12.17. Coccidioidomycosis. The large spherule containing spores is best seen with the Papanicolaou stain (high magnification).

Protozoal Lymphadenitis

Toxoplasma

See Chap. 7. Toxoplasmosis is caused by *Toxoplasma gondii*, which is present in the cat intestine, the definitive host. Humans and other mammals are the intermediary hosts and are infected by ingestion of oocysts present in soil contaminated with cat feces. The trophozoites are released in the human intestine and are carried within macrophages in the circulation in the form of tachyzoites to other organs; the organisms are crescent shaped and measure 2–6 μm. Bradyzoites are slow multiplying forms within cysts that remain for long periods. In contrast to the life-threatening acute multiorgan form that affects immunocompromised patients, isolated toxoplasma lymphadenitis occurs in immunocompetent individuals, commonly affecting posterior cervical lymph nodes, and may be asymptomatic. Cytologic preparations show marked reactive lymphoid hyperplasia, monocytoid cells, scattered histiocytes, tingible-body macrophages, and rare plasma cells. Small granulomas are present in smears. However, multinucleated giant cells, necrosis, neutrophils, or eosinophils are not identified. The organisms, rarely found in immunocompetent individuals, are best seen in Romanovsky-stained preparations (Fig. 12.18). The findings must be correlated with serologic tests or confirmed by identification of the parasite. Other identification tests include immunoperoxidase or immunofluorescence with anti-Toxoplasma antibodies in tissue sections.

Leishmania

See Chap. 7. Leishmaniasis is endemic in South America, Africa, and Asia. *Leishmania donovani* is transmitted by sandflies (*Phlebotomus* sp.) that are the vectors. The natural reservoirs are various mammals, including dogs and cats. The promastigote, a flagellate form, is present in the insect and is transmitted to humans by sandfly bites. In human tissues, the promastigote is transformed into an amastigote and is phagocytosed by macrophages. Amastigotes are round or ovoid organisms measuring 1–3 μm and have a large nucleus and a characteristic rod-shaped kinetoplast. Both visceral (common in Africa) and cutaneous (common in South America)

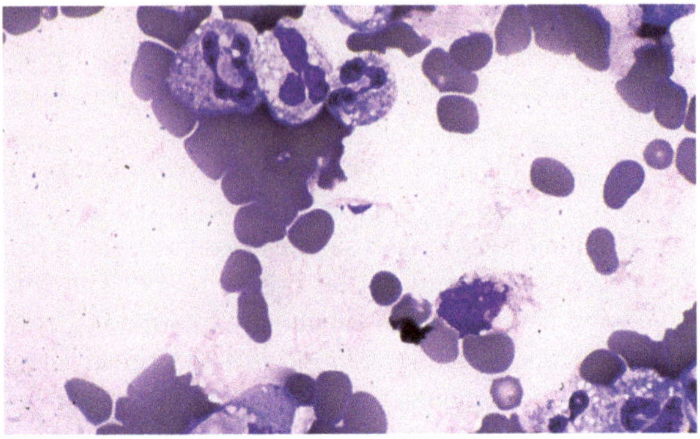

FIGURE 12.18. Toxoplasmosis. The crescent-shaped organism (center of frame) is best seen with Romanovsky-stained preparations (DiffQuik stain, high magnification).

leishmaniasis have regional lymphadenitis commonly affecting epitrochlear followed by inguinal and axillary lymph nodes that are slightly enlarged, firm, and nontender. Cytologic preparations show lymphoid hyperplasia, scattered epithelioid histiocytes, necrosis, and rare multinucleated giant cells. Small granulomas may be present in some cases. The amastigotes (Leishman–Donovan bodies) may be seen in the cytoplasm of histiocytes and giant cells, particularly in anergic conditions. The amastigotes can be detected in tissue sections by immunohistochemistry with monoclonal antibodies. However, cytology preparations have proved to have a higher diagnostic yield (Fig. 12.19).

Filaria

Wuchereria bancrofti (common in Africa and in Central and South America), *Onchocerca volvulus*, and *Brugia malayi* (common in Asia and South America), among others, are nematode worms that cause lymphatic filariasis. Mosquitoes are the intermediary hosts and vectors. The insect bite that penetrates the skin inoculates the infective larvae, enters the circulation, and settles in a suitable location to become an adult worm. In man, the filaria can live for years in the lymphatic system, including lymph nodes. Cervical, axillary,

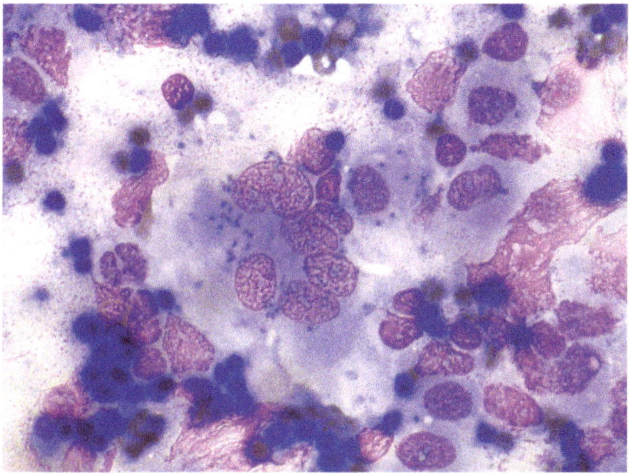

FIGURE 12.19. Leishmaniasis. The amastigotes (Leishman–Donovan bodies) are seen in the cytoplasm of histiocytes. Cytology preparations have proved to have a higher diagnostic yield than tissue sections. (Giemsa stain, high magnification). Courtesy of Dr. Yahya Daneshbod, Hematopathologist, Department of Pathology, Dr Daneshbod Laboratory, Shiraz, Iran.

and inguinal lymph nodes may be affected and tender. Cytology preparations show reactive lymphoid hyperplasia, histiocytes, small granulomas, necrosis, giant cells, and numerous eosinophils. Fragments of dead calcified organisms may be identified.

Non-neoplastic, Noninfectious Lymphadenopathies

Reactive Lymphoid Hyperplasia

This process has been treated in Chap. 7.

Kimura Lymphadenopathy

See Chap. 7. This inflammatory disorder is endemic in Asian countries and is characterized histologically by angiolymphoid hyperplasia with peripheral-blood eosinophilia. It involves the subcutaneous tissue and lymph nodes in the head and neck region of young adults, with a male predominance. High levels of serum IgE are a feature of this process. No pathogen has been demonstrated. The lymph nodes are enlarged and matted, simulating a neoplastic process. Cytology preparations show a reactive follicular hyperplasia, endothelial cells, eosinophils, and giant cells with a grape-like nuclear arrangement (Warthin–Finkeldey type). Occasionally, the pattern resembles that in Hodgkin lymphoma. Thus, lymph node excision is suggested for definitive diagnosis. The process may involve the adjacent salivary gland.

Kikuchi Disease

This subacute necrotizing lymphadenitis of unknown etiology is particularly common in young Asian individuals, with a slight female predominance. It is rare in Western countries. The cervical lymph nodes are often involved, and less commonly the axillary and inguinal lymph nodes. Involvement of deep lymph nodes and extranodal sites is rare. The process is self-limited and resolves spontaneously in weeks to months. Cytology preparations show necrosis, scattered histiocytes, some with eccentrically placed nuclei (plasmacytoid monocytes), tingible-body macrophages, and plasma cells (Fig. 12.20). The lesional cells show an immature dendritic-cell phenotype.

Rosai–Dorfman Disease

The etiology of this disease, also called massive lymphadenopathy with sinus histiocytosis, remains unknown. It is geographically widespread in all races and occurs at any age, although it predominates in young males with a ratio 3:2 for females; it may involve extranodal sites, frequently in the head and neck. The patients remain healthy despite the massive matted lymphadenopathy that commonly involves the cervical region. Cytologic preparations show lymphocytes, plasma cells, and large histiocytes with abundant cytoplasm, a single nucleus, and an occasional nucleolus. The cytoplasm contains vacuoles with engulfed lymphocytes

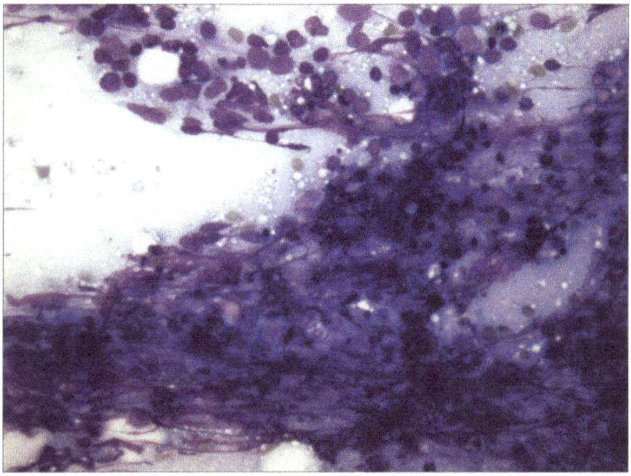

FIGURE 12.20. Kikuchi disease. Extensive necrosis and scattered reactive lymphocytes are seen in this case (Giemsa stain, medium magnification).

(emperipolesis), red blood cells, and plasma cells in various numbers (Figs. 12.21 and 12.22). Histiocytes may be large and atypical with hyperchromatic nuclei. Granulomas or necrosis are absent. The histiocytes are positive for S100 protein and CD68. T-cell and B-cell antigen receptor genes are germline, and HHV-6 and -8 as well as EBV by ISH are negative.

Sarcoidosis

Sarcoidosis is a multisystem disease of unknown etiology. It is widespread geographically although it predominates in African-Americans of any age, commonly affecting patients between the third and fifth decades of life. The organs affected include mediastinal lymph nodes, lungs, peripheral lymph nodes, liver, eyes, skin, and other organs in decreasing order of frequency. The patients commonly have chronic respiratory symptoms and mediastinal lymphadenopathy that may be sampled by endoscopic ultrasound-guided FNA. The smears are sparsely cellular and show damaged lymphoid cells and granulomas with no necrosis; however, small foci of necrosis may be present. The granulomas are

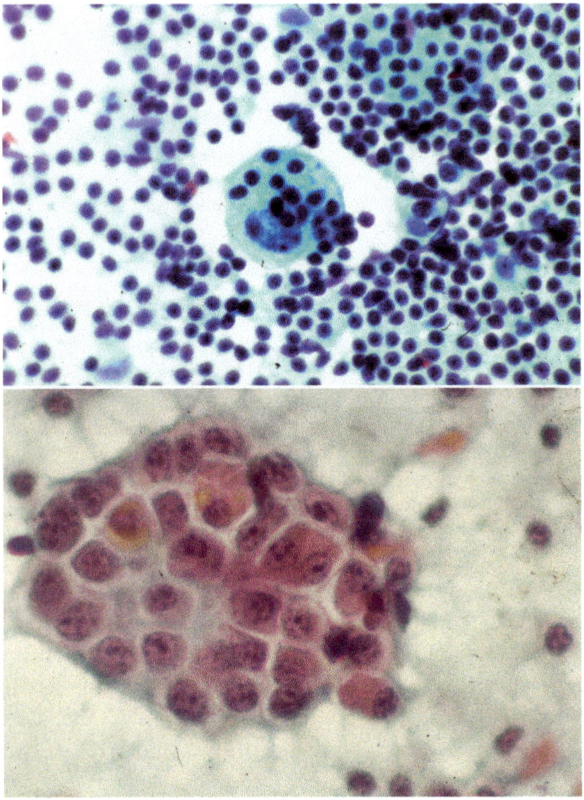

FIGURES 12.21–12.22. Rosai–Dorfman disease. Lymphocytes (Top) and plasma cells (bottom) have been engulfed in these two cases (*Top*, Diff-Quik stain and *bottom* hematoxylin and eosin stain, high magnification).

composed of tightly packed histiocytes (Fig. 12.23). Occasionally, Langhans-type multinucleated giant cells showing the characteristic Schaumann (basophilic concentrically laminated) and asteroid bodies (red spider-like inclusions) are present. The granulomas rapidly resolve after steroid therapy or spontaneously, leaving a small scar. The diagnosis of sarcoidosis is made after exclusion of granulomatous infectious processes. There are no specific confirmatory tests for sarcoidosis.

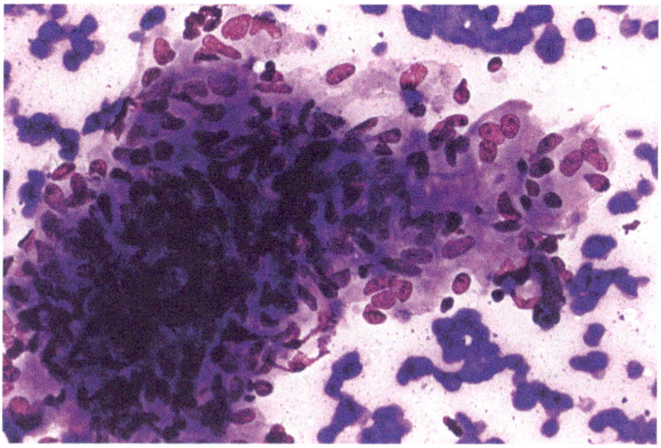

FIGURE 12.23. Sarcoidosis. Granulomas with tightly packed histiocytes and absence of necrosis are characteristic in sarcoidosis (DiffQuik stain, high magnification).

Collagen Vascular Diseases

Systemic lupus erythematosus (SLE) lymphadenopathy usually correlates with the severity of the disease, affects young individuals, and may be regional or generalized (12% of cases), involving cervical, mesenteric, axillary, inguinal, and retroperitoneal lymph nodes in decreasing order of frequency. The incidence of lymphadenopathy in SLE appears to have dropped in the last four decades. Indications for FNA include the exclusion of non-Hodgkin lymphoma or infection. Cytologic preparations show necrosis and plasma cells that may have Russell bodies, and no neutrophils or eosinophils. Reactive follicular hyperplasia and amorphous necrotic basophilic material (hematoxylin bodies) may be seen in the background. The smear pattern must be distinguished from the necrotizing lymphadenopathy of Kikuchi disease based on serology and the presence of hematoxylin bodies. See Chap. 7 for more details.

Rheumatoid arthritis lymphadenopathy (see Chap. 7) is present in up to 75% of patients and may be localized or generalized, commonly accompanied by constitutional symptoms. The lymph nodes are nontender and nonmatted. When localized, it affects mainly axillary, cervical, and supraclavicular lymph nodes, although it can occur in other regions. FNA is performed to exclude lymphoma, the risk of which is increased in these patients, and infections. Cytologic preparations show marked follicular hyperplasia and numerous plasma cells, as described in Chap. 7 (Fig. 12.24). Occasionally, an atypical immunoblastic and lymphoplasmacytic proliferation is identified.

Castleman Disease

The etiology of CD or angiofollicular lymph node hyperplasia is unknown. The hyaline vascular (HV-CD) and plasma-cell (PC-CD) variants can be unicentric or multicentric (MCD). There is no evidence of light-chain restriction in CD. The human herpes virus type 8 (HHV-8) or Kaposi sarcoma herpes virus has been shown in 50% of cases of PC-CD.

The HV-CD comprises most cases of CD and usually affects young patients, with equal incidence in males and females. The patients are usually asymptomatic and have mass-effect signs and symptoms due to massive mediastinal adenopathy, the mediastinum being the region most commonly affected. Other lymph nodes may

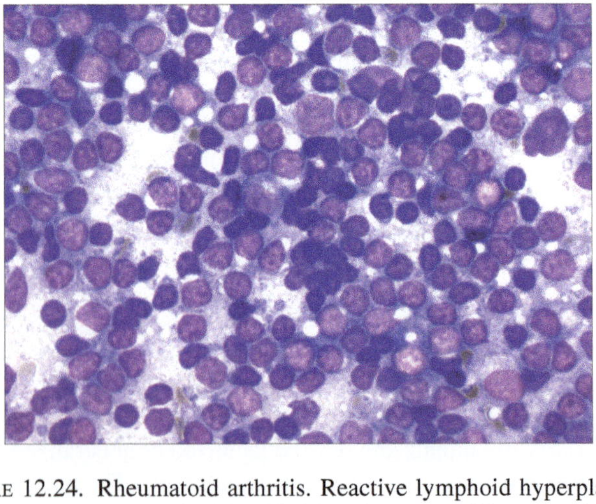

FIGURE 12.24. Rheumatoid arthritis. Reactive lymphoid hyperplasia is seen. Plasma cells may be identified in other cases (Giemsa stain, high magnification).

be affected. Cytology preparations show a predominance of small lymphocytes originating in the broad mantle zones and few germinal center cells as a result of the depleted germinal centers (Fig. 12.25). Plasmacytoid monocytes, immunoblasts, and rare plasma cells are also seen. See Chap. 8 for more details.

PC-CD comprises the minority of cases, equally affects males and females, and occurs in patients older than those affected by HV-CD. The patients may be asymptomatic or have constitutional symptoms. Any lymph node chain can be affected. Follicular hyperplasia and sheets of mature plasma cells, some binucleated, are seen in the cytology preparations from HHV-8-negative PC-CD. In contrast, in HHV-8 positive cases, the smears show follicular hyperplasia and plasma cells that range from mature, immature, to atypical cells.

Most cases of MCD have been under-recognized as PC-CD. The patients usually have constitutional symptoms and commonly are associated with HHV-8 positivity. Abdominal and peripheral lymphadenopathy is usually present. Coexistence of a chronic infectious process, including Kaposi sarcoma and HIV, is frequent in these patients.

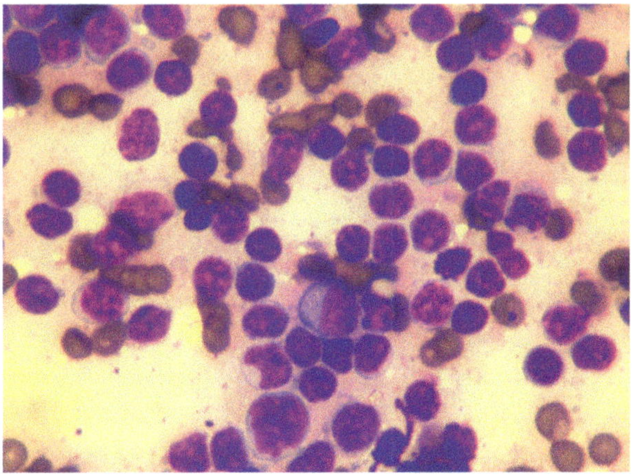

FIGURE 12.25. Castleman disease, hyaline vascular variant. Cytology preparations show a predominance of small lymphocytes originating in the broad mantle zones (DiffQuik stain, high magnification). Courtesy of Dr. Luis de las Casas, Pathologist, Department of Pathology, Texas Tech University, El Paso Texas.

Dermatopathic Lymphadenopathy

See Chap. 7. This is a reactive lymphadenopathy frequently associated with a benign or malignant dermatologic lesion that occurs in the territory of lymphatic drainage. The eliciting agents include drainage of melanin or other skin antigens into a lymph node, commonly axillary and inguinal. Histologically, the lymph node shows paracortical hyperplasia, and cytologic preparations show numerous interdigitating dendritic cells (IDCs) and Langerhans cells, small lymphocytes, scattered plasma cells, and eosinophils. Cytologically, the histiocytes may contain lipid vacuoles or pigment, mostly melanin, in the cytoplasm (Fig. 12.26). Both IDCs and Langerhans cells are positive for S100 protein and negative for CD68. Histiocytes are positive for CD68 and S100 protein. In contrast to IDC, Langerhans cells are positive for CD1a.

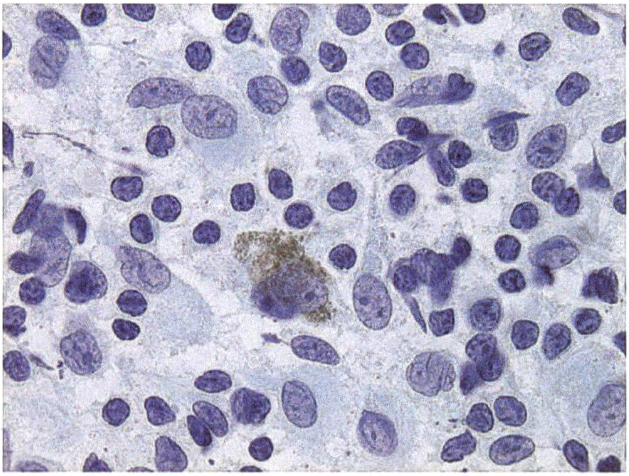

FIGURE 12.26. Dermatopathic lymphadenopathy. Cytologically, the histiocytes may contain lipid vacuoles or pigment, mostly melanin, in the cytoplasm and numerous Langerhans cells and lymphocytes. In this particular case, the lymphocytes have cerebriform nuclei corresponding to a coexistent Sezary syndrome (hematoxylin and eosin stain, high magnification). Courtesy of Dr. Javier Saenz de Santamaria, Pathologist, Department of Pathology, Complejo Universitario de Badajoz, Spain.

Lymphoepithelial Lesions

Cystic lymphoepithelial lesions are part of the spectrum of HIV-related lymphadenitis of the salivary gland lymph nodes. Patients usually have masses in the parotid gland area that represent lymph nodes with marked reactive lymphoid hyperplasia or cystically dilated, keratin containing lesions as a result of squamous metaplasia and duct obstruction. FNA smears show keratin and reactive lymphocytes (Fig. 12.27). Multinucleated giant cells of foreign body type may be present when the cystic lesions rupture into the surrounding lymphoid tissue. Oncocytic cells and macrophages are seen in Warthin tumor and distinguish it from a lymphoepithelial lesion.

Tumor-Associated Lymphadenopathy

Tumor-draining regional lymph nodes are usually enlarged and show paracortical and follicular hyperplasia and sinus histiocytosis. The smears reflect the various histologic patterns, including lymphocyte predominance, germinal-center predominance, sinus histiocytosis, lymphocyte depletion, and granulomatous reaction alone or in various combinations (Fig. 12.28).

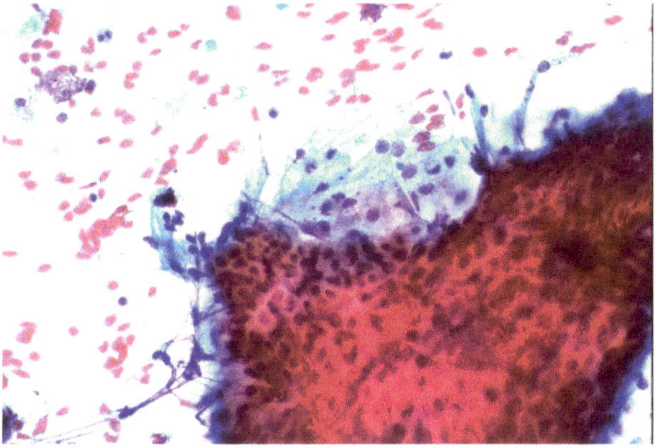

FIGURE 12.27. Lymphoepithelial cyst. An intact small fragment of squamous epithelium with rare crushed lymphocytes in the *left border* is seen. Numerous anucleated squamous cells were identified in other areas of the smear (Papanicolaou stain, high magnification).

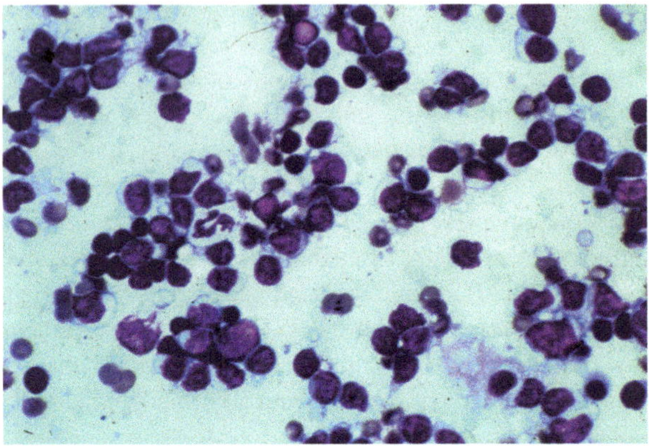

FIGURE 12.28. Tumor-associated lymphadenopathy. The cytology smears reflect the various histologic patterns, including reactive lymphoid hyperplasia as seen in this case. Metastatic melanoma was detected in adjacent lymph nodes (DiffQuik stain, high magnification).

Drug-Induced Lymphadenopathy

Drugs such as methotrexate, azathioprine, sulfasalazine, and cyclophosphamide have linked to the development of lymphoproliferative disorders. Methotrexate, often used in the treatment of rheumatoid arthritis and severe psoriasis, is the most common. This lymphoproliferative disorder, almost always of B-cell type, occurs from months to several years after initiation of therapy. In some cases, the process regresses after cessation of therapy. The cytologic preparation may show polymorphous reactive follicular cells, immunoblasts, histiocytes, and plasma cells or a monotonous population of immunoblasts or centroblasts. Other types of non-Hodgkin lymphoma and Hodgkin lymphoma, often extranodal, have also been described. EBV is common in methotrexate-related lymphoproliferative disorders. The clinical history is useful for the final diagnosis.

Anticonvulsant drugs such as phenytoin and carbamazepine can produce lymphadenopathy that mimics malignant lymphoma. Anticonvulsant lymphadenopathy can be regional or generalized, develops in 75% of patients, and occurs between 2 and 8 weeks after initiation of therapy, often accompanied by fever and skin rash. The clinical picture can regress after cessation of therapy. Histologically, there is paracortical hyperplasia. Cytologic preparations show a prominent immunoblastic proliferation (Fig. 12.29) and scattered lymphocytes, histiocytes, plasma cells, and eosinophils. Occasional Reed–Sternberg-like cells and focal necrosis may be seen. In equivocal cases, the absence of light chain restriction by flow cytometry and/or gene rearrangements by molecular analysis supports the diagnosis of drug-induced lymphadenopathy. Other responsible drugs include phenobarbital, propylthiouracil, methimazole, quinidine, indomethacin, phenylbutazone, gold, and methyldopa.

Foreign-Body Lymphadenopathy

Both endogenous (lipids and proteins) and exogenous (often therapeutic) agents draining into the lymph nodes are phagocytosed by transformed histiocytes, i.e., multinucleated giant cells, macrophages, and epithelioid cells.

Amyloid lymphadenopathy may be seen in primary (AL type) and secondary (AA type) amyloidosis and is almost always a part

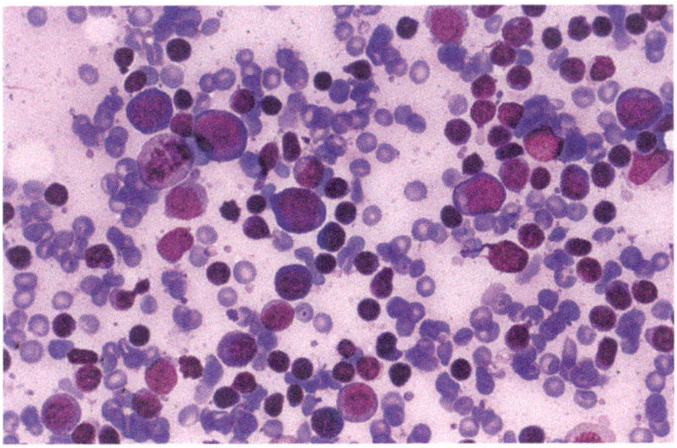

FIGURE 12.29. Anticonvulsant lymphadenopathy. Cytologic preparations show a prominent immunoblastic proliferation (DiffQuik stain, high magnification).

of the systemic process and not an isolated finding. The involved lymph nodes do not always follow the lymphatic drainage of the organ containing amyloid deposits. The presence of AL amyloidosis in the involved lymph node is associated with plasma-cell myeloma, lymphoproliferative disorder, or idiopathic amyloidosis, and further evaluation is indicated. The presence of AA amyloidosis is secondary to a chronic process such as rheumatoid arthritis, tuberculosis, osteomyelitis, or lymphoma, among others. The aspirates show amorphous and acellular material (Fig. 12.30). Small lymphocytes and multinucleated giant cells may be present. With Congo red stain, the amyloid stains slightly orange under light microscopy and apple green under polarized light. The amyloid deposits are composed of randomly distributed, nonbranching fine fibrils when examined by electron microscopy.

Silicone lymphadenopathy can mimic clinically metastatic cancer. In cases of breast implants, a microscopic leakage can cause axillary or a more distal lymphadenopathy or even a solid organ deposit. Cytologic preparations show multinucleated giant cells of the foreign-body type, laden with or surrounded by silicone particles that appear as fine and foamy vacuoles in the cytoplasm (Fig. 12.31).

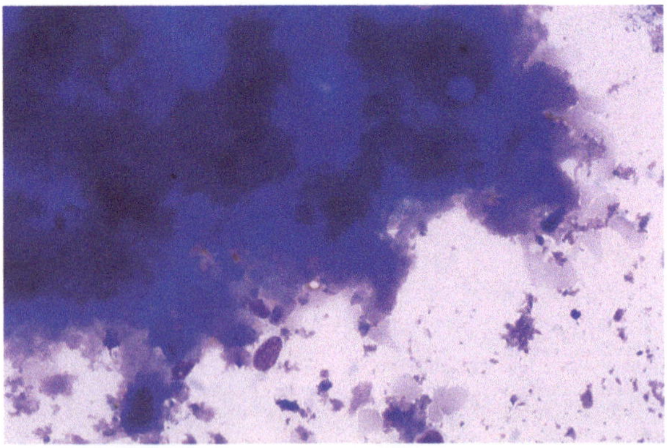

FIGURE 12.30. Amyloidosis. Cytologic preparations show amorphous and acellular material and granulomas and scattered histiocytes (not in this picture) (DiffQuik stain, high magnification).

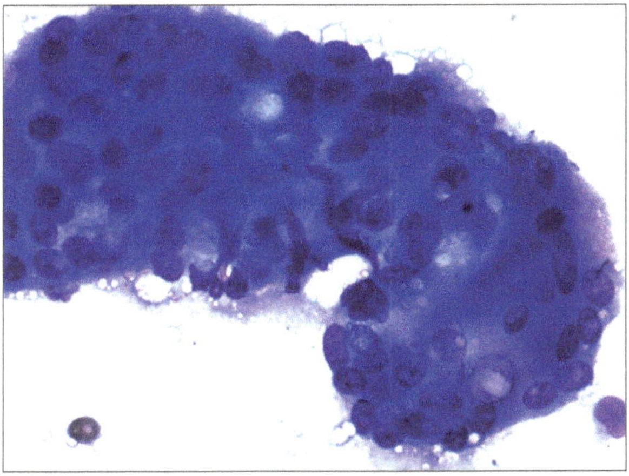

FIGURE 12.31. Silicone. Cytologic preparations show foreign-body-type multinucleated giant cells, laden with or surrounded by silicone particles that appear as fine and foamy vacuoles in the cytoplasm (Giemsa stain, high magnification).

The silicone is a nonstaining, refractile, and nonpolarizable material that is important for its recognition and differentiation from other material. A history of cosmetic or reconstructive surgery is important.

Lipid lymphadenopathy can be seen in obese patients and in patients who have diabetes mellitus, hyperlipidemia, long-term total parenteral nutrition, chronic cholecystitis, hematomas, or tumors. The characteristic finding is a foreign-body reaction to lipid or lipogranulomas; a pattern of histiocytes with small cytoplasmic vacuoles and multinucleated cells of the giant cell type.

In cases of lymphadenopathy associated with *joint prosthesis* such as the hip, the macrophages and multinucleated giant cells of foreign-body type contain needle-shaped metal particles that stain dark and are refringent under polarized light. *Gold* therapy for rheumatoid arthritis may cause a foreign-body-type giant cell reaction to cytoplasmic black or colorless crystalline nonpolarizable material in a background of follicular hyperplasia (Fig. 12.32).

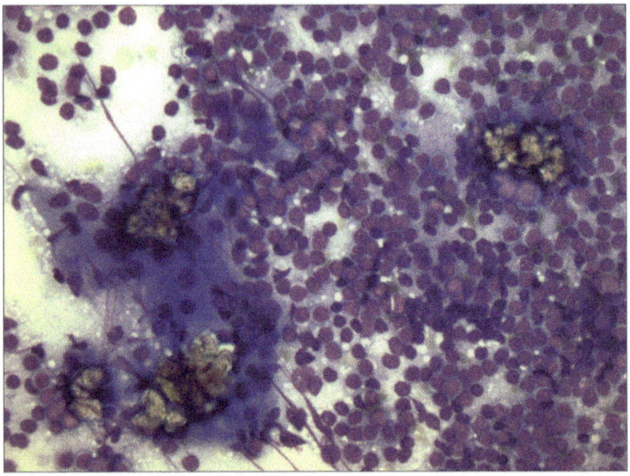

FIGURE 12.32. Gold therapy lymphadenopathy. Foreign-body-type giant cells, refractile crystalline material, and reactive lymphoid hyperplasia were seen in the lymph node cytology smears of a patient with rheumatoid arthritis undergoing therapy with gold salts (Giemsa stain, high magnification).

Suggested Reading

Annema JT, Veselic M et al (2005) Endoscopic ultrasound-guided fine-needle aspiration for the diagnosis of sarcoidosis. Eur Respir J 25(3):405–409

Chow LT, Yuen RW et al (1994) Cytologic features of Kimura's disease in fine-needle aspirates. A study of eight cases. Am J Clin Pathol 102(3):316–321

Daneshbod Y, Daneshbod K et al (2007) New cytologic clues in localized Leishmania lymphadenitis. Acta Cytol 51(5):699–710

Deschenes M, Michel RP et al (2008) Fine-needle aspiration cytology of Castleman disease: case report with review of the literature. Diagn Cytopathol 36(12):904–908

Donnelly A, Hendricks G et al (1995) Cytologic diagnosis of cat scratch disease (CSD) by fine-needle aspiration. Diagn Cytopathol 13(2): 103–106

Ellison E, Yuen SY et al (1995) Fine-needle aspiration diagnosis of extrapulmonary Pneumocystis carinii lymphadenitis in a human immunodeficiency virus positive patient. Diagn Cytopathol 12(3):251–253

Gonzalez-Peramato P, Jimenez-Heffernan JA et al (2002) Lipogranulomatous lymphadenopathy as a potential source of error in fine needle aspiration cytology. A case report. Acta Cytol 46(4):772–775

Hadfield TL, Lamy Y et al (1995) Demonstration of Chlamydia trachomatis in inguinal lymphadenitis of lymphogranuloma venereum: a light microscopy, electron microscopy and polymerase chain reaction study. Mod Pathol 8(9):924–929

Halliday BE, Silverman JF et al (1998) Fine-needle aspiration cytology of amyloid associated with nonneoplastic and malignant lesions. Diagn Cytopathol 18(4):270–275

Ioachim HL, Medeiros LJ (2009) Lymphadenitides. Ioachim's lymph node pathology. Wolters Kluwer Lippincott Williams & Wilkins, Philadelphia, 76–169, 172–291

Jackuliak P, Koller T et al (2008) Whipple's disease-generalized stage. Dig Dis Sci 53(12):3250–3258

Juskevicius R, Finley JL (2001) Rosai-Dorfman disease of the parotid gland: cytologic and histopathologic findings with immunohistochemical correlation. Arch Pathol Lab Med 125(10):1348–1350

Kondratowicz GM, Symmons DP et al (1990) Rheumatoid lymphadenopathy: a morphological and immunohistochemical study. J Clin Pathol 43(2):106–113

Meyer L, Gibbons D et al (1999) Fine-needle aspiration findings in Castleman's disease. Diagn Cytopathol 21(1):57–60

Miliauskas JR, Leong AS (1991) Localized herpes simplex lymphadenitis: report of three cases and review of the literature. Histopathology 19(4):355–360

Pai MR, Adhikari P et al (2000) Fine needle aspiration cytology in systemic lupus erythematosus lymphadenopathy. A case report. Acta Cytol 44(1):67–69

Raab SS, Silverman JF et al (1993) Fine-needle aspiration biopsy of pulmonary coccidiodomycosis. Spectrum of cytologic findings in 73 patients. Am J Clin Pathol 99(5):582–587.

Santos-Briz A Jr, Lopez-Rios F et al (1999) Granulomatous reaction to silicone in axillary lymph nodes. A case report with cytologic findings. Acta Cytol 43(6):1163–1165

Stanley MW, Horwitz CA et al (1990) Negative images of bacilli and mycobacterial infection: a study of fine-needle aspiration smears from lymph nodes in patients with AIDS. Diagn Cytopathol 6(2):118–121

Stanley MW, Steeper TA et al (1990) Fine-needle aspiration of lymph nodes in patients with acute infectious mononucleosis. Diagn Cytopathol 6(5):323–329

van Crevel R, Grefte JM et al (2009) Syphilis presenting as isolated cervical lymphadenopathy: two related cases. J Infect 58(1):76–78

Viguer JM, Jimenez-Heffernan JA et al (2005) Fine needle aspiration of toxoplasmic (Piringer-Kuchinka) lymphadenitis: a cytohistologic correlation study. Acta Cytol 49(2):139–143

Wright CA, van der Burg M et al (2008) Diagnosing mycobacterial lymphadenitis in children using fine needle aspiration biopsy: cytomorphology, ZN staining and autofluorescence – making more of less. Diagn Cytopathol 36(4):245–251

13 Unusual Neoplastic and Nonneoplastic Conditions of Lymph Nodes

Entities that clinically and/or cytologically mimic a lymphoproliferative disorder are described in this chapter.

Hairy Cell Leukemia

Hairy cell leukemia (HCL) is an uncommon mature B-cell neoplasm with cells showing characteristic cytoplasmic projections. HCL is more common in middle-age to elderly than in younger patients and occurs preferentially in men. Patients commonly have pancytopenia and marked splenomegaly and hepatomegaly in 50% of cases. Peripheral lymphadenopathy is mild and uncommon, although retroperitoneal, abdominal, and mediastinal lymph nodes may be involved. However, lymph node evaluation is not conducted regularly for diagnosing HCL.

Cytology preparations show cells of small to medium size with eccentric nuclei, absent or inconspicuous nucleoli, smooth nuclear contours, and light blue cytoplasm with spiculated borders. Characteristically, the cells retain acid phosphatase positivity after tartaric acid treatment; hence, TRAP is a characteristic marker for hairy cells. By flow cytometry, the neoplastic cells are gated in the monocytoid regions, and monotypic light chain, CD20, and CD22 are brightly expressed.

S.E. Pambuccian and R.H. Bardales, *Lymph Node Cytopathology*, Essentials in Cytopathology 10, DOI 10.1007/978-1-4419-6964-4_13,

No characteristic cytogenetic abnormalities have been detected in HCL. The clinical course of HCL is often indolent.

Plasma Cell Neoplasms

Monoclonal gammopathy of undetermined significance (MGUS), plasma cell myeloma, plasmacytoma, primary amyloidosis, and light- and heavy-chain deposition disease are included in this category.

Monoclonal GUS may be associated with connective-tissue disorders, peripheral neuropathies, and with endocrine, dermatologic, and liver diseases. The clinical diagnostic criteria for MGUS include monoclonal protein <30 g/L, <10% bone marrow clonal plasma cells, no lytic lesions, no myeloma-related or tissue impairment, and absence of a B-cell proliferative disorder. The clonal plasma cell proliferation that produces IgM MGUS involves the bone marrow, spleen, and lymph nodes. The clinical course in most patients is stable, with no progression to plasma cell myeloma or amyloidosis (in non-IgM MGUS) or other lymphoproliferative disorder (in IgM MGUS).

Plasma cell myeloma is associated with generalized bone marrow involvement and lytic bone lesions. Extramedullary involvement is a manifestation of advanced disease.

Extramedullary plasmacytomas arise in tissues other than bone. Eighty percent occur in the upper respiratory tract; other sites include the gastrointestinal tract, lymph nodes, bladder, CNS, and breast (Figs. 13.1–13.3).

Lymph node involvement is exceedingly rare in primary amyloidosis and in monoclonal light- and heavy-chain deposition disease.

Myeloid Sarcoma (Figs. 13.4–13.7)

Myeloid sarcoma or chloroma is a tumor of immature myeloid cells that occurs in extramedullary sites and can precede, occur simultaneously, or follow the diagnosis of acute myeloid leukemia. It affects elderly adults especially, with no gender predominance. Myeloid sarcoma can occur in sites such as the subcortical bone

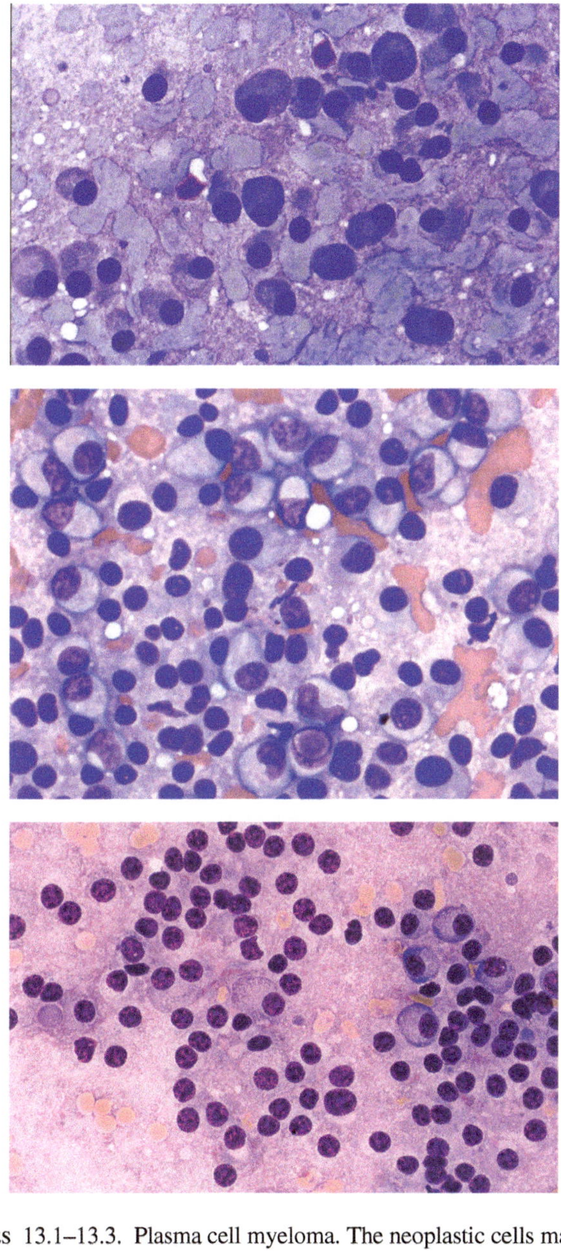

FIGURES 13.1–13.3. Plasma cell myeloma. The neoplastic cells may show various stages of differentiation and the typical cytomorphology may not be that evident in some cases. Figure 13.3 shows aggregates of amyloid in the background. (DiffQuik stain, High magnification).

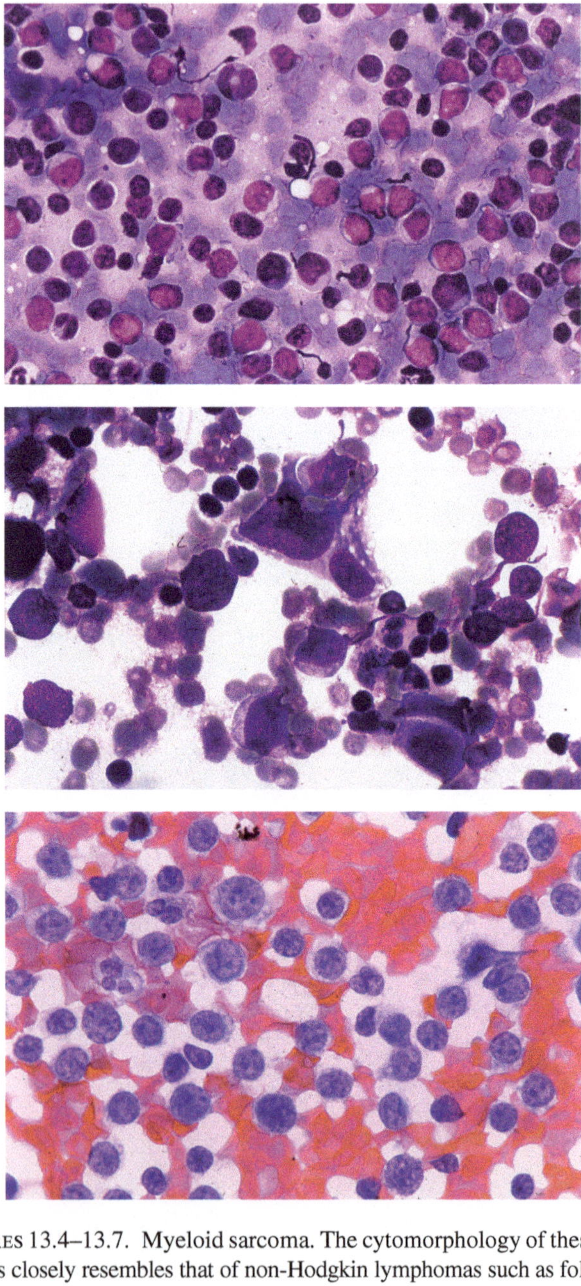

FIGURES 13.4–13.7. Myeloid sarcoma. The cytomorphology of these neoplasms closely resembles that of non-Hodgkin lymphomas such as follicular

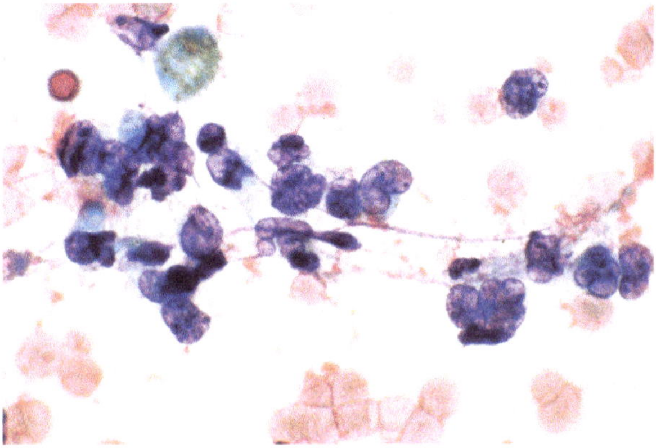

FIGURES 13.4–13.7. (continued) (Fig. 13.4), immunoblastic (Fig. 13.6), and anaplastic (Fig. 13.7) lymphomas or epithelial malignancies (Fig. 13.5, that shows immature megakaryocytes in a case of chronic myelogenous leukemia involving lymph nodes). (DiffQuik and Papanicolaou stains, High magnification).

of the skull, sternum, ribs, and vertebrae, as well as the paranasal sinuses, lymph nodes, skin, and internal organs. The tumor has abundant myeloperoxidase that gives it a green color. Cytology preparations stained with Giemsa show myeloid blasts with cytoplasmic azurophilic granules and Auer rods. Cytochemical stains such as myeloperoxidase, butyrate esterase, PAS, and chloroacetate esterase used for differentiating among the various FAB types of acute myeloid leukemia can be used in cytology specimens. Lysozyme, myeloperoxidase, CD117, CD13, CD33, and CD43 are positive in more than 90% of cases of myeloid sarcoma. Patients with AML and t(8;21)(q22;q22), inv(16)(p13q22), and monocytic leukemias have the greatest frequency of occurrence of myeloid sarcoma.

The main differential diagnosis is that with large cell lymphoma; cytomorphology and flow cytometry are helpful in the diagnosis. Cases of monocytic myeloid sarcoma need to be distinguished from anaplastic large cell lymphoma. Undifferentiated carcinomas and small round cell sarcomas should be included in the differential diagnosis.

Histiocytic Sarcoma

Histiocytic sarcoma is a rare malignant neoplasm composed of cells with histology and immunophenotype similar to those of mature tissue histiocytes. The relative frequency of this neoplasm is 0.15% among hematopoietic neoplasms. It occurs at any age, but most cases are found in adults. A subset of cases is seen in association with mediastinal germ cell tumors, malignant lymphoma, and myelodysplasia and leukemia. Most cases have involvement of extranodal sites, and others have lymphadenopathy. This is usually an aggressive neoplasm with a poor response to therapy.

The neoplastic cells are large, round, and often pleomorphic, with ample eosinophilic cytoplasm that may show fine vacuoles. Erythrophagocytosis and emperipolesis may be seen, but usually are not prominent. Occasional multinucleated cells may be present. Nonneoplastic cells including lymphocytes, plasma cells, eosinophils, and neutrophils may be seen. In essence, the neoplastic population is indistinguishable from that with large cell lymphoma, melanoma, or carcinoma, without the use of marker studies.

The neoplastic cells are CD45, CD45RO, HLA-DR, lysozyme, CD163, and CD68 positive. Langerhans cell (CD1a, langerin), follicular dendritic cell (CD21, CD35), and myeloid cell (CD33, CD13, myeloperoxidase) markers are negative. T-cell and B-cell markers, HMB45, keratin, and epithelial membrane antigen are also negative.

Dendritic Cell Neoplasms

Neoplasms included in this category are derived from follicular dendritic cells, interdigitating dendritic cells, and Langerhans cells. A degree of histomorphology and immunophenotypic overlap exists among these neoplasms, and a precise distinction may not be possible.

The *follicular dendritic cell sarcoma* shows spindle to ovoid cells with an immunophenotype similar to that of follicular dendritic cells. It occurs mainly in adults, and males and females are affected equally. Castleman disease, hyaline vascular variant, appears to be a precursor lesion in some cases. Lymph nodes, often cervical, are usually markedly enlarged and cause no pain. Extranodal sites such as the tonsils, oral cavity, mediastinum, and gastrointestinal tract may be involved. The cells show indistinct cytoplasmic borders and moderate eosinophilic cytoplasm. The nuclei are oval or elongated, with finely granular chromatin and small distinct nucleoli. Binucleated and multinucleated cells are often seen. Cellular pleomorphism with scattered mitosis and necrosis may be seen in some cases. The background shows small lymphocytes. The immunophenotype is positive for one or more of the follicular dendritic markers CD21, CD35, CD23, KiM4p, and CAN 42. Clusterin, a marker that is usually negative in other dendritic cell tumors, is almost always strongly positive in follicular dendritic cell sarcoma.

Interdigitating dendritic cell sarcoma is a very rare neoplasm that contains spindle to ovoid cells with an immunophenotype similar to that of interdigitating dendritic cells. The neoplasm usually involves the lymph nodes, but involvement of extranodal sites may occur. The cytoplasm is usually abundant and slightly eosinophilic, and has indistinct borders. The nuclei are ovoid to elongated, the chromatin is vesicular, and the nucleoli are of variable size. Cytologic atypia may be present. Scattered small lymphocytes and rare plasma cells are seen in the background. The neoplastic cells are S100 protein-positive and langerin, CD1a, and vimentin-negative. They are negative for the follicular dendritic cell markers CD21, CD23, and CD35.

Langerhans cell histiocytosis is a neoplastic proliferation of cells that express CD1a, langerin, and S100 protein and shows Birbeck granules on electron microscopy. It is more common in children than in adults, with male predominance. The disease can be localized to a single site (eosinophilic granuloma), multiple sites within a single system, usually bone (Hand–Schuller–Christian disease), or more disseminated and multisystem (Letter–Siwe disease). The lymph nodes may be affected in the localized form. Bone and adjacent soft tissue are commonly affected in the multifocal form. Hepatosplenomagaly is present in the multisystem form. The cells are oval with grooved nuclei, powdery chromatin, inconspicuous nucleoli, and a thin nuclear membrane. Cellular atypia is minimal, and mitotic figures are variable in presence. The background shows eosinophils, histiocytes, multinucleated cells, neutrophils, and small lymphocytes. The neoplastic cells are CD1a, langerin, S100 protein, vimentin, HLA-DR, and CD68-positive (Figs. 13.8 and 13.9).

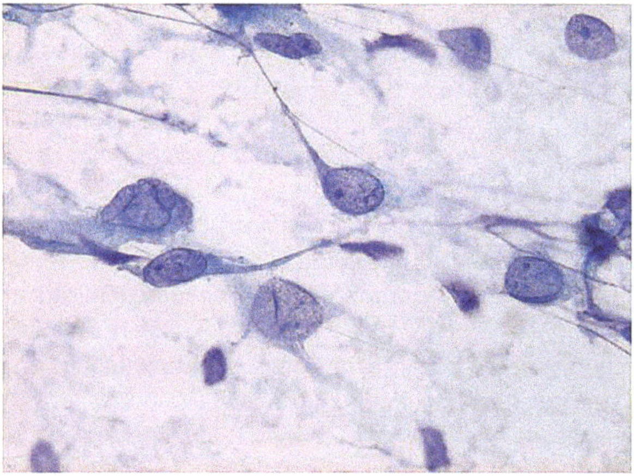

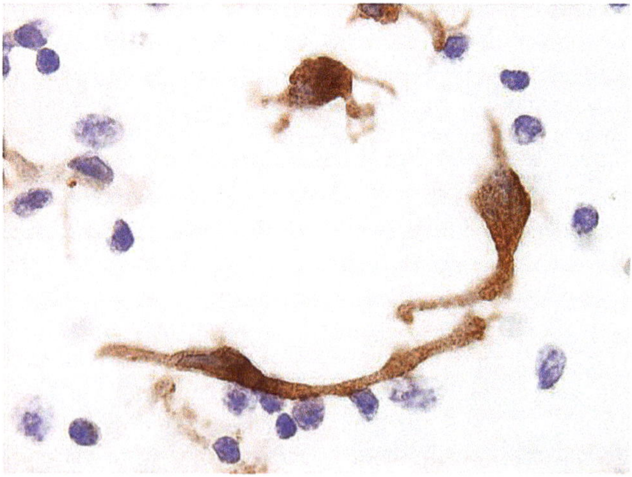

FIGURES 13.8–13.9. Langerhans cell histiocytosis. The cells have bland cytologic features, nuclear grooves, may have slender cytoplasmic processes, and are CD1a-positive as seen in Fig. 13.9. (Hematoxylin and eosin, and immunocytochemistry, High magnification) Courtesy Dr. Javier Saenz de Santamaria, Pathologist, Department of Pathology, Complejo Universitario de Badajoz, Spain.

Langerhans cell sarcoma is a rare high-grade neoplasm that occurs in adults and shows a malignant cytology and a Langerhans cell immunophenotype with focal stain positivity. The patients show skin, soft tissue, lymph node, and multiorgan involvement.

Spindle Cell Neoplasms

Palisaded myofibroblastoma is a unilateral, painless, benign mesenchymal lymph node tumor that shows deposits of collagen (amianthoid fibers) and hemorrhage. Most patients have a solitary and painless nodule in the inguinal area. The spindle cells lack atypia, and the background shows fragments of amorphous eosinophilic material (Figs. 13.10–13.12). The neoplasm is smooth-muscle actin, vimentin, and myosin-positive, but desmin-negative. The S100 protein-positive stain helps to distinguish neurilemmoma from this tumor.

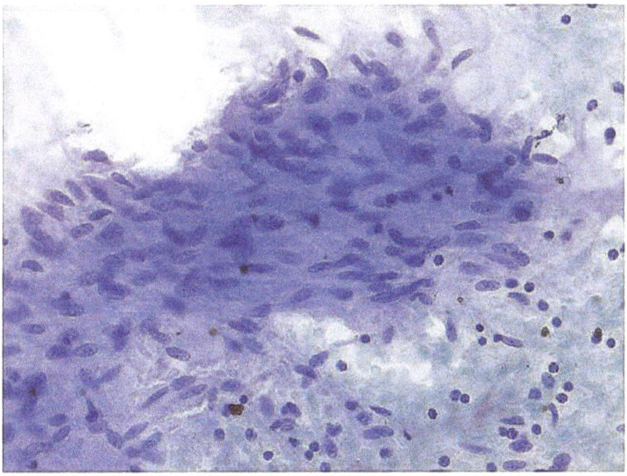

FIGURES 13.10–13.12. Palisaded myofibroblastoma. Aggregates of spindle cells with bland cytologic features (Fig. 13.10) and fragments of amorphous eosinophilic material (Fig. 13.11) reflect the histologic features (Fig. 13.12). (Hematoxylin and eosin, High magnification). Courtesy Dr. Javier Saenz de Santamaria, Pathologist, Department of Pathology, Complejo Universitario de Badajoz, Spain.

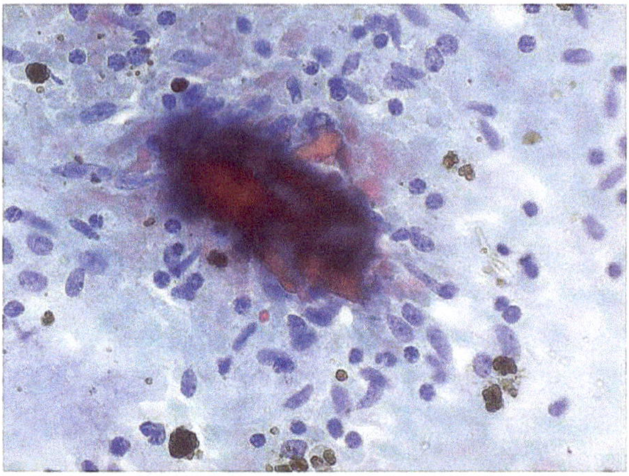

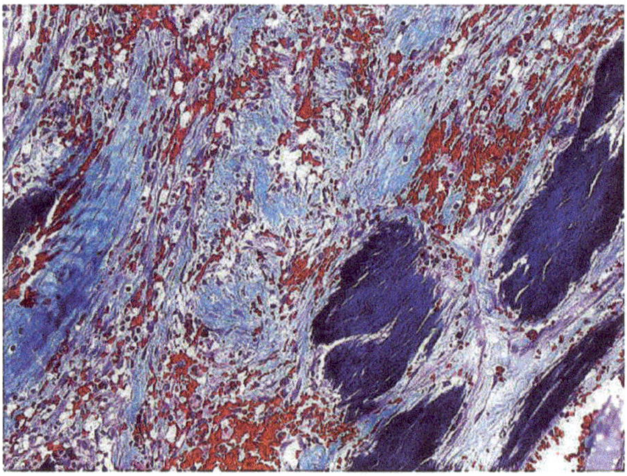

FIGURES 13.10–13.12. (continued).

Inflammatory myofibroblastic tumor or inflammatory pseudotumor (Fig. 13.13) is an inflammatory proliferative process of histiocytic and fibroblastic origin involving the lymph node connective tissue. The patients may complain of systemic symptoms including fever, night sweats, and anemia and localized or generalized lymphadenopathy involving cervical, axillary, mediastinal, retroperitoneal, or inguinal regions and the surrounding soft tissue.

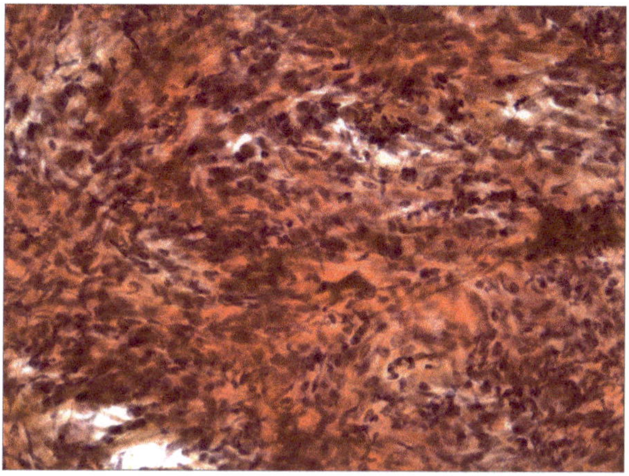

FIGURE 13.13. Inflammatory myofibroblastic tumor. Aggregates of bland appearing spindle cells are admixed with inflammatory cells. (Papanicolaou stain, High magnification) Courtesy Edward Stelow, MD Associate Professor of Pathology. University of Virginia, Charlottesville, VA.

Cytologic preparations are similar to those seen in similar lesions in other locations, and they show spindle cells of endothelial and fibroblastic origin, neutrophils, plasma cells, and neutrophils with no necrosis or eosinophils. The spindle cells have reactive cytologic features and rare nonatypical mitoses and lack nuclear pleomorphism. The spindle cells show strong vimentin positivity. Endothelial and histiocytic/macrophage markers are negative. The differential diagnosis includes mycobacterial spindle cell pseudotumor, anthracotic and anthracosilicotic spindle cell pseudotumors in the mediastinal nodes (see Fig. 5.14), follicular dendritic cell tumor, and spindle cell malignancies including melanoma.

Small Blood Vessel Proliferations

Primary vascular neoplasms or proliferative angioformative lesions may be found in the lymph nodes.

Bacillary angiomatosis (see Chap. 12). The smears show a proliferation of blood vessels lined with plump endothelial cells, neutrophils, debris, and clumps of amphophilic granular material. The Warthin–Starry silver stain shows clusters of the diagnostic gram-negative bacilli.

Kaposi sarcoma. Similar to bacillary angiomatosis, Kaposi sarcoma also occurs in a state of immunodeficiency, particularly in patients with AIDS. The smears show spindle-shaped endothelial cells in a background of blood and scattered plasma cells (Figs. 13.14 and 13.15).

HIV lymphadenopathy, involutional stage. Lymphoid cells are involuted, the background shows red blood cells and spindle cells with small fragments of stroma corresponding to the thick-walled vessels seen in tissue preparations.

Castleman disease, hyaline vascular variant (See Chap. 8). The lymph nodes are massively enlarged and the smears show scattered spindled cells in a background of polymorphous mature lymphocytes.

Angioimmunoblastic lymphadenopathy. The smears show scattered immunoblasts in a background of red blood cells (Fig. 13.16). Small fragments of stroma and spindled cells corresponding to blood vessels may be seen.

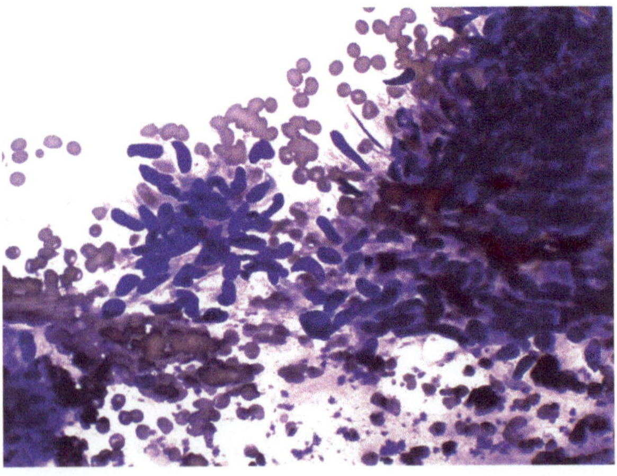

FIGURES 13.14–13.15. Kaposi sarcoma. Bloody aspirates and clusters of spindle cells in a background of blood are characteristic in the appropriate clinical setting. (DiffQuik stain, High magnification).

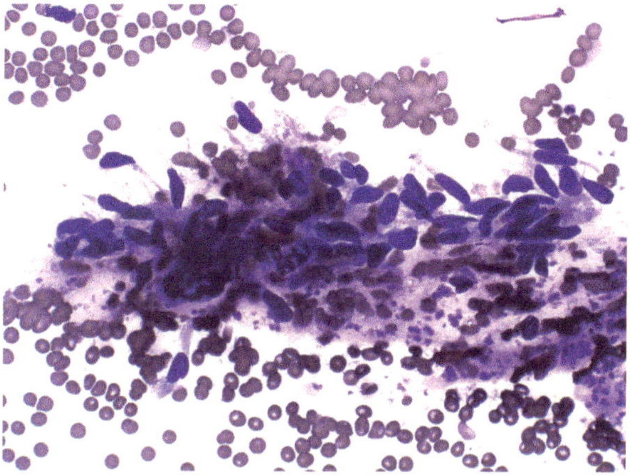

FIGURES 13.14–13.15. (continued).

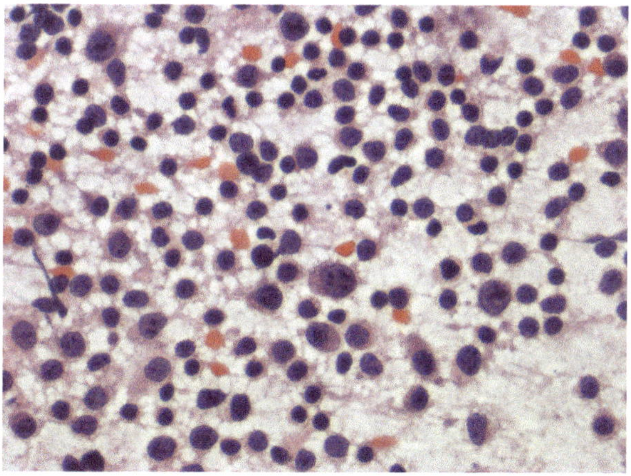

FIGURE 13.16. Angioimmunoblastic lymphadenopathy. Immunoblasts are seen in this case of angioimmunoblastic T-cell lymphoma. (Hematoxylin and eosin stain, High magnification) Courtesy Roberto Miranda MD, Associate Professor, Department of Pathology. MD Anderson Cancer Center.

Vascular transformation of sinuses. The lymph node is moderately enlarged, found in any location, and is usually an incidental finding. Histologically, the lymph node architecture is preserved. The smears show blood and rare spindled cells.

Hemangiomas/hemangioendotheliomas. These are primary benign vascular tumors of lymph nodes, usually found incidentally. The cytologic findings are identical to the counterpart in the soft tissues. Smears show rare spindle cells in a background of abundant blood. The definitive diagnosis is usually made on lymph node excision.

Angiosarcoma. The smears show atypical spindled or epithelioid cells with pleomorphic nuclei and scattered mitoses in a background of blood (Figs. 13.17 and 13.18).

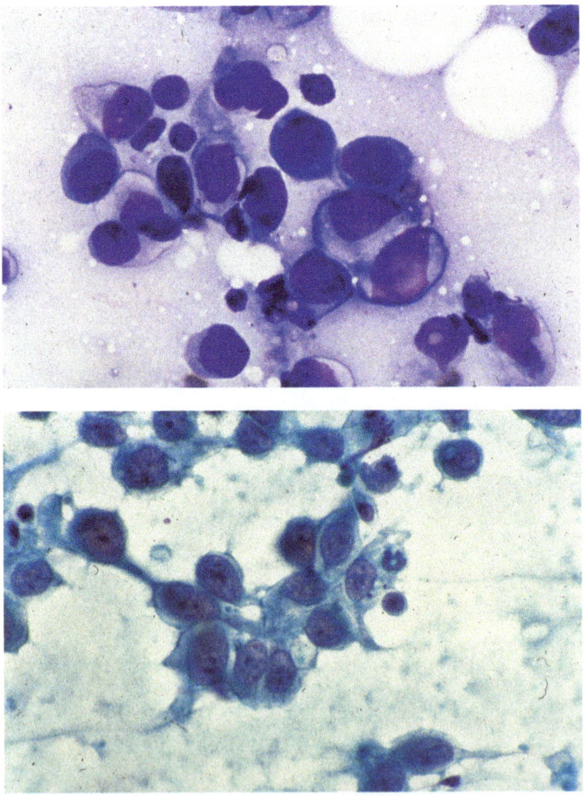

FIGURES 13.17–13.18. Angiosarcoma. Cuboidal and elongated cells are arranged in loose aggregates. (*top* DiffQuik and *bottom* Papanicolaou stains, High magnification).

Epithelial Cell Inclusions

Benign epithelial elements may be seen in lymph nodes. They have bland cytologic features and lack nuclear pleomorphism or mitotic activity. The pathogenesis is unclear and may be the result of developmental heterotopias. The epithelial cell inclusions are rare, and when encountered, they must be distinguished from a metastatic deposit of a well-differentiated malignancy. Clinical correlation including a history of malignancy and careful evaluation of the cytomorphology are crucial for a correct interpretation in tissue and cytology samples.

Salivary gland tissue may be seen in the upper cervical lymph nodes. Thyroid tissue in the lower cervical lymph nodes should be considered as evidence of metastasis of an occult thyroid-gland primary tumor, although there have been occasional reports of thyroid follicles in lymph nodes with no thyroid primary. Axillary lymph nodes may harbor benign breast elements such as ductal epithelial cells with myoepithelial cells; their presence seem to be related to a vigorous breast examination. Pleural mesothelial cells may be present in mediastinal lymph nodes, colonic glands in mesenteric lymph nodes, renal tubular cells in perirenal lymph nodes, and glandular elements from fallopian-tube and ovarian origin in pelvic and paraoartic lymph nodes. Aggregates of benign melanocytes may be seen occasionally, and they lack nucleolar prominence and nuclear pleomorphism; furthermore, they are HMB 45- and Ki67-negative.

Infarction

Massive coagulative necrosis may be seen in malignant processes such as lymphoma, metastatic carcinoma, melanoma, and granulocytic sarcoma (Fig. 13.19). In some cases, the cause of infarction is not obvious. Clinically, the necrotic lymph nodes are usually larger than those with viable tumor deposits. Thus, in the presence of necrosis, the aspiration biopsy should be performed in a smaller lymph node. Necrosis has also been reported in nonmalignant processes such as infectious mononucleosis, collagen vascular disease including systemic lupus erythematosus and rheumatoid

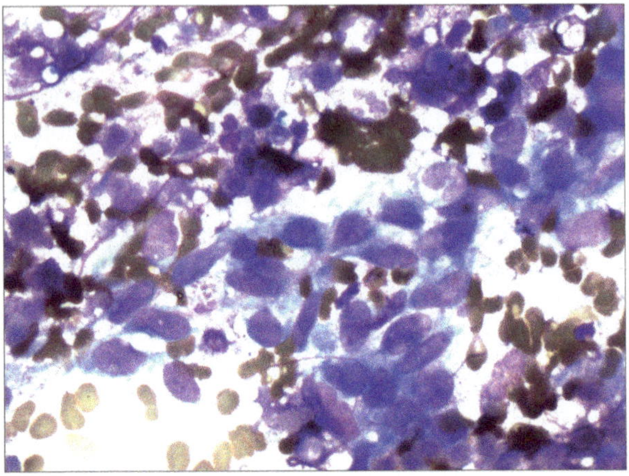

FIGURE 13.19. Lymph node necrosis. Lymphoma is the most common underlying malignant process. Necrotic stromal and lymphoid cells are seen. Further cytologic evaluation can not be made. (Giemsa stain, High magnification).

arthritis after gold therapy, cholesterol atheromatous emboli, and Kikuchi disease. Infectious lymphadenitis such as fungal and mycobacterial infections may produce marked necrosis. In such cases, a silver stain may show the fungal organisms, particularly in histoplasmosis. Necrosis following lymph node FNA has also been reported.

Suggested Reading

Bangerter M, Hildebrand A et al (2000) Diagnosis of granulocytic sarcoma by fine-needle aspiration cytology. Acta Haematol 103(2):102–108

Iacobuzio-Donahue CA, Clark DP et al (2002) Reed-Sternberg-like cells in lymph node aspirates in the absence of Hodgkin's disease: pathologic significance and differential diagnosis. Diagn Cytopathol 27(6):335–339

Ioachim HL, Medeiros LJ (2009) Lymphadenopathies. Ioachim's lymph node pathology. Wolters Kluwer Lippincott Williams & Wilkins, Philadelphia, pp 172–291

Ioachim HL, Medeiros LJ (2009) Granulocytic, histiocytic, and dendritic cell neoplasms. Ioachim's lymph node pathology. Wolters Kluwer Lippincott Williams & Wilkins, Philadelphia, pp 517–544

Ioachim HL, Medeiros LJ (2009) Spindle cell neoplasms of lymph nodes. Ioachim's lymph node pathology. Wolters Kluwer Lippincott Williams & Wilkins, Philadelphia, pp 569–575

Jaffe R, Pileri S et al (2008) Histiocytic and dendritic cell neoplasms. In: Swerdlow S, Campo E, Harris N et al (eds) WHO classification of tumors of hematopoietic and lymphoid tissues. WHO OMS, Lyon, pp 354–367

Lopez-Ferrer P, Jimenez-Heffernan JA et al (2008) Fine needle aspiration cytology of Langerhans cell sarcoma. Cytopathology 19(1):59–61

Pugh JL, Jhala NC et al (2006) Diagnosis of deep-seated lymphoma and leukemia by endoscopic ultrasound-guided fine-needle aspiration biopsy. Am J Clin Pathol 125(5):703–709

14 Pitfalls and Limitations of FNA of Lymph Nodes

Pitfalls or diagnostic errors in the interpretation of lymph node aspirates frequently have their origin in inadequate diagnostic material on the aspirate smears, inadequate triage of the aspirate during the initial on-site evaluation, lack of clinical data, cytologic, screening and interpretative errors or to pitfalls in the interpreta-tion of ancillary methods used.

Inadequate Diagnostic Material, Either Due to Changes Caused by the Pathologic Process Involving the Lymph Node or to Technical Problems

Focal Involvement of the Lymph Node

Diagnostic errors can occur because the sample does not contain the neoplastic cells, as may occur in partial involvement of the lymph node by Hodgkin lymphoma (interfollicular HL), ALCL and rarely by other lymphomas and in metastatic malignancies.

S.E. Pambuccian and R.H. Bardales, *Lymph Node Cytopathology*, Essentials in Cytopathology 10, DOI 10.1007/978-1-4419-6964-4_14,

The Presence of Extensive Necrosis

Necrosis is frequently the result of an infectious or inflammatory process but may also accompany a malignancy. The necrotic background may obscure the rare neoplastic cells that are present in the sample, especially in smears stained with Romanowsky-type stains. Aspirates from a completely necrotic lymph node in which an infectious etiology cannot be demonstrated by cultures, special stains, or other methods should not be diagnosed as negative for malignancy, but rather as atypical and an excisional biopsy should be recommended.

Spontaneous infarction of lymph nodes is rare and may be associated with a variety of benign conditions that compromise the vascular supply of the lymph node. Lymph node infarction or necrosis of tumor cells may also occur in lymphomas and metastatic malignancies. Immunoperoxidase stains on cell block sections may sometimes demonstrate the characteristic markers of metastatic malignancies or a predominance of B cells within the cell "ghosts" present in the necrotic aspirate, as immunoreactivity may be preserved in the necrotic cells. Sometimes the initial lymph node excisional biopsy may fail to diagnose lymphoma; biopsy of any additional enlarged lymph nodes is recommended to exclude lymphoma. Lymphomas are eventually found in at least one-third of patients presenting with infarcted lymph nodes.

Cystic Aspirates

Lymph node aspirates may yield cyst fluid. The smears of such aspirates show a cystic background of proteinaceous fluid with debris, cholesterol crystals, and foamy macrophages with a variable number of lymphocytes. The differential diagnosis of such aspirates obtained from masses clinically believed to be enlarged lymph nodes includes a variety of benign conditions, such as lymphoepithelial cysts, Warthin tumor, developmental cysts, thyroid, and parathyroid cysts. However, such cystic aspirates may also represent malignancies, especially metastatic malignancies. The metastatic malignancies most likely to appear cystic in fine-needle aspirates are metastatic squamous cell carcinomas and metastatic papillary carcinomas of the thyroid. Metastatic cystic squamous cell carcinomas may show only mature-appearing squamous cells with mild atypia in aspirates and may be misdiagnosed as developmental cysts (branchial cleft cysts). Such cystic metastatic squamous cell carcinomas frequently originate in the oropharynx and tonsils, and are HPV-positive. Careful examination of the smears for squamous atypia and correlation with clinical findings, especially the age of the patient and imaging findings will frequently allow a diagnosis of suspicious for a metastatic squamous cell carcinoma. In addition, detection of HPV by in-situ hybridization or molecular methods or staining for p16, a surrogate marker of HPV infection may support the diagnosis of metastatic cystic squamous cell carcinoma. Cystic metastases from papillary carcinomas of the thyroid may show no tumor cells or only degenerated tumor cells that resemble macrophages. Chemical determination of thyroglobulin levels in the FNA needle rinses can be diagnostic. Demonstration of thyroglobulin and/or TTF1 reactivity in cell block sections may also be helpful. Ultrasound-guided FNA of such cystic neoplasms is able to direct the needle to sample the solid component and obtain material adequate for diagnosis.

Technical Problems

Aspirates may be paucicellular and the smears may be too thick or show too much crush artifact, or fixation and staining artifacts which preclude an accurate diagnosis. Such aspirates should be diagnosed as unsatisfactory rather than negative for malignancy and a repeat FNA or excisional biopsy recommended in order to elucidate the cause of the lymphadenopathy.

Inadequate Triage of the Aspirate for Ancillary Studies

Errors may arise because the inappropriate work-up was initiated during the initial on-site evaluation of the sample. Cultures should be initiated in samples showing necrosis, neutrophils or granulomas; flow cytometry in most aspirates from adults and a cell block should be prepared from aspirates showing predominance of aggregates or a pleomorphic pattern. When the appropriate ancillary tests were not performed it is better to defer a definitive diagnosis to a repeat FNA or an excisional biopsy.

Inadequate Clinical Information

Clinical correlation of morphologic findings and the data provided by ancillary tests is critical in the accurate interpretation of fine-needle aspirates of lymph nodes. Clinical information such as the patient's history, the size, palpation characteristics, and exact location of the mass aspirated as well as the "feel of the needle" during the aspiration are known when aspirates are performed by the pathologist, but most of this information may not be available in FNAs performed by radiologists, endoscopists, or surgeons. Frequently, aspirates are received by the pathologist with only minimal information such as the age and sex of the patient and a vague location of the aspiration target, such as "neck mass." Close collaboration with clinicians and the presence of the pathologist to assess adequacy and triage the specimen on-site during imaging-guided fine-needle aspirations is essential to obtain adequate clinical information.

Screening and Interpretative Errors

Rare Reed-Sternberg cells may be missed, especially in suboptimal aspirates where most of the cells are stripped of their cytoplasm. Rare neoplastic cells may be similarly missed in metastatic malignancies, especially in those characterized by a single cell pattern and resemblance of tumor cells to lymphocytes, such as metastatic lobular carcinomas of the breast and metastatic neuroendocrine carcinomas, including Merkel cell carcinoma.

Interpretative errors occur most often in look-alikes, i.e., in primary lymphoid neoplasms that show features of metastatic malignancies or the other way around. Lymphoid neoplasms may show extensive crush artifact, thereby mimicking metastatic small-cell carcinomas or apparently cohesive sheets of neoplastic cells, thereby mimicking metastatic carcinomas and melanoma. Lymphoid neoplasms may also show a variety of unusual features that we associate with non-lymphoid malignancies, such as the presence of Homer-Wright rosettes, typically found in neuroblastomas, in large-cell lymphomas, of both B- and T-cell lineage or the presence of signet-ring cells in follicular lymphomas. Metastatic malignancies with a single cell pattern, especially metastatic neuroendocrine carcinomas and small blue cell tumors, such as rhabdomyosarcomas may closely mimic the cytomorphology of lymphomas.

Interpretative errors may be minimized by considering the clinical context of the lymph node aspirate and performing the appropriate ancillary studies.

Pitfalls in the Interpretation of Ancillary Studies

Pitfalls in the Interpretation of Flow Cytometry Data

Flow cytometry is a powerful tool to determine both the clonality of the lymphoid proliferation and its immunophenotype, which is helpful in the classification of the lymphoid neoplasm. However, sometimes flow cytometry is unable to detect the clonality of a lymphoid proliferation, or may be falsely negative. This is especially prone to occur in lymphomas with a small number of neoplastic cells, such as Hodgkin lymphoma, in lymphomas with very large neoplastic cells, such as ALCL and in large-cell lymphomas, where the cytoplasm of the fragile neoplastic cells are lost during the preparation of the sample. Such false negativity may occur in 15–25% of DLBCL cases.

Fortunately, smears from these types of lymphoid neoplasms most often show morphologic evidence of an abnormal lymphoid proliferation; therefore diagnostic errors are unusual. Immunoperoxidase stains performed on the cell block material, if available, can be helpful to support the morphologic impression of lymphoma. Fortunately, such false negativity is uncommon in small-cell lymphoid neoplasms where the morphologic diagnosis is most difficult.

Pitfalls in the Interpretation of Immunohistochemistry

Since almost no antibody shows complete specificity, it should be taken into consideration that antibodies typically used in the work-up of lymphoid proliferations may cross-react with non-lymphoid cells and neoplasms.

Lymphomas and normal lymphoid elements may sometime stain for markers used to demonstrate the presence of metastatic malignancies.

- Cytokeratin expression, usually indicating a metastatic carcinoma, may be present in normal dendritic cells and has been reported in malignant lymphomas of B-cell lineage, plasma cell tumors and rarely in T-cell lymphomas as well as in metastatic melanomas. Dendritic cells expressing cytokeratin have a characteristic elongated or dendritic pattern, which is helpful in distinguishing them from metastatic carcinoma cells.
- p63 staining, usually performed to document metastatic squamous cell carcinoma may be positive cells in a subset of normal lymphocytes as well as in B-cell lymphomas, particularly in DLBCL, SLL/CLL, and FL.
- CD99 and FLI-1, markers used to document metastatic Ewing sarcoma/peripheral neuroectodermal tumors may also be expressed in lymphoid neoplasms that enter the differential diagnosis of small blue cell tumors, such as lymphoblastic lymphomas, small-cell variant of anaplastic large-cell lymphoma and angioimmunoblastic T-cell lymphoma.

Conversely, lymphohematopoietic markers may be expressed in metastatic malignancies, some of which may enter the differential diagnosis of lymphoid neoplasms.

- PAX-5, a transcription factor which is almost completely restricted to the B-cell lineage may be expressed in alveolar rhabdomyosarcoma.
- CD30 expression may occur in a variety of metastatic malignant neoplasms that enter the differential diagnosis of cHL and ALCL, such as leiomyosarcomas, rhabdomyosarcomas, undifferentiated sarcomas (malignant fibrous histiocytomas), osteosarcoma, Ewing sarcomas, embryonal carcinoma, and malignant melanomas.
- ALK expression may occur in inflammatory myofibroblastic tumors.
- Terminal deoxynucleotidyl transferase (TdT) a marker used to document the presence of lymphoblastic lymphoma may be expressed in metastatic Merkel cell carcinomas, neoplasms that may also show "blastic" tumor cells.

- CD5, a marker frequently used to characterize lymphoid proliferations is expressed in thymomas.
- CD138, a marker used to document plasma cell differentiation, is also expressed in metastatic carcinoma cells of various types and in metastatic mesenchymal neoplasms and melanomas.
- CD56, a marker used to document NK cell differentiation can be expressed in metastatic small cell and Merkel cell carcinomas.
- Cyclin D1 staining, which among lymphomas is specific for mantle cell lymphoma can be seen in parathyroid adenomas and a variety of carcinomas as well as in a subset of plasma cell tumors.

Correlation with clinical data and morphologic features and the use of panels of immunostains minimizes the potential for misdiagnosis.

Pitfalls in the Interpretation of Molecular Data

Clonality assessment by molecular techniques is an important tool in the diagnosis of lymphoproliferations, especially in T-cell lymphomas, where flow cytometry may not be able to demonstrate clonality. It is important to consider that clonality, as determined by molecular studies does not always imply malignancy, since some reactive lymphoid proliferations may contain clonal populations. This occurs especially in conditions where there is an exaggerated immune response with a dominant specificity to a small number of antigens.

Technical difficulties, related to degraded DNA and few B or T cells in the sample may give rise to spurious clonal peaks (pseudoclonality). Conversely, lymphoid clones that are present in the sample may not be demonstrated due to technical problems. Correlation with clinical, immunophenotyping, and morphologic findings is essential to avoid overdiagnosis.

Limitations of Fine-Needle Aspiration of Lymph Nodes

Some conditions are very difficult if not impossible to accurately diagnose on fine-needle aspirates. In some of these conditions, a diagnosis of a lymphoid neoplasm is possible but the exact type of lymphoma cannot be determined with accuracy. These include conditions where the histologic pattern is essential for the diagnosis:

- Grade 3 (especially grade 3B) follicular lymphomas versus DLBCL with centroblastic morphology.
- Subtyping of Hodgkin lymphoma.
- Diagnosis of marginal zone lymphomas, especially extranodal marginal zone lymphomas of mucosal-associated lymphoid tissue.

In other conditions, there are cases in which there is an extensive morphologic and immunophenotyping overlap between different entities that may make the differential diagnosis difficult or impossible even on adequate excisional biopsy specimens. Such grey-zone lymphomas include:

- Classical Hodgkin lymphoma versus primary mediastinal large B-cell lymphoma.
- Burkitt lymphoma versus diffuse large B-cell lymphoma.
- Nodular lymphocyte predominant Hodgkin lymphoma versus T-cell/histiocyte-rich large B-cell lymphoma.
- ALK-negative anaplastic cell lymphoma (ALCL) versus peripheral T-cell lymphoma, not otherwise specified.

In other lymphoid proliferations, the diagnosis of malignancy is very difficult due to either the small number of neoplastic cells, as in T-cell/histiocyte-rich B-cell lymphomas and nodular lymphocyte predominant Hodgkin lymphoma or to difficulties in the demonstration of clonality, as frequently occurs in peripheral T-cell lymphomas.

In such cases, it is important to convey the diagnostic uncertainty in the cytopathology report. It is also important to acknowledge the potential limitations of fine-needle aspiration of lymph nodes and to recommend excisional biopsy of the lymph node if an unexplained lymphadenopathy persists over 1–3 months after a fine-needle aspiration interpreted as negative for malignancy.

Suggested Reading

Bertram HC, Check IJ, Milano MA (2001) Immunophenotyping large B-cell lymphomas. Flow cytometric pitfalls and pathologic correlation. Am J Clin Pathol 116(2):191–203

Fathallah L, Tulunay OE, Feng J, Husain M, Jacobs JR, Al-Abbadi MA (2006) Histopathologic and cytopathologic diagnostic discrepancies in head and neck region: pitfalls, causes, and preventive strategies. Otolaryngol Head Neck Surg 134(2):302–308

Geisinger KR (1995) Differential diagnostic considerations and potential pitfalls in fine-needle aspiration biopsies of the mediastinum. Diagn Cytopathol 13(5):436–442

Groenen PJ, Langerak AW, van Dongen JJ, van Krieken JH (2008) Pitfalls in TCR gene clonality testing: teaching cases. J Hematop 1(2):97–109

Hummel M, Stein H (2003) Clonality and malignancy. PCR assays for the diagnosis of clonal B- and T-cell proliferations: potentials and pitfalls. Verh Dtsch Ges Pathol 87:102–108

Katz RL (1997) Pitfalls in the diagnosis of fine-needle aspiration of lymph nodes. Monogr Pathol 39:118–133

Kroft SH (2004) Monoclones, monotypes, and neoplasia pitfalls in lymphoma diagnosis. Am J Clin Pathol 121(4):457–459

Young NA, Moriarty AT, Haja JC, Wilbur DC (2006) Fine-needle aspiration biopsy of lymphoproliferative disorders – interpretations based on morphologic criteria alone: results from the College of American Pathologists Interlaboratory Comparison Program in Nongynecologic Cytopathology. Arch Pathol Lab Med 130(12):1766–1771

Zhao XF (2009) Pitfalls in diagnostic hematopathology: part I. Int J Clin Exp Pathol 2(1):11–20

Zhao XF (2009) Pitfalls in diagnostic hematopathology – part II. Int J Clin Exp Pathol 3(1):39–46

Index

N

P

R

S

T

Kolibri 360 GmbH
Ferdinand-Jühlke-Straße 7
99095 Erfurt, Deutschland
produktsicherheit@kolibri360.de